DISABILITY IN THE TIME OF PANDEMIC

RESEARCH IN SOCIAL SCIENCE AND DISABILITY

Series Editors: Sharon N. Barnartt and Barbara M. Altman

Recent Volumes:

Volume 1:	Expanding the Scope of Social Science Research on Disability – Edited by Sharon N. Barnartt and Barbara M. Altman
Volume 2:	Exploring Theories and Expanding Methodologies: Where We Are and Where We Need to Go – Edited by Sharon N. Barnartt and Barbara M. Altman
Volume 3:	Using Survey Data to Study Disability: Results From the National Health Interview Survey on Disability – Edited by Barbara M. Altman, Sharon N. Barnartt, Gerry E. Hendershot and Sheryl A. Larson
Volume 4:	International Views on Disability Measures: Moving Toward Comparative Measurement – Edited by Barbara M. Altman, Sharon N. Barnartt, Gerry E. Hendershot and Sheryl A. Larson
Volume 5:	Disability as a Fluid State – Edited by Sharon N. Barnartt
Volume 6:	Disability and Community – Edited by Allison C. Carey and Richard K. Scotch
Volume 7:	Disability and Intersecting Statuses– Edited by Sharon N. Barnartt and Barbara M. Altman
Volume 8:	Environmental Contexts and Disability – Edited by Sharon N. Barnartt and Barbara M. Altman
Volume 9:	What Did We Know and When Did We Know It – Edited by Sara E. Green and Sharon N. Barnartt
Volume 10:	Factors in Studying Employment for Persons with Disability: How the Picture Can Change – Edited by Barbara M. Altman and Sharon N. Barnartt
Volume 11:	New Narratives of Disability: Constructions, Clashes, and Controversies – Edited by Sara E. Green and Donileen R. Loseke
Volume 12:	Disability Alliances and Allies: Opportunities and Challenges – Edited by Allison C. Carey, Joan M. Ostrove and Tara Fannon

RESEARCH IN SOCIAL SCIENCE AND DISABILITY
VOLUME 13

DISABILITY IN THE TIME OF PANDEMIC

EDITED BY

ALLISON C. CAREY
Shippensburg University, USA

SARA E. GREEN
University of South Florida, USA

And

LAURA MAULDIN
University of Connecticut, USA

emerald
PUBLISHING

United Kingdom – North America – Japan
India – Malaysia – China

Emerald Publishing Limited
Howard House, Wagon Lane, Bingley BD16 1WA, UK

First edition 2023

British Library Cataloguing in Publication Data
A catalogue record for this book is available from the British Library

ISBN: 978-1-80262-140-2 (Print)
ISBN: 978-1-80262-139-6 (Online)
ISBN: 978-1-80262-141-9 (Epub)

ISSN: 1479-3547 (Series)

Printed and bound by CPI Group (UK) Ltd, Croydon, CR0 4YY

CONTENTS

LIST OF FIGURES

LIST OF TABLES

ABOUT THE CONTRIBUTORS

Jihan Abbas, PhD, is an independent researcher and lecturer working with diverse organizations including government departments, the non-profit sector, community-based organizations, unions, startup companies, and universities. She has been involved in the disability movement for several years and has extensive advocacy and professional experiences related to access, exclusion, and equality (Canada).

Heather M. Aldersey, PhD, is an Associate Professor (Queen's National Scholar), Canada Research Chair (Tier 2), and the Director of the International Centre for the Advancement of Community Based Rehabilitation in the School of Rehabilitation Therapy at Queen's University in Canada. Her research focuses on family support in disability, community-based rehabilitation, and disability-inclusive development.

Pamela Block, PhD, is a Professor of Anthropology at Western University (Canada). She is a Fellow of the Society for Applied Anthropology and is a former president of the Society for Disability Studies (2009–2010). Her books include co-authored *Allies and Obstacles: Disability Activism and Parents of Children with Disabilities* (2020) and co-edited *Occupying Disability: Critical Approaches to Community, Justice, and Decolonizing Disability* (2016).

Madeline Burghardt has a PhD in Critical Disability Studies from York University and is the author of *Broken: Institutions, Families, and the Construction of Intellectual Disability*. She teaches at York and Western Universities (Canada). Her research interests include geopolitical constructions and histories of difference and disability. Madeline is a long-time friend and contributor to the creative arts group Sol Express.

Allison C. Carey, PhD, is a Professor of Sociology and Chair of the Department of Sociology & Anthropology at Shippensburg University in Pennsylvania (USA). She is co-author of *Allies and Obstacles: Disability Activism and Parents of Children with Disabilities* (2020) and author of *On the Margins of Citizenship: Intellectual Disability and Civil Rights in Twentieth Century America* (2009). She has co-edited several volumes, including two other volumes of RSSD.

Lei Chai is a PhD candidate in Sociology at the University of Toronto, Canada. His research focuses on health and mental health, work and family, and social stratification.

Jayajit Chakraborty, PhD, is a Professor in the Department of Sociology and Anthropology, and the Founding Director of the Socio-Environmental and Geospatial Analysis Lab at the University of Texas at El Paso, USA. He is currently serving as a member of the US Environmental Protection Agency (EPA) Science Advisory Board and the inaugural EPA Environmental Justice Science Committee.

Colleen M. Davison, PhD, is an Associate Professor of Public Health Sciences and Global Development Studies and Associate Dean for Equity and Social Accountability at Queen's University, Kingston, Canada. Her research interests include equity-oriented research methodologies, child and adolescent health and rights, and social justice in the realms of public health, global health and health sciences training.

Nelly De Arcos was an undergraduate student at Brown University (USA), majoring in Education Studies and Psychology at the time of writing this manuscript. She is now completing her master's degree in School Psychology at Loyola Marymount University.

Kim Fernandes is a joint doctoral candidate in Anthropology and Human Development at the University of Pennsylvania (USA). They are interested in questions of disability, data, and governance in South Asia. Their dissertation is focused on the processes and practices of identifying and enumerating disability in Delhi, India.

Rachel Elizabeth Fish, PhD, is an Assistant Professor in the Department of Teaching & Learning at New York University, USA. Her research examines racialized and gendered constructions of disability and giftedness, and how these processes relate to educational inequality.

Grace L. Francis, PhD, is an Associate Professor of Special Education at George Mason University, USA. Her research interests include transition to adulthood and family support policies and practices that result in a high quality of life for individuals with significant support needs.

Olivia Friend was an undergraduate at Brown University (USA), majoring in Education Studies, at the time of writing this manuscript. She is now pursuing a teaching career in Greenwich Connecticut as a fourth grade teacher. In addition, she is working toward her master's degree in elementary and special education at Bank Street College of Education in New York City.

Sharon Gabison, PhD, is an Assistant Professor in the Department of Physical Therapy at the University of Toronto, Canada, and an Affiliate Scientist at the KITE Research Institute at Toronto Rehabilitation Institute – University Health Network. Her research is focused on the development and evaluation of tools and technologies to support caregivers. At the time of the study, she was a representative of Family Alliance Ontario.

Navjit Gaurav is a Rehabilitation Science doctoral student at Queen's University, Canada. He has extensive community work experience in the informal settlements of Mumbai's M-East ward. His research aims to explore the Community schools' design in Indian slums to promote meaningful participation and social interaction of children with disabilities.

Ewa Giermanowska is an Associate Professor and Sociologist at the Institute of Applied Social Sciences at the University of Warsaw, Poland, and the author of expert analyses for government, NGOs, and scientific publications dealing with disability and employment. She is a member of the Polish Sociological Association, Section of Sociology of Work, and Section of Sociology of Disabilities.

Robert Gould, PhD, is an Associate Clinical Professor in the Department of Disability and Human Development and is the Director of Research for the Great Lakes ADA Center at the University of Illinois at Chicago, USA. His research interests lie in social policy, employment, knowledge translation, rights, and social justice.

Valérie Grand'Maison is a doctoral candidate in the Department of Sociology and Anthropology at the University of Guelph, Canada. Her areas of research include violence against women and girls with disabilities, feminist disability activism, and intersectionality.

Sara E. Green, PhD, is Professor and Chair of the Department of Sociology and Interdisciplinary Social Sciences at the University of South Florida, USA, past chair and career award recipient of the American Sociological Association (ASA) Section on Disability & Society, and past co-chair of the ASA Committee on the Status of Persons with Disabilities in Sociology. Her work focuses on narrative constructions of disability, stigma, and disability in family life.

Andy Holmes is a PhD student in Sociology at the University of Toronto, Canada. His research focuses on sexuality, social movements, and media framing of contemporary LGBTQ2+ issues.

Srishti Jaitely is a Counsellor-Programme Manager with M-iCall Psycho-Social Helpline under the Transforming M-ward Project of TISS, Mumbai. Her areas of interest include mental health and well-being, implementing community-led and community-based interventions with marginalized groups, the interaction of urban local bodies with informal settlements in public health and education.

Julia Jansen-van Vuuren is a doctoral candidate in the School of Rehabilitation Therapy at Queen's University in Kingston, Canada. Her research focuses on family quality of life for families of children with disabilities in low-income contexts, specifically in Ethiopia.

Robin Jones is the Director of the Great Lakes ADA Center in the Department of Disability and Human Development at the University of Illinois at Chicago, USA. Her areas of expertise include employment, architectural accessibility, community integration, educational accommodations and accessibility of information technology.

Michelle Maroto, PhD, is an Associate Professor of Sociology at the University of Alberta, Canada. Her research interests include social stratification, gender and family, race and ethnicity, labor and credit markets, and disability studies.

Laura Mauldin, PhD, is Associate Professor of Women's, Gender, and Sexuality Studies at the University of Connecticut, USA. She is the author of *Made to Hear: Cochlear Implants and Raising Deaf Children* (University of Minnesota Press, 2016) which won honorable mention for the Outstanding Publication Award from the American Sociological Association's Disability in Society Section. Her work appears in journals such as *Journal of Health and Social Behavior*, *Social Science and Medicine, Gender & Society* and others. She is currently working on a second book about spousal caregivers.

Joana Milan Lorandi is an undergraduate student in Psychology at the Universidade Federal de Santa Catarina, Brazil, and an Assistant Researcher at the Western University in Canada through the Emerging Leaders of America program (ELAP). Her areas of research include disability studies in relation to intersectional feminist studies and gender-based violence.

Courtney Mullin is a doctoral candidate in the Department of Disability and Human Development at the University of Illinois at Chicago, USA. Her research focuses on disability inclusion and workplace diversity, equity, and inclusion strategies, knowledge translation, and social policy.

Sarah Parker Harris, PhD, is a Professor in the Department of Disability and Human Development at the University of Illinois at Chicago, USA. Her research areas of focus broadly touch on disability policy and law, social entrepreneurship and disability, knowledge translation, and international human rights and social justice.

David Pettinicchio, PhD, is an Associate Professor of Sociology and affiliated faculty in the Munk School of Global Affairs and Public Policy at the University of Toronto, Canada. He is the author of *Politics of Empowerment* and co-editor of the *Oxford Handbook of the Sociology of Disability*. His research lies at the intersection of policy, politics, inequality, health, and disability.

Laura Pin, PhD, is an Assistant Professor in the Department of Political Science at Wilfrid Laurier University, Canada. Her research examines how social inequality intersects with policy-governance regimes and how political scientists can use community-engaged research to understand participation in public policy beyond formal political institutions.

Mariola Racław is an Associate Professor and Sociologist at the Institute of Applied Social Sciences at the University of Warsaw, Poland. She is a member of the Government Population Council and the Co-Founder and Vice-President of the Sociology of Disabilities Section of the Polish Sociological Association.

David Enrique Rangel, PhD, is an Assistant Professor of Education at Brown University, USA. His research examines the relationship between education and social inequality, with emphasis on the Latinx experience in the United States.

Kathryn Reinders is a doctoral student in the Social Practice and Transformational Change program at the University of Guelph, Canada. Her areas of research include sovereignty, public policy, human rights, and political action.

Danielle Roberts is a master's student in Occupational Therapy in the School of Rehabilitation Therapy at Queen's University, Kingston, Canada. Danielle is interested in occupational engagement for people with disabilities and barriers that are present internationally.

Tanushree Sarkar is a doctoral candidate in Community Research and Action at the Peabody College of Education and Human Development, Vanderbilt University (Nashville, USA). Her research interests include inclusive and social justice pedagogy, teacher agency, and education policy for equity and inclusion in the Global South.

Deborah Stienstra, PhD, holds the Jarislowsky Chair in Families and Work at the University of Guelph, the Director of the Live Work Well Research Centre and Professor of Political science (Canada). Her research explores the intersections of disabilities, gender, childhood, and Indigenousness, identifying barriers to, and possibilities for, engagement and transformative change.

Dorota Szawarska is an Anthropologist working at the Institute of Applied Social Sciences at the University of Warsaw, Poland. Currently, she is engaged in a research project being carried out at Warsaw University Policies for independent living in Poland and Norway, funded by a Norway grant.

LIST OF CONTRIBUTORS

Jihan Abbas	DisAbled Women's Network of Canada, Canada
Heather M. Aldersey	Queen's University, Canada
Pamela Block	Western University, Canada
Madeline Burghardt	York and Western Universities, Canada
Allison C. Carey	Shippensburg University, USA
Lei Chai	University of Toronto, Canada
Jayajit Chakraborty	University of Texas at El Paso, USA
Colleen M. Davison	Queen's University, Canada
Nelly De Arcos	Brown University, USA
Kim Fernandes	University of Pennsylvania, USA
Rachel Elizabeth Fish	New York University, USA
Grace L. Francis	George Mason University, USA
Olivia Friend	Brown University, USA
Sharon Gabison	University of Toronto and Family Alliance, Canada
Navjit Gaurav	Queen's University, Canada
Ewa Giemanowska	University of Warsaw, Poland
Robert Gould	University of Illinois at Chicago, USA
Valérie Grand'Maison	University of Guelph, Canada
Sara E. Green	University of South Florida, USA
Andy Holmes	University of Toronto, Canada
Srishti Jaitely	Tata Institute of Social Sciences, India
Julia Jansen-van Vuuren	Queen's University, Canada
Robin Jones	University of Illinois at Chicago, USA
Michelle Maroto	University of Alberta, Canada
Laura Mauldin	University of Connecticut, USA
Joana Milan Lorandi	Federal University of Santa Catarina, Brazil
Courtney Mullin	University of Illinois at Chicago, USA
Sarah Parker Harris	University of Illinois at Chicago, USA
David Pettinicchio	University of Toronto, Canada

Laura Pin	Wilfrid Laurier University, Canada
Mariola Racław	University of Warsaw, Poland
David E. Rangel	Brown University, USA
Kathryn Reinders	University of Guelph, Canada
Danielle Roberts	Queen's University, Canada
Tanushree Sarkar	Vanderbilt University, USA
Deborah Stienstra	University of Guelph, Canada
Dorota Szawarska	University of Warsaw, Poland

INTRODUCTION TO DISABILITY IN THE TIME OF PANDEMIC

Laura Mauldin[1], Sara E. Green and Allison C. Carey

In March 2020, as the pandemic arrived in the United States and generated a new reality of fear and anxiety, disability scholars and disabled people got to work.[1] From past experience of pandemics and national emergencies more broadly, they expected that disabled people, particularly disabled people of color, would be the most likely to die from COVID-19 and among the least likely to be protected from it. Their expectations proved to be true. The United States Centers for Disease Control quickly learned that those with chronic illnesses or disabilities, as well as those over the age of 65, occupy the highest risk categories for COVID-19 (CDC, 2019). Indeed, COVID-19 disproportionately affects disabled, chronically ill, and elderly people across the globe.

DISABILITY IN THE TIME OF PANDEMIC: DIFFERENTIAL HEALTH OUTCOMES

The expectation that people with disabilities and chronic health conditions would be disproportionately affected by the pandemic was confirmed from the start and solidified as the pandemic unfolded. Cloaked in the language of "pre-existing conditions," "underlying conditions," or "co-morbidities," studies found that people in those categories, that is, disabled people, died at four times the rate of able-bodied people (e.g., Choi, 2021). Congregate settings – a broad category including sites of long-term care like nursing homes, rehabilitation facilities, elderly housing facilities, shelters for unhoused people, and prisons – were hit the hardest due in part to being unable to isolate, often combined with inadequate access to protective equipment and poor overall conditions. Here again, disabled

[1]Laura Mauldin is lead author on this introduction. The author order for the volume is alphabetical and denotes equal contributions by the three authors to the overall volume.

Disability in the Time of Pandemic
Research in Social Science and Disability, Volume 13, 1–12

Published under exclusive licence by Emerald Publishing Limited
ISSN: 1479-3547/doi:10.1108/S1479-354720230000013001

people were disproportionately vulnerable because they are far more likely to be institutionalized in some way than able-bodied people (Landes et al., 2020). Indeed, in 2020, more than 41 percent of all COVID-19 deaths in the US were linked to nursing home residents or care workers (Centers for Medicaid and Medicare Services, 2020).

Demonstrating the intersecting disadvantages associated with race and disability that pre-dated the pandemic (e.g., Frederick & Shifrer, 2019), nursing homes with higher populations of non-white residents fared worse than those with primarily white residents (Gebeloff et al., 2020; Kim, 2020). Meanwhile, disabled residents (and their care workers) in smaller congregate care settings like group homes were "dying from the virus at a higher rate than the wider populations" (MacDonald, 2020), although not all governmental bodies kept statistics on these locations (Knezevich, 2020). Tsaplina and Stramondo (2020) reported that "Congregate housing for disabled people in New York other than nursing homes also shows infection and death rates far above average that may equal or even exceed those of nursing facilities" (Tsaplina & Stramondo, 2020). In New York State, residents of group homes for people with intellectual and developmental disabilities were far more likely than the general population to develop COVID-19 and far more likely to die from it (Landes et al., 2020).

Once infected, disabled people faced additional barriers, such as discrimination in healthcare. Multiple states in the US released "triage plans" for rationing care during the crisis and disabled people as a category were planned targets of treatment denial (Ne'eman, 2020). This was evidenced in "Alabama's Emergency Operations Plan that would deny ventilators to folks with severe or profound intellectual disabilities, or Tennessee, where those with spinal muscular atrophy who require help with activities of daily living would be denied treatment in a pandemic" (Stramondo, 2020). Like the general population, many medical professionals carry with them ableist perceptions that the quality of life for disabled people is invariably and necessarily low (Iezzoni et al., 2021). Drawing implicitly and explicitly on eugenics, some politicians and other public figures advocated letting disabled and elderly people die. The Lieutenant Governor of Texas suggested that older people should sacrifice themselves so the economy would not get destroyed (Levin, 2020), and a California official suggested that the virus be left to take its natural course on "the sick, the old, the injured" (Ormseth, 2020).

Around the world, general healthcare also became more inaccessible, threatening the well-being of disabled people. Many health services went online, but access to computers and the internet are unequally distributed. Medical care that was not COVID-19 related was deprioritized, leaving many people who are dependent on treatments and therapies in the lurch. The combination of high need and limited resources created a "thin margin of health" for people with disabilities, such that accessing even vital health care became uncertain (Kennedy et al., 2020, p. 5; see also Lederer, 2020; Prior, 2020).

As we write this in the spring of 2022, over 1 million people in the US have died and, according to the National Center for Health Statistics, the majority of these have been elderly people (CDC, 2022). In a recent National Council for Disability report on the impact of COVID-19 on disabled people, they write that "disability status as a demographic fact is not required or asked on death certificates, it is extremely difficult to establish even the bare fact of how many people with disabilities died from COVID-19" (2021, p. 40). They also argue that various studies of different disability populations indicate that disabled people were far more likely to die than nondisabled people. There "…is still not, however, an actual count of the numbers of COVID-19 infections or deaths of people with disabilities who have died directly as a result of contracting COVID-19" (NCD, 2021, p. 40).

But there are clues from one study in the UK: one study found that 17% of the population had a disability, but disabled people made up nearly 60% of COVID-19 deaths (Bosworth et al., 2021). On its face, the fact that more disabled than non-disabled people may have been affected by the COVID-19 pandemic might seem easily explainable by purely biological factors. Our goal as social scientists, and the goal of this volume, however, is to produce scholarship that improves our understanding of the social causes and consequences of the unequal distribution of disease. A social scientific approach to disability during the pandemic starts with the premise that while there may be physiological reasons for the particularly deadly effects of the virus on disabled people once they are exposed, the disproportionate spread of COVID-19, risk of infection, and other negative distal effects in these populations are the result social arrangements in which disabled people are disadvantaged.

DISABILITY IN THE TIME OF PANDEMIC: DIFFERENTIAL SOCIAL AND EMOTIONAL OUTCOMES

While evidence on the social effects of the pandemic is still accumulating, early research suggests that COVID-19 has had ramifications that reverberated throughout the economy, education, community life, and the social world. In the process, the pandemic revealed the economic and social marginality of disabled people. Economically, disabled people lost their jobs at higher rates, despite their already low employment rates. Between March and April 2020, employment fell by 24% for disabled people compared to 18% for the general population (Brooks, 2020; Maroto & Pettinicchio, 2020). Job loss was particularly severe for White and Black disabled women who tend to work in industries hit hardest by the pandemic (Schur & Kruse, 2020; Schur et al., 2021). Because recipients of disability benefits are often prohibited from saving because of program limits, they are also uniquely unprepared for economic emergencies.

Education was transformed, and these transformations were often unresponsive to the needs to disabled children and/or parents. Some disabled students needed the health protections afforded by the shift to online education, but were disadvantaged by the social isolation. Other students needed educational services that required face-to-face interaction, and even hands-on activities, in order to be successful. The individualized nature of meeting student needs often were cast aside as districts implemented hastily constructed emergency plans. Many students lost key components of their individualized education plans (Sonnenschein et al., 2022). Children and adults with disabilities also lost access to disability services outside of the school system. Many programs, such as arts and recreational programs and worship services, went online or into hiatus. Community-based direct care staffing became perilously unstable. Rarely did disabled people and their families have input into how their services and supports transformed (Schormans et al., 2021).

Early evidence also suggests that social and economic upheaval associated with the pandemic had serious consequences for the psychological health and emotional well-being of many people (Pfefferbaum & North, 2020; Rajkumar, 2020; Usher et al., 2020; Vindegaard & Benros, 2020). There is some evidence that the pandemic has increased discrimination toward people who were already targets of stigma before the pandemic – including people with disabilities and chronic health conditions (Abrams & Abbott, 2020; Bagcchi, 2020; Chen & McNamara, 2020; Maroto et al., 2021). Discrimination and stigma are known to have negative psychological consequences for people with disabilities (Brown, 2017; Ciciurkaite et al., 2021; Namkung & Carr, 2020). Lack of participation in social and recreational activities has also been shown to be negatively associated with well-being among people with disabilities (Green & Vice, 2017). Thus, the pandemic is likely to have decreased well-being through increased discrimination and social isolation.

DISABILITY IN THE TIME OF PANDEMIC: A ROAD MAP TO THIS VOLUME

The social and emotional effects of the pandemic noted above are variable, complex, and likely to extend far into the future in novel ways. As we live through the radical transformation of work, school, and family life, we need to understand how such transformations affect social arrangements that are already precarious for people with disabilities. Understanding the disproportionate effects of the pandemic on disabled people in their varied communities and across their complex identities requires that a variety of disciplinary and interdisciplinary lenses and analytic tools be put to use with data from around the world.

Authors in this volume approach their research using the insights, perspectives, and methods of a variety of social science disciplines and related areas of professional expertise. These include Anthropology, Disability Studies, Education, Physical and Rehabilitation Therapies, Public Health, Psychology, Sociology, and Women's and Gender Studies. They are affiliated with institutions in both the Global North and the Global South, and the data on which the research presented in this volume is based come from Canada, India, Poland, and the United States. The chapters in this volume also include collaborations across disciplines, among students and seasoned academics, among people in and outside of academic institutions, and among people with and without lived experience of disability. The volume includes both quantitative analysis of large data sets suitable for testing hypotheses about the relationship between disability status and various kinds of pandemic-related outcomes, and qualitative analysis of interviews, case studies, observations, and textual data to uncover nuanced patterns of pandemic experiences within the context of disability. A number of chapter authors explore complex social locations and intersectional identities that interact with disability and the pandemic in people's lives.

We have organized the volume around two broad inter-related themes. Chapters in Part 1, *Implications of the Pandemic for the Health, Well-being, and Care of People with Disabilities and their Families,* address differential vulnerability to negative pandemic-related outcomes such as access to services; social, emotional, and economic well-being; and opportunities for meaningful social interaction. In Part 2, *Implications of the Pandemic for People with Disabilities in Educational and Workplace Settings,* we turn our attention to how the pandemic affected people with disabilities in two specific contexts. Educational and workplace settings are particularly interesting because they are known to be spaces in which people with disabilities experience significant discrimination and stigma and yet they are also spaces in which inclusive programs have been intentionally developed and accommodations have been mandated.

Part 1: Implications of the Pandemic for the Health, Well-Being, and Care of People With Disabilities and Their Families

In Chapter 1, Jayajit Chakraborty reports results of a large scale quantitative study examining the relationship between county-level pandemic vulnerability and disability distribution in the United States. Findings show that not only is the percentage of disabled people in the population higher in counties that are more vulnerable to the pandemic, the most vulnerable counties also contain the highest percentage of people whose disability identity intersects with other disadvantaged social locations such as being a member of a racial/ethnic minority group, being female, living in poverty, and being unemployed. This chapter establishes a theme that runs through the entire volume – preexisting disadvantages were exacerbated during the pandemic. In Chapter 2, Valérie Grand'Maison and colleagues explore the impact of pandemic-related public policies on people with disabilities in Canada. Findings suggest a mechanism through which the pandemic reproduced preexisting inequalities. The chapter argues that pandemic-response policies that overlooked the social, economic, and housing precarity in which disabled people often live can worsen preexisting disadvantages – especially among people with disabilities from historically marginalized groups. In Chapter 3, Michelle Maroto and colleagues examine the positive and negative outcomes of social distancing – one particular pandemic response – in a mixed methods study of Canadians who live with disabilities and chronic health conditions. They found that people with disabilities felt that while social distancing measures such as avoiding contact with non-household members, avoiding public places, and transitioning to remote work/school offered vital protection against the disease, they also often resulted in increased loneliness and anxiety.

In Chapter 4, Srishti Jaitely and Gaurav turn our attention to pandemic experiences of people living in informal settlements in Mumbai, India. Using a qualitative case study approach including observations and interviews, the authors found that pre-pandemic disadvantages such as social and economic difficulties, environmental inaccessibility, limited transportation, and lack of disability-specific training among healthcare workers interacted with the pandemic in important ways and created significant barriers to the success of pandemic-related resource mobilization. In Chapter 5, Fernandes and Sarkar also address pandemic experiences in India through a critical discourse analysis of the media constructions of disabled children's lives, needs, and desires during the pandemic. They show how the disaster framing of the pandemic masked preexisting inequality and neglect and contributed to a narrative construction of disabled children as vulnerable and burdensome.

Chapter 6 ends the first part of the volume by bringing us back to the United States. Joana Milan Lorandi and Pamela Block explore the experiences of people with complex health conditions before and during the pandemic through 12 in-depth interviews with six participants. They draw particular attention to the ways in which participants imagined post-pandemic futures based on experiences before and during the pandemic. They conclude that participants felt they had been targets of ableism in the health system before the pandemic and feared that barriers to fair treatment and access to health care had been pushed to new heights by the pandemic.

Taken together, the six chapters in Part 1 tell a story in which pre-existing social, and economic disadvantages experienced by people with disabilities in Canada, India, and the United States interacted in complex ways with public policies, media coverage, and the virus to create additional layers of disadvantage and barriers to well-being for people with disabilities that may persist in a post-pandemic world. These chapters also suggest that pandemic-exacerbated inequalities intersect with those associated with other disadvantaged social locations – leaving the lives of those at the intersections in particularly precarious post-pandemic positions.

Part 2: Implications of the Pandemic for People With Disabilities in Educational and Workplace Settings

Previous research suggests that educational and workplace settings are sites in which people with disabilities often encountered disadvantages prior to the pandemic (Maconi et al., 2019; Maroto & Pettinicchio, 2014). These are also social institutions in which intentional, though far from perfect, accommodations, adaptations, and protections have been developed and/or legally mandated.

In Chapter 7, Rachel Fish and colleagues report findings of a US-based qualitative study of changes in the school experiences of disabled children as well as changes in the ways in which families engaged with schools and advocated for and/or supported their children during the pandemic. As in previous chapters, findings suggest that disability interacted with other axes of inequality in shaping these processes and that the pandemic exacerbated preexisting disadvantages at the intersections of class, disability, gender, linguistic status, and race in ways that created an uneven distribution of pandemic-related negative outcomes for children and families.

In Chapter 8, Julia Jansen-van Vuuren and colleagues explore how family-school partnerships in Canada were affected by the pandemic through interviews with 18 parents in Ontario. Findings suggest that parents value frequent, open, personalized communication about their children, and felt that they experienced a less than optimal degree of this kind of communication during the pandemic. They also expressed hope and optimism about the potential for developing effective future partnerships with their children's schools in the future.

In Chapter 9, Madeline Burghardt and colleagues report on a highly creative emancipatory research project conducted in collaboration with staff and participants of a disability-based arts program in Ontario, Canada. Findings suggest that social distancing and the pivot to online activities within the arts program created barriers to social inclusion for program participants that were not equally distributed. While many participants found that the pandemic provided opportunities for learning and growth, others remained disengaged and "lost" due to lack of technological access and personal support.

In Chapter 10, Giermanowska and colleagues report on a qualitative study based on interviews with 25 university students from across Poland who use assistant support services provided in private and public universities. Again, findings indicate that the negative effects of the pandemic were unequally distributed and that the pandemic exacerbated preexisting segregation and inequality in ways that heightened the social isolation of students who rely on personal supports for social engagement and community participation. As in other chapters in this section, however, the authors point out that some students found value in the pivot to online education in that it provided them with a sense of self-reliance and independence.

In the final chapter in this section and the book (Chapter 11), we move from the classroom to the workplace. Courtney Mullin and colleagues explore the role of disability-based employee resource groups in implementing disability inclusion strategies within large organizations and corporations in the United States, and the ways in which the pandemic changed the workplace experiences of disabled employees. Interviews with members of disability-based employee resource groups and diversity, equity, and inclusion officers suggest that the responsibility for disability inclusion shifted to employee resource groups at the start of the pandemic and that these groups played an important role in enhancing disability awareness and responding to instances of ableism. Findings also suggest that, as in the classroom, there were unequally distributed benefits and costs of pandemic-related changes. Some participants reported that the pandemic created a heightened awareness of disability issues that resulted in a growth in inclusive policies and practices, but others reported a near erasure of disability-inclusion efforts during the pandemic.

Taken together, chapters in Part 2 provide evidence that even within social institutions in which disability accommodations and support services have been mandated and in which programs specifically designed to enhance disability inclusion have developed, measures taken to reduce the spread of the physical disease had unequal consequences for people with disabilities. Some students and workers found that changes and challenges associated with the pandemic provided opportunities for individual and collective growth, while others lacked the support or infrastructure needed to take advantage of these opportunities.

DISABILITY IN THE TIME OF PANDEMIC: SUMMARY AND DISCUSSION

While this volume is being produced at a time in which social science understandings of the consequences of this ongoing pandemic are just beginning to develop, the research reported in this volume tells a compellingly consistent story. Far from a narrative in which the COVID-19 pandemic is a natural disaster or universal phenomenon that united the world through shared adversity, the research presented in this volume provides a narrative of differential access and differential impact. The narrative is remarkably similar across research settings, geographic locations, disciplinary backgrounds of authors, and epistemological and methodological approaches. The disadvantages and barriers experienced by people with disabilities before the pandemic tended to be heightened by the policies and practices designed to reduce its impact, but the pandemic and related changes also brought some opportunities for enhanced inclusion for some people with disabilities. Disabled people with other marginatized identities, however, were the hardest hit and the least likely to be able to benefit from the opportunities the pandemic provided. Chapter authors offer some clear and specific policy implications and make suggestions for future research that will enhance our understanding of how disability operates as a social location and axis of inequality around the world - as well as a deeper understanding of disability in the time of pandemic.

Our premise is that the disproportionate effects of the pandemic on disabled people that are described in this volume and other early work aren't inherent or "natural." Rather, these social patterns are symptoms of systemic ableism at work. Understanding this system and its effects on disabled people and communities in the context of the pandemic are what prompted the idea for this volume. Ableism, similar to and in conjunction with other "isms" such as racism and sexism, involves discrimination toward members of a social group, but it goes beyond discrimination to also encompass the value placed on certain attributes (Wolbring, 2008) and ways in which these values are codified in the daily doings of programs and institutions (Lewis, 2022). The idea that disabled lives are less valuable than other lives is codified in policies that deprioritize funding for homecare that would enable disabled people to live in their homes rather than institutions. It is reflected in the failure to prioritize mental healthcare so disabled people could receive treatment rather than incarceration. During the pandemic, the devaluation of disabled lives was blatantly reflected in "triage plans" that were proposed around the world in which disabled people *as a category* would be allowed to die in order to ration care, saving treatment for those whose lives were deemed to be more worthwhile.

The need to take up disability as a category of social experience worthy of analysis cannot be overstated; this must be the starting point if we want to uncover the mechanisms by which ableism operates (Green & Barnartt, 2017). As Mauldin and Brown (2021) write, "Like other minority groups, people with disabilities experience health disparities that are not functions of their condition but that derive from ableism that often goes unrecognized" (2021, p. 482). Thus, we proceed from the fundamental assertion that disability should not be "solely constituted as a medical classification; rather, it is positioned as an axis of inequality decoupled from any particular impairment" (Mauldin & Brown, 2021, p. 479).

While there is a wealth of evidence that disabled people experience ableism, they are not passive victims and they and their allies have engaged in disability activism throughout the twentieth and twenty-first centuries (Barnes, 2000; Barnett & Scotch, 2001; Carey et al., 2020; Pettinicchio, 2019). The pandemic was no exception. While under threat of greater vulnerability to the physical consequences of the COVID-19 virus, disabled people and their allies collectively organized and built community in response to the pandemic and its impacts. Disability justice communities have been steadfastly organizing in unique ways. For example, groups like the Disability Justice Culture Club in the San Francisco Bay Area and Crip Fund have been providing direct assistance and money to those facing serious needs. Disability rights organizations such as the American Association of People with Disabilities and the National Council of Independent Living have mobilized nationally to advocate for the passage of legislation that ensures that the needs of people with disabilities are included in every aspect of social and political response to the pandemic. Activists created the #NoBodyIsDisposable and #HighRiskCA hashtags, and quickly shared resources (Wong, 2022). Chapters included in this volume provide further evidence of the agency of people with disabilities during the time of pandemic. Disabled artists in the Sol Express program collaborated with program staff and chapter author Madeline Burghardt (Chapter 9) to provide evidence of the impact of the pandemic on people with disabilities and make suggestions of ways to improve disability inclusion in the future. Members of the disability-based employee resource groups interviewed by Mullin et al. (Chapter 11) promoted disability inclusion and responded to ableist incidents in large corporations across the United States, despite their own challenges as employees with disabilities in the midst of a pandemic. The will and ability to organize in the face of a frightening pandemic with the certain knowledge that its consequences would fall heavily on the shoulders of people with disabilities demonstrates the resilience and tenacity of people who are living with disability in the time of pandemic and we are pleased that their voices and experiences are reflected in the pages of this volume.

ACKNOWLEDGMENTS

We wish to thank the external reviewers who provided valuable suggestions for the chapters included in this volume, the chapter authors who served as blind reviewers for each other's work, series editors Barbara Altman and Sharon Barnartt, and the Emerald team.

NOTE

1. Following the social model of disability (Barnes, 2000), we differentiate between impairment and disability. We associate "impairment" with bodily differences currently conceived to be outside of the range of "normal" variation, recognizing that "normal" is also a social construct that varies with social, cultural, and historical context. We associate "disability" with social, cultural, and physical environments that impose layers of disadvantage on people whose bodies do not conform to current concepts of normality. Further, there are ongoing debates about how to refer to disabled people, reflecting what is called "identity first" language and "person first" language. According to Emily Ladau (2015), the latter has its origins in service providers rather than disability communities, while the former is often preferred by disabled people. We therefore alternate between "people with disabilities" and "disabled people" in this introduction and provided leeway for chapter authors to use whichever they find most comfortable.

REFERENCES

Abrams, T., & Abbott, D. (2020). Disability, deadly discourse, and collectivity amid coronavirus (COVID-19). *Scandinavian Journal of Disability Research*, *22*(1), 168–174.

Bagcchi, S. (2020). Stigma during the COVID-19 pandemic. *The Lancet Infectious Diseases*, *20*(7), 782.

Barnartt, S., & Scotch, R. (2001). *Disability protests contentious politics 1970 – 1999*. Gallaudet University Press.

Barnes, C. (2000). A working social model?: Disability, work, and disability politics in the 21st century. *Critical Social Policy*, *20*(4), 441–457.

Bosworth, M. L., Ayoubkhani, D., Nafilyan, V., Foubert, J., Glickman, M., Davey, C., & Kuper, H. (2021). Deaths involving COVID-19 by self-reported disability status during the first two waves of the COVID-19 pandemic in England: A retrospective, population-based cohort study. *The Lancet Public Health*, *6*(11), e817–e825. https://doi.org/10.1016/S2468-2667(21)00206-1

Brooks, J. (2020). Workers with disabilities may remain unemployed long after the Covid-19 pandemic. Lerner Center for Public Health Promotion, Issue Brief #30. Syracuse University.

Brown, R. L. (2017). Functional limitation and depressive symptomatology: Considering perceived stigma and discrimination within a stress and coping framework. *Stigma and Health*, *2*(2), 98–109.

Carey, A. C., Block, P., & Scotch, R. (2020). *Allies and obstacles: Disability activism and parents of children with disabilities*. Temple University Press.

Centers for Disease Control. (2019). *COVID-19: People with certain medical conditions*. Centers for Disease Control and Prevention. https://www.cdc.gov/coronavirus/2019-ncov/need-extra-precautions/people-with-medical-conditions.html. Accessed on June 14, 2022.

Centers for Disease Control. (2022). COVID-19 mortality overview. https://www.cdc.gov/nchs/covid19/mortality-overview.htm. Accessed on June 14, 2022.

Centers for Medicaid and Medicare Services. (2020). *COVID-19 nursing home data*. Department of Health and Human Services, Baltimore, MD.

Chen, B., & McNamara, D. M. (2020). Disability discrimination, medical rationing and COVID-19. *Asian Bioethics Review*, *12*(4), 511–518.

Choi, W. (2021). Mortality rate of patients with COVID-19 based on underlying health conditions. *Disaster Medicine and Public Health Preparedness*, 1–6. https://doi.org/10.1017/dmp.2021.139

Ciciurkaite, G., Marquez-Velarde, G., & Brown, R. L. (2021). *Stressors associated with the COVID-19 pandemic, disability, and mental health: Considerations from the Intermountain West*. Stress and Health. https://doi.org/10.1002/smi.3091

Frederick, A., & Shifrer, D. (2019). Race and disability: From analogy to intersectionality. *Sociology of Race and Ethnicity*, *5*(2), 200–214.

Gebeloff, R., Ivory, D., Richtel, M., Smith, M., Yourish, K., Dance, S., Fortiér, J., Yu, E., & Parker, M. (2020). The striking racial divide in how covid-19 has hit nursing homes. *The New York Times*. May 21.

Green, S. E., & Barnartt, S. (Eds.). (2017). *Sociology looking at disability: What did we know and when did we know it, research in social science and disability* (*Vol. 9*). Emerald Publishing Limited.

Green, S. E., & Vice, B. (2017). Disability and community life: Mediating effects of work, social inclusion, and economic disadvantage in the relationship between disability and subjective well-being. In B. Altman (Ed.), *Factors in Studying Employment for Persons with Disability* (*Vol. 10*, pp. 225–246). Emerald Publishing Limited.

Iezzoni, L. I., Row, S. R., Rssalam, J., Blocic-Jankovic, D., Agarronnik, N., Donelan, K., Lagu, T., & Campbell, E. G. (2021). Physicians' perceptions of people with disabilities and their health care. *Health Affairs*, *40*(2), 297–306.

Kennedy, J., Frieden, L., Dick-Mosher, J., & Curtis, B. (2020). COVID-19 related needs of centers for independent living, CIL staff, and consumers. Collaborative on Health Reform and Independent Living. https://www.chril.org/

Kim, E. T. (2020). When you are paid 13 hours for a 24-hour shift. *The New York Times*. June 30.

Knezevich, A. (2020). Invisible care aides: They serve the vulnerable, but many low-wage home care workers are overlooked in pandemic, Baltimore area advocates say. *The Baltimore Sun*, p. 1. June 8.

Ladau, E. (2015). Person-first language doesn't always put the person first. Think Inclusive. http://www.thinkinclusive.us/why-person-first-language-doesnt-always-put-the-person-first/

Landes, S. D., Turk, M. A., Formica, M. K., McDonald, K. E., & Stevens, J. D. (2020). COVID-19 outcomes among people with intellectual and developmental disability living in residential group homes in New York State. *Disability and Health Journal*, *13*(4), 100969. https://doi.org/10.1016/j.dhjo.2020.100969

Lederer, E. (2020, May 6). UN leader says 1B people with disabilities hard hit by virus. Associated News. https://apnews.com/c753de7283390477e007b0aeb4d09e3c

Levin, B. (2020). Texas Lt. Governor: Old people should volunteer to die to save the economy. *Vanity Fair*. Retrieved August 6, 2020 https://www.vanityfair.com/news/2020/03/dan-patrick-coronavirus-grandparents.

Lewis, T. (2022). Working definition of ableism - January 2022 update. TALILA A LEWIS. http://www.talilalewis.com/1/post/2022/01/working-definition-of-ableism-january-2022-update.html

MacDonald, A. (2020, June 11). Pandemic hits forgotten profession: Special-needs careworkers. *Wall Street Journal*.

Maconi, M. L., Green, S. E., & Bingham, S. C. (2019). It's not all about coursework: Narratives of inclusion and exclusion among university students receiving disability accommodations. In K. Scorgie & C. Forlin (Eds.), *Promoting social inclusion: Co-Creating environments that foster equity and belonging, international perspectives on inclusive education* (*Vol. 13*, pp. 181–194). Emerald Publishing Limited.

Maroto, M., & Pettinicchio, D. (2014). Disability, structural inequality, and work: The influence of occupational segregation on earnings for people with different disabilities. *Research in Social Stratification and Mobility*, *38*, 76–92.

Maroto, M., & Pettinicchio, D. (2020). An unequal labor market means that COVID-19 has been especially harmful for vulnerable groups including people with disabilities. London School of Economics US Centre. https://blogs.lse.ac.uk/usappblog/2020/05/21/an-unequal-labor-market-means-that-covid-19-has-been-especially-harmful-for-vulnerable-groups-including-people-with-disabilities/

Maroto, M. L., Pettinicchio, D., & Lukk, M. (2021). Working differently or not at all: COVID-19's effects on employment among people with disabilities and chronic health conditions. *Sociological Perspectives*. https://doi.org/10.1177/07311214211012018

Mauldin, L., & Brown, R. L. (2021). Missing pieces: Engaging sociology of disability in medical sociology. *Journal of Health and Social Behavior*, *62*(4), 477–492.

Namkung, E. H., & Carr, D. (2020). The psychological consequences of disability over the life course: Assessing the mediating role of perceived interpersonal discrimination. *Journal of Health and Social Behavior*, *61*(2), 190–207.

National Council on Disability. (2021). The impact of COVID-19 on people with disabilities. Washington, DC.

Ne'eman, A. (2020, March 23). I will not apologize for my needs. *New York Times*. https://www.nytimes.com/2020/03/23/opinion/coronavirus-ventilators-triage-disability.html

Ormseth, M. (2020). Northern California official ousted after saying elderly, ill, homeless should be left to die in pandemic. *Los Angeles Times*. May 1.

Pettinicchio, D. (2019). *Politics of empowerment: Disability rights and the cycle of American policy reform*. Stanford University Press.

Pfefferbaum, B., & North, C. S. (2020). Mental health and the Covid-19 pandemic. *New England Journal of Medicine*, *383*(6), 510–512.

Prior, R. (2020, April 8). Coping with disease and disability in the time of coronavirus. CNN. https://www.cnn.com/2020/04/08/health/coronavirus-disability-and-chronic-illness-wellness/index.html

Rajkumar, R. P. (2020). COVID-19 and mental health: A review of the existing literature. *Asian Journal of Psychiatry*, *52*, 102066. https://doi.org/10.1016/j.ajp.2020.102066

Schormans, A. F., Hutton, S., Blake, M., Earle, K., & Head, K. (2021). Social isolation continued: COVID-19 shines a light on what self-advocates know too well. *Qualitative Social Work*, *20*(1/2), 83–89.

Schur, L., & Kruse, D. (2020). Coronavirus could revolutionize work opportunities for people with disabilities. The Conversation. https://theconversation.com/coronavirus-could-revolutionize-work-opportunities-for-people-with-disabilities-137462

Schur, L., van der Meulen Rodgers, Y., & Kruse, D. (2021). *COVID-19 and employment losses for workers with disabilities: An intersectional approach*. The Center for Women and Work Working Paper Series. Rutgers University. http://smlr.rutgers.edu/sites/default/files/Documents/Centers/CWW/Publications/draft_covid19_and_disability_report.pdf

Sonnenschein, S., Stites, M. L., Grossman, J. A., & Galczyk, S. H. (2022). "This will likely affect his entire life": Parents' views of special education during COVID-19. *International Journal of Educational Research*, *112*. https://doi.org/10.1016/j.ijer.2022.101941

Stramondo, J. (2020). COVID-19 triage and disability: What NOT to do. Bioethics.Net. http://www.bioethics.net/2020/03/covid-19-triage-and-disability-what-not-to-do/?fbclid=IwAR1h8RcueMcdn6spIPnhjVXz0Sn08-ir2LfUwCB5aeS0bzdEK9XNbpLU8yM

Tsaplina, M., & Stramondo, J. A. (2020). #WeAreEssential: Why disabled people should be appointed to hospital triage committees. The Hastings Center. https://www.thehastingscenter.org/weareessential-why-disabled-people-should-be-appointed-to-hospital-triage-committees/

Usher, K., Durkin, J., & Bhullar, N. (2020). The COVID-19 pandemic and mental health impacts. *International Journal of Mental Health Nursing*, *29*(3), 315–318.

Vindegaard, N., & Benros, M. E. (2020). COVID-19 pandemic and mental health consequences: Systematic review of the current evidence. In *Brain, Behavior, and Immunity* (*Vol. 89*, pp. 531–542). Academic Press.

Wolbring, G. (2008). The politics of ableism. *Development*, *51*(2), 252–258. https://doi.org/10.1057/dev.2008.17

Wong, A. (2022). High-risk pandemic stories: A syllabus. Disability Visibility Project. https://disabilityvisibilityproject.com/2022/01/09/high-risk-pandemic-stories-a-syllabus/

PART I

IMPLICATIONS OF THE PANDEMIC FOR THE HEALTH, WELL-BEING, AND CARE OF PEOPLE WITH DISABILITIES AND THEIR FAMILIES

Chapter 1

COVID-19 AND PEOPLE WITH DISABILITIES: SOCIAL INEQUALITIES IN THE DISTRIBUTION OF PANDEMIC VULNERABILITY

Jayajit Chakraborty

ABSTRACT

Purpose: *This chapter addresses the growing need to analyze the relationship between COVID-19 vulnerability and disability status at the national scale in the US. It presents a quantitative study that seeks to determine whether US counties more vulnerable to the COVID-19 pandemic contain significantly higher percentages of people with disabilities (PwDs), in general, and socially disadvantaged PwDs (based on their ethnicity/race, biological sex, age poverty, and employment status), in particular.*

Methods/Approach: *Vulnerability to COVID-19 is measured using the COVID-19 Pandemic Vulnerability Index (PVI) model developed by the National Institute of Environmental Health Sciences, which integrates multiple variables into relevant indicators that are weighted and combined to formulate a county-level PVI score. These scores are linked to a wide range of disability-related variables from the 2019 American Community Survey five-year estimates. Statistical analyses are based on multivariable generalized estimating equations that extend the generalized linear model to account for spatial clustering.*

Findings: *US counties more vulnerable to the COVID-19 pandemic are characterized by significantly higher percentages of PwDs, when vaccination is*

Disability in the Time of Pandemic
Research in Social Science and Disability, Volume 13, 15–29

Published under exclusive licence by Emerald Publishing Limited
ISSN: 1479-3547/doi:10.1108/S1479-354720230000013002

considered in estimating the PVI. These counties also contain significantly higher percentages of ethnic/racial minority, female, below poverty, and unemployed PwDs, in multiple timeframes of the pandemic.

Implication/Value: *The findings provide important insights and new knowledge on the relationship between COVID-19 vulnerability and socially disadvantaged PwDs in the US. The county-level associations highlight the need for additional data and more detailed analysis to examine the differential impacts of this pandemic on PwDs, as well as formulate appropriate intervention strategies.*

Keywords: COVID-19; disability; generalized estimating equations; intra-categorical analysis; pandemic vulnerability; social inequality

INTRODUCTION

People with disabilities (PwDs) may be four times more likely to be injured or die than non-disabled persons during the COVID-19 pandemic and other recent emergencies caused by climate change and natural disasters, in part, because their needs have not been considered in public health policy, planning, and practice (Izutsu, 2020; Pineda & Corburn, 2020). The social vulnerability of PwDs is also amplified by their lower socioeconomic status, since almost 62% of PwDs in the US are unemployed and 27% live below the poverty line (Houtenville & Boege, 2019). The urgent need to examine increased risks faced by PwDs from the COVID-19 pandemic was first emphasized as a research priority in a World Health Organization report (WHO, 2020). Compared to the non-disabled population, PwDs face higher risks of contracting COVID-19 because of barriers in implementing basic hygiene measures, enacting social distancing, and accessing health information, as well as the need to touch objects to obtain information or for physical support (Boyle et al., 2020; Turk & McDermott, 2020; WHO, 2020). PwDs are also at greater risk of developing severe disease if they become infected because of pre-existing health conditions underlying their disability and barriers to accessing health care (Pendo, 2020). Additionally, PwDs may be negatively impacted by the COVID-19 outbreak because of disruptions to services they depend on (Turk & McDermott, 2020; WHO, 2020). PwDs who reside in places facing greater exposure or vulnerability to the COVID-19 pandemic are more likely to experience these adverse consequences and challenges (Bosworth et al., 2021; Chakraborty, 2021).

While recent studies have reported greater COVID-19 infection and mortality rates in US counties containing higher proportions of racial/ethnic minorities, people in poverty, and other socially disadvantaged groups (Finch & Hernández Finch, 2020; Hendryx & Luo, 2020; Karaye & Horney, 2020; Karmakar et al., 2021; Mahajan & Larkins-Pettigrew, 2020), the relationship between disability status and COVID-19 vulnerability has not been systematically investigated in adequate detail at the national scale. The only county-level study to focus specifically on PwDs found higher COVID-19 incidence to be negatively associated with the overall percentage of PwDs, but positively related to the presence of PwDs who are minority, female, and below poverty level (Chakraborty, 2021). Since this study used COVID-19 cases as the only measure of pandemic vulnerability, more detailed analyses are necessary to examine spatial and social inequalities in the distribution of COVID-19 for PwDs and specific subgroups of PwDs.

This chapter addresses the growing need to analyze the relationship between COVID-19 vulnerability and disability status at the national scale in the US, as well as contribute to an emerging body of research that recommends an intra-categorical approach for quantitative analysis of socio-spatial inequalities experienced by PwDs (Chakraborty, 2020, 2021). McCall (2005) termed an intra-categorical approach as a component of her work on intersectionality, which focused more broadly on the life experiences of multiple marginalized groups. Following McCall (2005), an intra-categorical analysis focuses on characterizing differences of experience for subgroups within a category based on other axes of marginality (Allain & Collins, 2021; Chakraborty, 2020). The study presented in this chapter applies an intra-categorical approach to explore the ways in which disability status combines with other socio-demographic characteristics to shape disproportionate exposure to higher pandemic vulnerability. Since all PwDs may not be equally disadvantaged, an important premise of this work is that factors such as ethnicity, race, gender, age, poverty, and employment status can intersect differently with disability to amplify or attenuate COVID-19 vulnerability for specific subgroups within the broader disability category.

This study seeks to examine whether PwDs and socio-demographically disadvantaged PwDs, in particular, are disproportionately located in US counties that are more vulnerable to the COVID-19 pandemic. The key goal is to determine if counties characterized by greater pandemic vulnerability contain significantly higher proportions of ethnic/racial, minority, female, older-aged, below poverty, and unemployed PwDs, after controlling for relevant contextual factors and spatial clustering. An additional goal is to examine how statistical associations between COVID-19 vulnerability and socio-demographic characteristics of PwDs have changed over time, during the first 18 months of the pandemic.

Vulnerability to COVID-19 for this study is measured using the Pandemic Vulnerability Index (PVI) model that was recently developed through a collaborative effort that included scholars and scientists from the National Institute of Environmental Health Sciences (NIEHS), North Carolina State University, and Texas A&M University (NIEHS, 2021a). The PVI is a comprehensive and robust indicator that combines well-established social vulnerability factors for public health with emerging factors relevant to the pandemic. Statistical analysis is based on multivariable generalized estimating equations that account for spatial clustering of US counties and provide statistically reliable inferences regarding relationships between pandemic vulnerability and socio-demographic characteristics of PwDs.

DATA AND METHODS

Dependent Variables: Measuring Pandemic Vulnerability

The recently developed US COVID-19 PVI model integrates multiple variables into relevant indicators that are weighted and combined to formulate an overall county-level PVI score (Marvel et al., 2021; NIEHS, 2021b). These indicators or data components comprise a variety of well-documented vulnerability factors for public health and pandemic-relevant factors that encompass four domains: (1) infection rates; (2) baseline population concentration; (3) intervention measures; and (4) health and environmental vulnerabilities. These domains and data components associated with the two current models (PVI Model 11.2 and PVI Model 12.4), as well as the weights assigned to each domain and data component, are listed in Table 1. The key difference between the two PVI models is the inclusion of vaccine data (i.e., percentage of unvaccinated residents in the county) and subsequent reweighting applied to Model 12.4.

PVI Models 11.2 and 12.4 are referred to as *Original PVI Mod*el and *PVI with Vaccine Model*, respectively, in subsequent sections of this paper. For both models, the overall PVI profile for each US county is calculated using the Toxicological Prioritization Index (ToxPi) framework for data integration within

Table 1. Pandemic Vulnerability Index (PVI) Models: Domains, Data Components, and Weights.

Model 11.2: Original PVI		Model 12.4: PVI with Vaccine	
Major Domains	Data Components	Major Domains	Data Components
Infection rate (24%)	Transmissible cases (20%)	Infection rate (25%)	Transmissible cases (20%)
	Disease spread (4%)		Disease spread (5%)
Population concentration (16%)	Population mobility (8%)	Population concentration (15%)	Population mobility (10%)
	Residential density (8%)		Residential density (5%)
Intervention measures (16%)	Social distancing (8%)	Intervention measures (25%)	Unvaccinated rate (15%)
	Testing rate (8%)		Social distancing (5%)
			Testing rate (5%)
Health and environment (44%)	Population demographics (8%)	Health and environment (35%)	Hospital beds (10%)
	Air pollution (8%)		Hospital ventilators (10%)
	Age distribution (8%)		Population demographics (3%)
	Co-morbidities (8%)		Air pollution (3%)
	Health disparities (8%)		Age distribution (3%)
	Hospital beds (4%)		Co-morbidities (3%)
			Health disparities (3%)

Source: National Institute of Environmental Health Sciences (NIEHS), 2021b.

a geospatial context (Bhandari et al., 2020; Marvel et al., 2018). Data sources used to derive the various components/indicators and methodological details associated with the integration of data streams, including the daily time series of all source data since February 2020 and resultant PVI scores, are available on the public PVI GitHub project page [https://github.com/COVID19PVI/data]. Visual representations of PVI profiles for each US county are provided in the interactive COVID-19 PVI Dashboard (NIEHS, 2021c) maintained by the NIEHS and the Centers for Disease Control and Prevention (CDC).

For this study, PVI scores for all 3,142 counties in the US were downloaded from the *Original PVI Model* for three specific dates: August 1 2020, February 1 2021, and August 1, 2021. These dates were chosen to examine the relationship between pandemic vulnerability with disability status across three equally-spaced timeframes (every six months), during the first 18 months since COVID-19 cases were officially recorded in the US. For the *PVI with Vaccine Model*, the same data were downloaded for two of these three dates (February 1 2021 and August 1 2021), since vaccination information was not included in the PVI Model prior to February 2021. The use of multiple PVI datasets for each model allows us to examine if the statistical results are sensitive to the choice of timeframe associated with COVID-19 case, intervention, and vaccination data. Descriptive statistics for all PVI-related variables are provided in Table 1.

Independent Variables: Social Characteristics of PwDs

Data on the total number and socio-demographic characteristics of PwDs were extracted from the latest (2019) American Community Survey (ACS) five-year estimates. While disability is a complex and multidimensional concept, this research uses the US Census definition that has been used by the ACS and federal government agencies since 2008. PwDs include members of the civilian non-institutionalized population who reported having serious self-care, hearing, vision, independent living, ambulatory, or cognitive difficulties on the ACS form (US Census Bureau, 2021). The ACS disability estimates allow disaggregation of PwDs based on six socio-demographic categories (ethnicity, race, biological sex, age, poverty level, and employment status) that were used for the intra-categorical analysis. For each county, the total number of PwDs was used to estimate the percentage of the civilian non-institutionalized population who are PwDs, as well as the population density of PwDs (total number per square mile) which was included as a control variable. All remaining variables are specific to PwDs, and comprise relevant subgroups of PwDs.

To examine ethnicity and race, the analysis included variables for the percentage of PwDs in each county who self-identified as Hispanic/Latino (of any race) and each of the following subgroups: Black or African-American, Asian, American Indian/Alaskan, and multi-racial/other minority race (comprised Hawaiian/Pacific Islander, some other race, and two or more races). The percentage of non-Hispanic White PwDs was excluded from multivariable models to allow results for the minority ethnic/racial categories to be interpreted relative to non-Hispanic White PwDs. The percentage of PwDs who are female was used to examine gender-based inequalities. The percentage of PwDs aged 17 years or less and 65 years or more were included to serve as age-related variables, with those aged 18–64 years serving as the reference group. To evaluate socioeconomic status, the analysis included the percentage of PwDs below poverty level and those who are unemployed. Unlike the other PwD-specific variables that utilize the total number of PwDs in the county as denominator, the percentage of PwDs below poverty is based on PwDs for whom poverty status is determined and the percentage of unemployed PwDs is based on PwDs in the labor force (aged 18–64 years). Summary statistics for all independent variables are provided in Table 2.

Statistical Methodology

To analyze the relationship between pandemic vulnerability and disability status, this study utilizes generalized estimating equations (GEEs) – a multivariable modeling technique that extends the generalized linear model to accommodate clustered data (Garson, 2013; Nelder & Wedderburn, 1972). GEEs are particularly suitable for this analysis because they account for clustering in the data, relax several assumptions of traditional regression models, and provide multiple advantages compared to other techniques such as spatial regression or multilevel modeling (Chakraborty, 2020).

For estimating a GEE, clusters of analytic units must be defined based on the assumption that units within a cluster are correlated, while units from different

Table 2. Descriptive Statistics for Variables Analyzed.

	Min	Max	Mean	SD
Dependent variables:				
Original PVI: August 1, 2020	0.18	0.70	0.50	0.09
Original PVI: February 1, 2021	0.18	0.64	0.47	0.07
Original PVI: August 1, 2021	0.19	0.67	0.47	0.08
PVI with Vaccine: February 1, 2021	0.18	0.70	0.50	0.09
PVI with Vaccine: August 1, 2021	0.21	0.67	0.47	0.08
Independent variables:				
% People with disabilities (PwDs)	4.04	36.79	15.96	4.44
% PwDs: Hispanic or Latino	0.00	99.31	6.54	12.12
% PwDs: Black or African-American	0.00	90.52	8.88	14.75
% PwDs: Asian	0.00	48.43	0.83	2.38
% PwDs: American Indian and Alaskan	0.00	94.79	2.20	8.09
% PwDs: Multi-racial/Other minority	0.00	53.58	3.72	4.07
% PwDs: Female	17.15	75.24	49.42	4.67
% PwDs: Age 17 years or less	0.00	30.75	6.96	2.87
% PwDs: Age 65 year or more	20.78	84.31	44.28	7.51
% PwDs: Below poverty level	0.00	35.51	17.03	4.61
% PwDs: Unemployed	0.00	100.00	10.98	7.25
PwDs: population density (per sq. mi.)	0.01	7314.00	31.78	195.81

Note: N = 3,142 counties in the US (excludes Puerto Rico).

clusters are independent. A combination of two approaches was utilized to define county clusters for the GEE models. The state in which a county is located was first used to account for potential correlation in counties within the same state, because counties in a given state are likely to be similar in terms of various characteristics such as COVID-19 response and testing policies, sociocultural attributes, and healthcare systems. Since the use of states as the only clustering variable potentially ignores intra-state variations and urban-rural disparities, a second approach based on the county Rural-Urban Continuum (RUC) code was implemented. This classification scheme developed by the US Department of Agriculture (USDA, 2020) groups all counties into metropolitan and nonmetropolitan, and nonmetropolitan counties are further subdivided based on whether or not they are adjacent to a metropolitan area. This combination of 51 states and three RUC categories (metropolitan, nonmetropolitan adjacent, and nonmetropolitan non-adjacent) resulted in a total of 142 clusters, with the number of counties per cluster ranging from 1 to 98.

GEEs also require an intra-cluster dependency correlation matrix to be specified (Garson, 2013). After experimentation with several different specifications, the "exchangeable" correlation matrix was selected for GEEs that use scores from the *Original PVI Model* as the dependent variable and the "independent" correlation matrix was selected for GEEs that use scores from *PVI with Vaccine Model* as the dependent variable. These specifications were chosen because they yielded the best statistical fit based on the QIC (quasi-likelihood under the independence model criterion). To further improve model fit, the normal, gamma, and inverse Gaussian distributions with logarithmic and identity link functions were tested, since the PVI scores were not normally distributed. The gamma distribution with logarithmic link function was chosen for all five GEE models because this function indicated the best statistical fit based on the QIC.

All independent variables were standardized and standardized coefficients are provided in tables summarizing the GEE results. Potential multicollinearity among these variables were also examined using the multicollinearity condition index for the combination of all independent variables included in each GEE model. An index value of 10 or more suggests the presence of multicollinearity, while a value higher than 30 is indicative of severe multicollinearity (Belsley, 1991). The multicollinearity condition index for this combination of independent variables was 2.51, confirming that the multivariable GEEs are not affected by multicollinearity. Two-tailed *p*-values from the Wald chi-squared test were used to test the statistical significance of each variable coefficient.

RESULTS

Spatial patterns of pandemic vulnerability are depicted as classified choropleth maps in Fig. 1, where US counties are grouped into five classes with identical class intervals based on PVI scores from each of the two models (five dependent variables). Maps in the first or left column represent scores from the *Original PVI*

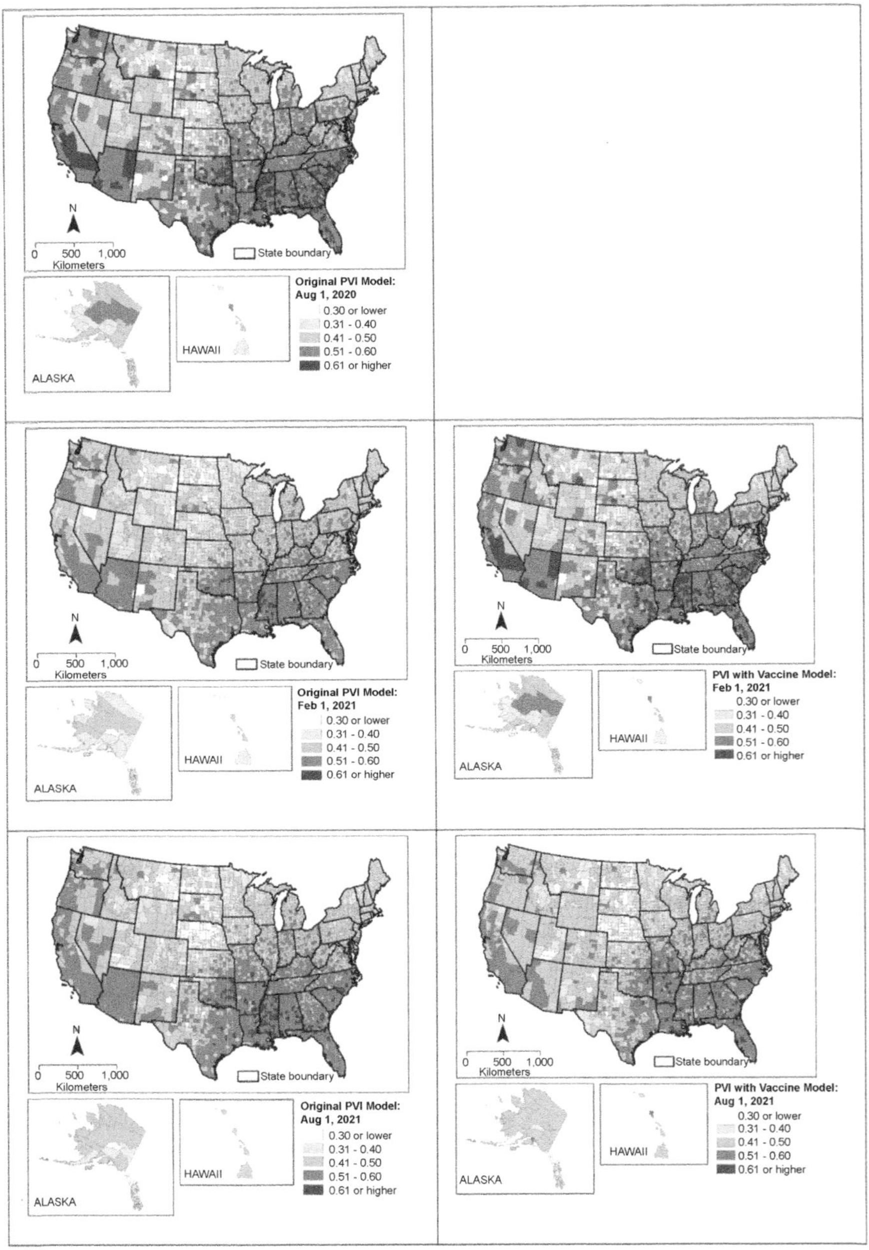

Fig. 1. County Level Distribution of Pandemic Vulnerability Index (PVI) Scores in the US.

Model in three timeframes, and those in second or right column shown PVI scores from the *PVI with Vaccine Model* in two timeframes. The county-level distribution patterns of the PVI appear to have changed over time, in specific regions of the US Counties in highest PVI category (i.e., PVI greater than 0.6), for example, can be observed in western states such as Arizona and California, as well as in southern states such as Mississippi, Texas, and Georgia, on August 1, 2020 (*Original PVI Model*). In subsequent timeframes, however, counties in the highest PVI category for this model are located only in southern states. Similar geographic shifts in PVI patterns can be seen in the two maps associated with the *PVI with Vaccine Model*, with counties in the highest PVI category concentrated only in the southern and southeastern states on August 1, 2021.

Results from the multivariable GEEs for scores obtained from the *Original PVI Model* are summarized in Table 3. In the GEE for August 1, 2020 (representing the first six months of the pandemic), the overall percentage of PwDs in the county indicates a statistically significant and negative relationship with the PVI ($p < 0.05$), after controlling for spatial clustering, population density, and other independent variables. However, the percentages of PwDs who are Hispanic, Black, American Indian/Alaskan, and female indicate a positive and significant association with the PVI. The percentages of PwDs below poverty level and PwDs who are unemployed also reveal a significantly positive relationship

Table 3. Multivariable Generalized Estimating Equations (GEEs) for Predicting PVI Scores From *Original PVI Model.*

	Aug 1, 2020		Feb 1, 2021		Aug 1, 2021	
	Beta	Wald Chi-Sq	Beta	Wald Chi-Sq	Beta	Wald Chi-Sq
% People with disabilities (PwDs)	−0.007	4.285*	−0.002	0.585	0.003	1.238
% PwDs: Hispanic or Latino	0.010	5.528*	0.006	2.339	0.003	0.894
% PwDs: Black	0.018	12.427**	0.016	10.442**	0.015	9.786**
% PwDs: Asian	0.002	0.256	0.003	1.079	0.008	5.157**
% PwDs: American Indian/Alaskan	0.018	24.421**	0.017	34.884**	0.015	12.138**
% PwDs: Multi-racial/Other minority	0.003	0.403	0.001	0.031	0.002	0.214
% PwDs: Female	0.015	21.929**	0.013	20.993**	0.012	18.300**
% PwDs: Age 17 years or less	0.001	0.000	0.001	0.165	0.002	0.909
% PwDs: Age 65 year or more	−0.034	86.864**	−0.029	65.027**	−0.030	44.956**
% PwDs: Below poverty level	0.027	55.890**	0.026	72.250**	0.028	63.702**
% PwDs: Unemployed	0.008	6.540*	0.005	5.151*	0.008	11.714**
PwDs: population density	0.001	0.004	0.002	4.518*	0.003	5.151*
Intercept	−0.726		−0.793		−0.779	
Quasi Likelihood under Independence Model Criterion (QIC)	155.24		140.08		155.90	

Note: GEEs are based on a gamma distribution with log link function and an exchangeable correlation matrix; $N = 3{,}142$.

with the PVI. The percentage of PwDs who are aged 65 or more years, in contrast, indicates a significantly negative association on August 1, 2020.

In the GEEs for February 1, 2021 and August 1, 2021, relationships between the independent variables and scores from the *Original PVI Model* are similar to those observed in the model for August 1, 2020, with two exceptions. In both these GEEs, the percentages of PwDs who are Black, American Indian/Alaskan, female, below poverty, and unemployed indicate a positive and significant association with the PVI, and the percentage of PwDs who are aged 65 or more years indicates a significantly negative association. The overall percentage of PwDs and the percentage of PwDs who are Hispanic, however, are not significant in the GEEs for both February 1, 2021 and August 1, 2021.

Table 4 summarizes the results from the multivariable GEEs for scores obtained from the *PVI with Vaccine Model.* In the GEE for February 1, 2021 (when vaccinations were available in all US states), the overall percentage of PwDs in the county indicates a positive and significant relationship with the PVI. The percentages of PwDs who are Black, Hispanic, female, below poverty, and unemployed also show significantly positive association with the PVI. In the GEE for August 1, 2021 (when vaccinations were available in all US states), a significantly positive relationship with PVI scores can be observed for the overall percentage of PwDs, as well as the percentages of PwDs who are Black, Asian, female, below poverty, and unemployed. The percentage of PwDs American Indian/Alaskan, however, indicates a negative and significant association with the

Table 4. Multivariable GEEs for Predicting PVI Scores From *PVI With Vaccine Model.*

	Feb 1, 2021		Aug 1, 2021	
	Beta	Wald Chi-Sq	Beta	Wald Chi-Sq
% People with disabilities (PwDs)	0.016	9.756**	0.019	12.676**
% PwDs: Hispanic or Latino	0.021	15.997**	0.007	1.096
% PwDs: Black	0.050	91.147**	0.042	58.677**
% PwDs: Asian	0.002	0.083	0.014	8.186**
% PwDs: American Indian/Alaskan	−0.002	0.081	−0.019	29.589**
% PwDs: Multi-racial/Other minority	0.004	0.363	0.003	0.250
% PwDs: Female	0.033	72.807**	0.027	50.228**
% PwDs: Age 17 years or less	−0.005	1.720	−0.005	2.949
% PwDs: Age 65 year or more	−0.053	64.000**	−0.058	52.362**
% PwDs: Below poverty level	0.028	24.263**	0.008	1.961*
% PwDs: Unemployed	0.015	13.679**	0.018	24.505**
PwDs: population density	−0.008	19.358**	0.000	0.041
Intercept	−0.700		−0.757	
QIC	167.33		177.57	

Note: GEEs are based on a gamma distribution with log link function and an independent correlation matrix; $N = 3{,}142$.

PVI. The percentage of PwDs who are aged 65 or more years is the only variable to indicate a significantly negative relationship in both GEE models.

CONCLUSION

This study sought to examine how vulnerability to the COVID-19 pandemic in the US is related to the overall proportion and socio-demographic characteristics of PwDs at the county level, using the most comprehensive and reliable measure of pandemic vulnerability currently available. When vaccination rates were not considered, the overall percentage of PwDs was significantly lower in counties with higher PVI in the first timeframe (August 2020) and not significantly related to the PVI in more recent timeframes (February and August 2021), after controlling for spatial clustering, population density of PwDs, and other relevant variables. These findings align with the first published study of the relationship between COVID-19 incidence and disability in the US (Chakraborty, 2021), which found a relatively weak but negative county-level correlation between COVID-19 infection rate and the overall disability percentage on August 1, 2020. However, when vaccination rates were incorporated to estimate the PVI in this study, significantly greater pandemic vulnerability was found in counties with higher percentages of PwDs, in both timeframes (February and August 2021). This finding could be a potential consequence of greater percentages of unvaccinated people in counties with higher PwD percentages, which can be partially explained by lower vaccination rates and limited access to vaccination for disabled residents. Although PwDs have reported less hesitancy in getting vaccinated compared to adults without disabilities, they have experienced a wide range of barriers that include difficulties in physically accessing vaccination sites and scheduling vaccination appointments online, as well as lack of training among vaccination providers on vaccinating PwDs (Heath, 2021; Ryerson et al., 2021).

The results demonstrate that all subgroups of PwDs are not equally likely to reside in counties with greater pandemic vulnerability, and highlight the benefits of an intra-categorical approach that elucidates how other sources of social disadvantage combine with disability status to amplify COVID-19 risk burdens for PwDs. The multivariable models provide strong evidence of ethnic/racial, gender-based, and socioeconomic inequalities in the distribution of pandemic vulnerability, after controlling for spatial clustering, population density, and other relevant factors. Counties with higher percentages of PwDs identifying as Black or African-American were found to have significantly greater pandemic vulnerability in all timeframes analyzed, both without and with the consideration of vaccines. This is an important but disturbing finding, because a large proportion of Black PwDs have been reported to have underlying health conditions such as obesity and diabetes that can lead to greater cardiovascular and respiratory problems in places with higher risks of COVID-19 exposure and increased pandemic vulnerability (Young, 2020).

Mixed results were observed for the other ethnic/racial subgroups of PwDs. For example, the percentage of PwDs identifying as Hispanic or Latino was significantly associated with greater pandemic vulnerability only in August 2020 (*Original PVI Model*) and February 2021 (*PVI with Vaccine Model*). PwDs who are American Indian or Alaskan are significantly more likely to reside in counties with higher PVI in all timeframes, except for August 2021 in the *PVI with Vaccine Model*. This underrepresentation of both Hispanic and American Indian PwDs in counties with greater pandemic vulnerability in the latest timeframe (August 2021) can be explained by their smaller percentages in southern and southeastern states characterized by considerably lower vaccination rates and larger percentages in western states where vaccination rates are relatively higher.

For both PVI models (without and with vaccines) and in all timeframes examined, the percentage of PwDs who are female is significantly greater in counties with higher PVI. This disproportionate overrepresentation of female PwDs in counties with greater pandemic vulnerability represents a major concern, since women with disabilities have been documented to face more discrimination and difficulties in attaining access to education, employment, housing, and healthcare, as well as higher risks of gender-based violence and sexual abuse (UN Department of Economic and Social Affairs, 2020; Wheaton & Crimmins, 2015). With regards to age, PwDs who are 65 years or older are significantly less likely to live in counties with higher PVI in all multivariable models. This finding could be related to the greater concentration of socioeconomically affluent and elderly retirees (self-identifying as PwDs in the ACS) in metropolitan or suburban counties with lower pandemic vulnerability because of better health infrastructure and implementation of intervention measures, as well as greater COVID-19 testing and vaccination rates.

In terms of socioeconomic status, both PwDs below poverty level and PwDs who are unemployed are consistently and significantly more likely to reside in US counties with greater pandemic vulnerability, in all multivariable models and timeframes. The significantly greater proportions of these socioeconomically disadvantaged PwDs in counties with higher COVID-19 infection rates, inadequate health infrastructure, and/or fewer testing and vaccination resources can only be expected to worsen their adverse experiences, since below poverty and unemployed PwDs are also likely to lack health insurance and financial resources necessary to address the negative impacts. Additionally, recent data and reports suggest that economic hardships have increased disproportionately for PwDs during the pandemic. For example, the number of employed working-age PwDs decreased by 20% from March to April 2020, while the number of employed working-age people without disabilities declined by only 14% (Kessler Foundation, 2020). Based on trends observed in previous recessions, it is also likely PwDs experiencing job losses will be slower to recover their previous employment status (Livermore & Hyde, 2020) and employed PwDs will face barriers to continue working (Cochran, 2020).

In summary, this study found US counties more vulnerable to the COVID-19 pandemic to be characterized by significantly higher percentages of PwDs when vaccination was considered and socio-demographically disadvantaged PwDs (based on their minority, female, below poverty, and unemployed status), with and without the consideration of vaccines. These county-level associations indicate an urgent need for more detailed analyses to document and understand the negative impacts of COVID-19 on PwDs and develop appropriate intervention strategies. A major impediment to such analyses is the unavailability of statistical data on COVID-19 infections, hospitalizations, deaths, testing rates, mitigation measures, vaccinations, and treatments for PwDs. Although COVID-19 Case Surveillance Data are now available in the US, these individual records do not provide disability-related information. The findings of this study emphasize the necessity for COVID-19 data collection and reporting systems to include disability indicators, in addition to existing demographic and socioeconomic indicators (i.e., age, ethnicity, race, and gender) than allow intra-categorical analysis.

In conclusion, it is important to consider that disability information in the ACS is collected and provided for only the civilian noninstitutionalized population. The excluded population includes people who reside in institutional group quarters such as adult correctional facilities, juvenile facilities, nursing facilities, in-patient hospice facilities, residential schools for the disabled, retirement homes, and hospitals with patients who have no usual home elsewhere (Chakraborty, 2019). While this exclusion is a limitation, the US Census Bureau and researchers have argued that people living in institutional group quarters tend to have their disability accommodation needs addressed by the services provided at the facilities in which they reside (Brault, 2008). However, several reports indicate that disproportionately large numbers of COVID-19 infections and deaths have occurred in adult group homes, nursing homes, psychiatric hospitals, and other congregate care settings where PwDs are significantly overrepresented (Greiman et al., 2021; National Council on Disability, 2021). Since the ACS does not provide detailed data on disability status of individuals in group quarters, future studies should explore the use of additional data sources and surveys that provide reliable information on institutionalized PwDs. To better address the needs of PwDs affected by the COVID-19 pandemic, more evidence-based research is urgently needed on their increased vulnerabilities and specific adverse impacts related to their physical and mental health, living conditions, access to health care, employment status, and self-care ability, as well as other negative consequences.

ACKNOWLEDGMENTS

This research is funded, in part, by the Geospatial Fellows Program supported by the US National Science Foundation (NSF) under grant number 1743184. Any opinions, findings, and conclusions or recommendations expressed in this paper are those of the author and do not necessarily reflect the views of the NSF. The author is also thankful to Jacob J. Aun, Master's student in Sociology at the University of Texas at El Paso, for his assistance with this study.

REFERENCES

Allain, M. L., & Collins, T. W. (2021). Differential access to park space based on country of origin within Miami's Hispanic/Latino population: A novel analysis of park equity. *International Journal of Environmental Research and Public Health, 18*, 8364. https://doi.org/10.3390/ijerph18168364

Belsley, D. A. (1991). *Conditioning diagnostics: Collinearity and weak data in regression*. Wiley.

Bhandari, S., Lewis, P. G., Craft, E., Marvel, S. W., Reif, D. M., & Chiu, W. A. (2020). HGBEnviroScreen: Enabling community action through data integration in the Houston–galveston–brazoria region. *International Journal of Environmental Research and Public Health*, *17*(4), 1130. https://doi.org/10.3390/ijerph17041130

Bosworth, M. L., Ayoubkhani, D., Nafilyan, V., Foubert, J., Glickman, M., Davey, C., & Kuper, H. (2021). Deaths involving COVID-19 by self-reported disability status during the first two waves of the COVID-19 pandemic in England: A retrospective, population-based cohort study. *The Lancet Public Health*, *6*(11), E817–E825. https://doi.org/10.1016/s2468-2667(21)00206-1

Boyle, C. A., Fox, M. H., Havercamp, S. M., & Zubler, J. (2020). The public health response to the COVID-19 pandemic for people with disabilities. *Disability and Health Journal*, *13*(3), 100943. https://doi.org/10.1016/j.dhjo.2020.100943

Brault, M. (2008). Disability status and the characteristics of people in group quarters. https://www.census.gov/library/working-papers/2008/demo/brault-01.html

Chakraborty, J. (2019). Proximity to extremely hazardous substances for people with disabilities: A case study in Houston, Texas. *Disability and Health Journal*, *12*(1), 121–125.

Chakraborty, J. (2020). Unequal proximity to environmental pollution: An intersectional analysis of people with disabilities in Harris County, Texas. *The Professional Geographer*, *72*(4), 521–534.

Chakraborty, J. (2021). Social inequities in the distribution of COVID-19: An intra-categorical analysis of people with disabilities in the U.S. *Disability and Health Journal*, *14*(1), 101007. https://doi.org/10.1016/j.dhjo.2020.101007

Cochran, A. L. (2020). Impacts of COVID-19 on access to transportation for people with disabilities. *Transportation Research Interdisciplinary Perspectives*, *8*, 100263. https://doi.org/10.1016/j.trip.2020.100263

Finch, W. H., & Hernández Finch, M. E. (2020). Poverty and Covid-19: Rates of incidence and deaths in the United States during the first 10 weeks of the pandemic. *Frontiers in Sociology*, *5*, 47. https://doi.org/10.3389/fsoc.2020.00047

Garson, G. D. (2013). *Generalized linear models and generalized estimating equations*. Statistical Associates Publishing.

Greiman, L., Traci, M., & Leopold, A. (2021). *People with disabilities still at risk in congregate care settings*. The University of Montana Rural Institute for Inclusive Communities. https://scholarworks.umt.edu/cgi/viewcontent.cgi?article=1054&context=ruralinst_health_wellness

Heath, S. (2021). COVID-19 vaccine care access barriers impact those with disabilities. Patient Care Access News. https://patientengagementhit.com/news/covid-19-vaccine-care-access-barriers-impact-those-with-disabilities

Hendryx, M., & Luo, J. (2020). Covid-19 prevalence and mortality rates in association with Black race and segregation in the United States April 1 to April 15, 2020. *The Lancet Public Health*. http://dx.doi.org/10.2139/ssrn.3582857

Houtenville, A., & Boege, S. (2019). *Annual report on people with disabilities in America*. University of New Hampshire: Institute on Disability. https://eric.ed.gov/?id=ED605685

Izutsu, T. (2020). Disability-inclusive disaster risk reduction and humanitarian action: An urgent global imperative. 29 November 2019. Paper presented at United Nations World Conference on disaster risk reduction and the progress thereafter. https://www.un.org/development/desa/disabilities/wpcontent/uploads/sites/15/2020/03/Final-Disabilityinclusive-disaster.pdf

Karaye, I. M., & Horney, J. A. (2020). The impact of social vulnerability on covid-19 in the U.S.: An analysis of spatially varying relationships. *American Journal of Preventive Medicine*, *59*(3), 317–325.

Karmakar, M., Lantz, P. M., & Tipirneni, R. (2021). Association of social and demographic factors with COVID-19 incidence and death rates in the US. *JAMA Network Open*, *4*(1). https://doi.org/10.1001/jamanetworkopen.2020.36462

Kessler Foundation. (2020). *May 2020 special report: Workers with disabilities in the COVID economy*. https://kesslerfoundation.org/press-release/ntide-may-2020-special-report-workers-disabilities-covid-economy

Livermore, G., & Hyde, J. S. (2020). Workers with disabilities face unique challenges in weathering the COVID-19 pandemic. https://www.mathematica.org/commentary/workers-with-disabilities-face-unique-challenges-in-weathering-the-covid-19-pandemic

Mahajan, U. V., & Larkins-Pettigrew, M. (2020). Racial demographics and COVID-19 confirmed cases and deaths: A correlational analysis of 2886 US counties. *Journal of Public Health, 42*(3), 445–447.

Marvel, S. W., House, J. S., Wheeler, M., Song, K., Zhou, Y., Wright, F. A., Chiu, W. A., Rusyn, I., Motsinger-Reif, A., & Reif, D. M. (2021). The COVID-19 pandemic vulnerability index (PVI) dashboard: Monitoring county level vulnerability. *Environmental Health Perspectives, 129*(1), 017701. https://doi.org/10.1101/2020.08.10.20169649

Marvel, S. W., To, K., Grimm, F. A., Wright, F. A., Rusyn, I., & Reif, D. M. (2018). ToxPi graphical user interface 2.0: Dynamic exploration, visualization, and sharing of integrated data models. *BMC Bioinformatics, 19*(80). https://doi.org/10.1186/s12859-018-2089-2

McCall, L. (2005). The complexity of intersectionality. *Signs, 30*, 1771–1800.

National Council on Disability. (2021). The impact of COVID-19 on people with disabilities. https://ncd.gov/sites/default/files/NCD_COVID-19_Progress_Report_508.pdf

National Institute of Environmental Health Sciences (NIEHS). (2021a). COVID-19 Pandemic Vulnerability Index quick start guide. https://www.niehs.nih.gov/research/programs/coronavirus/covid19pvi/index.cfm

Nelder, J. A., & Wedderburn, R. W. (1972). Generalized linear models. *Journal of the Royal Statistical Society: Series A, 135*(3), 370–384.

NIEHS. (2021b). Details of current models. https://www.niehs.nih.gov/research/programs/coronavirus/covid19pvi/details/index.cfm

NIEHS. (2021c). COVID-19 Pandemic Vulnerability Index (PVI) dashboard. https://covid19pvi.niehs.nih.gov/

Pendo, E. (2020). COVID-19 and disability-based discrimination in health care. https://www.americanbar.org/groups/diversity/disabilityrights/resources/covid19-disability-discrimination

Pineda, V. S., & Corburn, J. (2020). Disability, urban health equity, and the coronavirus pandemic: Promoting cities for all. *Journal of Urban Health, 97*(3), 336–341.

Ryerson, A. B., Rice, C. E., Hung, M., Patel, S. A., Weeks, J. D., Kriss, J. L., … Singleton, J. A. (2021). Disparities in COVID-19 vaccination status, intent, and perceived access for noninstitutionalized adults, by disability status — National Immunization Survey Adult COVID Module, United States, May 30–June 26, 2021. *Morbidity and Mortality Weekly Report, 70*(39), 1365–1371. http://dx.doi.org/10.15585/mmwr.mm7039a2

Turk, M. A., & McDermott, S. (2020). The COVID-19 pandemic and people with disability. *Disability and Health Journal, 13*(3), 100944. https://doi.org/10.1016/j.dhjo.2020.100944

United Nations Department of Economic and Social Affairs. (2020). Women and girls with disabilities. https://www.un.org/development/desa/disabilities/issues/women-and-girls-with-disabilities.html

US Census Bureau. (2021, October 08). How disability data are collected from The American Community Survey. https://www.census.gov/topics/health/disability/guidance/data-collection-acs.html

US Department of Agriculture (USDA). (2020). Rural-urban continuum codes. https://www.ers.usda.gov/data-products/rural-urban-continuum-codes/

Wheaton, F. V., & Crimmins, E. M. (2015). Female disability disadvantage: A global perspective on sex differences in physical function and disability. *Ageing and Society, 36*(06), 1136–1156. https://doi.org/10.1017/s0144686x15000227

World Health Organization (WHO). (2020). Disability considerations during the Covid-19 outbreak. https://www.who.int/publications/i/item/WHO-2019-nCoV-Disability-2020-1

Young, D. (2020). Black, disabled, and uncounted. National Health Law Program. https://healthlaw.org/black-disabled-and-uncounted/

Chapter 2

CUMULATIVE AND CASCADING IMPACTS OF INVISIBILITY: AN INTERSECTIONAL APPROACH TO UNDERSTANDING THE HOUSING EXPERIENCES OF CANADIANS WITH DISABILITIES DURING COVID-19

Valérie Grand'Maison, Kathryn Reinders, Laura Pin, Jihan Abbas and Deborah Stienstra

ABSTRACT

Purpose: *In this chapter, we examine the unique and heightened negative impacts of the COVID-19 pandemic through tracing how the preexisting social conditions of exclusion and precarity in which many disabled people live, effected access to safe, affordable, and accessible housing in Canada. We then illustrate the reverberating impacts housing choices have on how people with disabilities lived, lived well, and how they faced barriers to living well during the COVID-19 pandemic.*

Methods/Approach: *Using an intersectional livelihoods approach, we analyzed semi-structured interviews and focus groups with 32 diverse people with disabilities, 12 key informant semi-structured interviews, as well as academic and community literature and a social media scan of key disability advocacy organizations in Canada.*

Disability in the Time of Pandemic
Research in Social Science and Disability, Volume 13, 31–48

Published under exclusive licence by Emerald Publishing Limited
ISSN: 1479-3547/doi:10.1108/S1479-354720230000013003

Findings: *Pandemic-related policies in Canada often excluded people with disabilities, either overlooking barriers to access and safety, which exacerbated the already precarious livelihoods of people with disabilities or over-emphasized the usefulness of social adaptions such as work from home. These exclusions had more profound consequences for people with disabilities from historically marginalized groups, as they often faced increased barriers to livelihoods pre-pandemic, and disability- or care-specific policies failed to consider intersectional experiences of discrimination. People with disabilities formed communities of care to meet their needs and those of their loved ones.*

Implications/Values: *To achieve a responsive policy response that addresses the cascading impacts of risk and care, it is necessary for governments to engage, early and often, with people with disabilities, disability leaders and organizations in emergency planning and beyond.*

Keywords: Disability; housing; livelihoods; intersectionality; income; care

INTRODUCTION

People with disabilities are disproportionately affected by crises in comparison to people without disabilities (Handicap International, 2015; Mitchell & Karr, 2014; Pearce, 2014; UNHCR, 2016). The current COVID-19 pandemic is no exception, where people with disabilities experienced unique and heightened negative impacts of the pandemic. These negative impacts further exacerbate the conditions of exclusion and precarity in which many disabled people live (Stienstra et al., 2021). In Canada, crowdsourced data and community surveys revealed some of the barriers and discrimination that people with disabilities faced during the pandemic, including loss of employment, education and social supports, decreased access to care, decreased access to safe, affordable, and accessible housing, and increased mortality (Abilities Centre & CDPP, 2020; Egale Canada, African-Canadian Civic Engagement Council, & Innovative Research Group., 2020; Kraus De Camargo et al., 2020; Pettinicchio et al., 2021; Statistics Canada, 2020, 2021). Historically, people with disabilities have struggled to access affordable, accessible, and safe housing and are more likely to live alone than people without disabilities (Berrigan et al., 2020; DisAbled Women's Network of Canada, 2019; Plouin et al., 2021). To date, little research has examined the impact of COVID-19 on the housing experiences of disabled people in Canada (Ndumbe-Eyoh et al., 2021; Stienstra et al., 2021).

In this chapter, we start from the lived experiences of diverse Canadians with disabilities to expose the multiple and intersecting sites of exclusion related to housing and how housing choices impacted their ability to live well during the pandemic. Guided by a livelihoods framework (Levine, 2014; Stienstra & Lee, 2019), we examine the ways Canadians with disabilities navigated their housing situation to meet their needs and ensure their well-being and that of their family. We ask how people have survived and thrived during disruptions to housing engendered by the pandemic, how the pandemic changed the choices they feel they have with respect to housing and what helped them live well. With a commitment to building back a more inclusive and just society, we argue that the COVID-19 situation in Canada exacerbated existing housing inequalities for people with disabilities and they responded by creating alternatives through fostering relationships, building community support, and being advocates for policy change. Governments must engage with diverse people with disabilities and disability leaders early and often during a crisis in order to build responsive policy mechanisms that allow them to live well.

METHODOLOGY

This chapter shares knowledge gathered as part of a larger project conducted during the fall of 2020 that investigated the impacts of COVID-19 government measures on Canadians with disabilities across five provinces (British Columbia, Alberta, Ontario, Québec, and New Brunswick).[1] These provinces were chosen to enable comparative data given that the funder required a policy analysis of these provincial health authorities.

Intersectional Livelihoods Framework

In this research we combine intersectionality and livelihoods frameworks to examine how people's choices and access to basic needs are shaped by multiple structures of oppression which come together in unique ways in their lives. We approach intersectionality as an analytical tool and a practice for social change (Cho et al., 2013; Hankvisky et al., 2014; Hill Collins & Bilge, 2016), supporting both the analysis of the cumulating and cascading impacts of the pandemic on diverse Canadians with disabilities and recommendations for building back better. Intersectionality was first articulated by Black feminists and feminists of color who denounced single-axis analyses, which effectively erased their lived experiences and perpetuated their marginalization (Hill Collins & Bilge, 2016). An intersectional analysis details how multiple structures of domination shape the lives of differentially located people in specific ways (Crenshaw, 1991; Hill Collins & Bilge, 2016). It helps us start with the recognition that people with disabilities have a wide range of experiences, barriers, and choices depending on their race, gender, disability, Indigenous status, class, sexuality, citizenship, and other identities as well as how these interact. As such, we value the situated knowledge our participants bring when understanding and addressing the impacts of the COVID-19 pandemic on disabled people.

Livelihoods are the means through which life necessities are ensured, and they shape how individuals, families, and communities live (Stienstra & Lee, 2019).

[1]Disability Inclusion Analysis of Lessons Learned and Best Practices of the Government of Canada's Response to the COVID-19 Pandemic can be accessed at: https://liveworkwell.ca/sites/default/files/pageuploads/DisabilityInclusionAnalysisCOVID-19_Final_031621_protected.pdf.

A livelihoods approach makes visible the multiple forces that influence the options people perceive to have, the choices they make, and how they find meaning. These forces can facilitate or hinder paths to livelihoods and act together in cascading or cumulative ways to affect the livelihoods of certain groups of people more intensely depending on the context. These forces include power relations, policies and processes, institutions, and unexpected situations or crises. A livelihoods analysis challenges the mainstream emphasis on capitalistic forms of subsisting, for example, through employment or social assistance (Stienstra & Lee, 2019). The sustainable livelihoods framework is well developed and used in the global South (Collins, 2004; De Haan, 2017; Levine, 2014) and to examine the experiences of people with disabilities (Adams et al., 2014; Hanass-Hannock & Mitra, 2016; Srijuntrapun, 2018) but has not been applied to the same extent in the global North or in conjunction with intersectionality.

Taken together, an intersectional livelihoods framework brings attention to how the specific co-constitution of multiple structures of domination, such as ableism, racism, heterosexism, capitalism, and colonialism, shape the livelihood options people feel are available to them and inform the choices people make to survive and thrive. These approaches lead to rich analytical questions, such as: what are the facilitators and barriers to living well for diverse people with disabilities? What is at the root of these barriers for diverse people with disabilities? What power relations do diverse people with disabilities perceive to be most influential in shaping the choices that they make? The value of an intersectional livelihoods framework is that it highlights how multiple and intersecting social structures uniquely shape the lived experiences of diverse people, thus allowing for the development of strategies that better meet complex, and sometimes divergent, needs of disabled people.

Data Collection and Analysis

For the project undertaken to develop this chapter, we gathered qualitative data through semi-structured interviews and focus groups with 32 diverse people with disabilities from five provinces and 12 key informants, academic and community literature, and a social media scan of key disability advocacy organizations in Canada. The key informants represented provincial and federal governmental agencies and disability civil society organizations representing diverse groups of people with disabilities. We use the term "diverse people" to refer to our commitment to intersectionality, and we ensured diversity by using an intersectional recruitment matrix, where we asked participants to share demographic information, including type(s) of disability, gender, age group, Indigeneity, race, citizenship status, sexuality, caregiving and support relationships, living and housing arrangements, presence of children, and whether they live in a rural, urban, or remote location (Stienstra et al., 2021). Three housing contexts were represented among our interviewees: independent private market residential settings like rented apartments or living within the family home, self-contained apartments that were part of larger supportive housing units, and congregate supportive housing settings, with shared common areas and facilities.[2]

We analyzed data using reflexive thematic analysis which identifies, analyzes, and interprets patterns of meaning in qualitative data. This approach recognizes the situatedness and subjectivities of the researchers as generative of complex, yet partial interpretation (Braun & Clarke, 2019; Clarke & Braun, 2017), while qualitative research is particularly valuable to create knowledge from the margins and to reveal the nuances of lived experiences (Christensen & Jensen, 2012; Denzin & Lincoln, 2018). We conducted three collaborative data analysis sessions between researchers and community partners, co-producing knowledge based on our particular insights and emotions in response to the data gathered. This method generated complex analyses of the factors that shape the choices of diverse people with disabilities, and thus provides necessary insights into the policies, programs, and practices that may support diverse people with disabilities to live well (Stienstra et al., 2021).

In the following sections, we first explore how Canada's neoliberal policy approaches to affordable housing and social assistance combine with under/un-employment to shape the incomes of diverse Canadians with disabilities during the pandemic, further restricting access to safe, affordable, and accessible housing. Second, we explore how the housing situation of people with disabilities effects their livelihoods, including the choices people feel they have, the care they receive, their relationships, and their well-being. We conclude by highlighting implications of our research for building back better.

AFFORDABLE HOUSING, LIVELIHOODS, AND PANDEMIC HOUSING CHOICES

> I relied very much on babysitting because that is just so easy for me to turn down when someone asks me, "hey, can you take this job?" I can say, "unfortunately not." And also, community work and both of those things have been thrown off the table because of COVID. So I have virtually no income right now. I'm fortunate that I live with my parents and that I do have their support for certain things like obviously shelter and food and stuff. But I have no money right now to be able to save for school. I have no money to be able to save for recreation or anything. It's taken away some choices in terms of like not only what I can do to receive income but what that income allows me to choose to do. I don't have those choices anymore – *A white non-binary person from Ontario with mental health disabilities, living with at least one other person with a disability*. (Stienstra et al., 2021, p. 43)

The housing situation in which people live is linked to the availability of housing, housing policies, and income. There is a well-established relationship between disability and poverty (Groce et al., 2011; Ingstad & Eide, 2011). In Canada approximately 16% of people with disabilities live in poverty, and 25% of

---

[2]We were unable to conduct interviews with people living with disabilities in carceral situations or who were unhoused.

those are people with cognitive and mental health disabilities. People with disabilities disproportionately live in "deep income poverty," with income below 75% of Canada's Official Poverty Line (Employment and Social Development Canada, 2021). Poverty is further exacerbated by neoliberal policy approaches which privilege self-reliance in meeting individual needs while restricting government social safety nets, including income supports and public housing (Chouinard, 2006; Hulchanski, 2006). Lack of access to housing and insufficient income supports combine with un/der employment to restrict the housing options available to people with disabilities. As a result, many people with disabilities live in poverty and experience unmet housing needs (Employment and Social Development Canada, 2021). COVID-19 policies further exacerbated these livelihood conditions, with many of our participants discussing how preexisting housing challenges along with income limitations restricted the housing choices they felt were available to them. In this section, we illustrate how the housing situation of people living with disabilities is shaped by lack of access to safe, affordable, and accessible housing and/or the conditions of poverty which many people with disabilities in Canada live. We highlight some additional challenges experienced by diverse people with disabilities during the COVID-19 pandemic, and the limited impact of federal COVID-19 income support policies in meeting their needs during the pandemic.

Housing and Employment

> I was initially going to move out for the summer just to find a place just for myself...when COVID came down that immediately eliminated the new prospect of that happening and I'm forced to live at home. – *A racialized, urban man with disabilities, living with family members including caregiving responsibilities for other family members.*

While both the Canadian federal government's National Housing Strategy and the United Nations recognize housing as a human right, access to appropriate housing for the 6.2 million people living with a disability in Canada has been fraught both before and during the COVID-19 pandemic (Morris et al., 2018; DisAbled Women's Network of Canada, 2019; Employment and Social Development Canada, 2021). Before the pandemic, people with disabilities were more likely to be living in housing need than nondisabled Canadians, especially those with developmental disabilities (Berrigan et al., 2020), Autistic people (Tint & Weiss, 2018), women with disabilities living Canada's North (Manning et al., 2016) and Indigenous women (DisAbled Women's Network of Canada, 2019). These groups face particular barriers to livelihoods and experience discrimination when accessing housing, employment, or community supports. This means that they often have to live with aging family members, who may not have the available resources to support them, which in turn, may result in homelessness or institutionalization (Inclusion Canada, 2018; DisAbled Women's Network of Canada, 2019). This lack of safe, affordable, and accessible housing is characterized by long housing waitlists for affordable units and/or overrepresentation of people with disabilities among unhoused populations: "I have applied for low-income housing for two locations in Montreal. I'm 178 [178th on the waitlist] for one area of the city, and 150 for one area another area of the city, but the waiting list is 15 years… like for me to get into low-income housing, you know, even though my, my income allows me to get… But it ain't going to happen. Look I'm 64 years old. You know where am I going to be in 15 years' time," explains a white man who is blind (Stienstra et al., 2021, p. 64).[3] This chronic lack of affordable and accessible housing has resulted in a housing crisis for people with disabilities.

The crisis has been further exacerbated by the COVID-19 pandemic, where people living with disabilities were more likely to become unemployed or have reduced employment than other Canadians. Disability experts highlighted that people with disabilities were more likely to lose their employment due to various public health measures to combat the spread of COVID-19. Statistics Canada (2020) data reveals that people with disabilities were two times more likely than people without disabilities to have experienced temporary and permanent job loss. Job loss was further compounded with age, gender, lower levels of education attainment, and number of/severity of impairment or condition. A disability leader in the field of employment shared that approximately 30% of the jobs held by people with disabilities could be pivoted online (compared to close to 40% for the general Canadian population (Deng et al., 2020)), because the other 70% of people with disabilities held jobs that required their physical presence such as food service, warehousing, and retail.

Several of our participants discussed being unable to find employment during the pandemic, being laid off from paid-employment, or having their employment contracts not renewed. Other participants relied on disability income support because they were unable to meet their needs solely through employment income. During our research, participants told us that the impact of unemployment and/or reduced employment during the pandemic had consequences on their housing choices or led to additional stress upon the people who they shared housing with. While the relationship between housing and employment was present for all participants, the relationship was often shaped by contextual factors such as disability type, race, and their current housing situation. Participants concerned about their ability to rent on the private market or meet their existing rent during the pandemic were often non-racialized people with physical disabilities who either relied on government income assistance or contract work to meet their housing needs. Some of these participants also noted that service disruptions due to COVID-19 also affected access to housing subsidies. A white woman with physical disabilities explained that, pre-pandemic employment changes required them to apply for housing subsidy to maintain residency within their current unit but their city had stopped accepting applications due to the pandemic.

---

[3]Canadians with multiple disabilities are four times more likely to experience temporary homelessness than Canadians without disabilities (Rodrigue, 2016); while a 2017 submission to the UN Special Rapporteur on the Right to Housing estimated that 45% of those unhoused identified as having a disability or mental health illness (Alzheimer Society of Canada et al., 2017).

Participants who were racialized or lived with intellectual or mental health disabilities tended to live in multi-generational family homes or congregate settings and had a different relationship with COVID-19 and housing. While their housing situation was stable, they reported concern about additional financial pressures placed upon other family members after job loss, their ability to eventually move out of the family home post-pandemic, or isolation from their intimate partners due to restrictions placed by their congregate living homes. One of our participants was unable to live with their intimate partner pre-pandemic due to the rules of their congregate living situation combined with maintaining access to disability support. A white woman from Québec explained, "we can't live together because of you know legal reasons first of all, this is a one person dwelling there cannot be [more than] one person living here. But, financially, we can't live together because I would lose my disability, and I would lose part of my widow's pension." They experienced a period of isolation from their husband due to the visitor-policy in their congregate unit, which affected their feelings of home. These responses foreground the importance of understanding how different social locations and material forces combined to shape the living situations, barriers and facilitators to living well and accessing housing and home during the pandemic.

Income and Livelihoods

Further complicating access to housing, the pandemic entrenched many people with disabilities deeper in poverty. In our research, participants who held stable, full-time employment pre-pandemic, or lived in multi-generational housing tended to report that increased costs and reduced income were not a barrier. However, for the majority of our participants – regardless of race, age, or impairment type – the reality of increased costs combined with reduced or insufficient income complicated access to housing and their ability to meet their needs during the pandemic. Increased costs included food, transportation, health supports, and the cost of personal protective equipment. Increases combined with insufficient income support and loss of employment created conditions of further uncertainty surrounding the housing situation of many people with disabilities. "I've never had this much uncertainty in my life... It's very hard to plan for the next week, let alone the future... If I don't get things together in the next 30 days and have a little bit of certainty on where rent is coming from, I could be homeless" (MacLean, 2020). These consequences were more severe for people who already faced additional barriers to accessing social assistance and a heightened likelihood of living in poverty pre-pandemic, such as Indigenous people, racialized people, women, and people with lower levels of education.

However, consistent with neoliberal policy logics which reward labor market participation while restricting access to social programs for others, initial COVID-19 income support measures were tied to employment or student status pre-pandemic. Since many of our participants relied on government assistance or part-time and/or contract employment prior to the pandemic these policies did little to address the complex and cascading effects of COVID-19 on their income and housing situation. This was particularly true for those with more severe or multiple impairments. This is consistent with Statistics Canada data, which indicates that 40% of people aged 25–64 living with disabilities lacked employment, and of the 60% of individuals employed, people with disabilities were more likely to report working part-time (Morris et al., 2018). As a result, many people with disabilities were ineligible for federal COVID-19 income supports. For people who were eligible, those supports often conflicted with their existing provincial income supports, triggering clawbacks. While the federal government did eventually announce a one-time $600 payment to people with disabilities, it was linked to Canada's Disability Tax Credit (DTC), which is under-used by people with disabilities due to restrictive eligibility criteria and employment focused benefits (Canada Revenue Agency, 2019; Zwicker & Dunn, 2018). Many people with disabilities and disability advocates in our study claimed that this was "too little, too late," and insufficient to cover the increased costs caused by the pandemic (Stienstra et al., 2021, pp. 43–44). For our participants, this erasure of lived experiences in policy discussions is par for the course – as one blind man from Ontario told us, "the one thing that that policymakers have always, where we've always fallen down through the cracks, is that they're never, they never talked to people with disabilities."

Combined, insufficient additional income support measures along with limited employment opportunities for people with disabilities during the pandemic reinforced barriers to the inclusion of people with disabilities (den Houting, 2020) and solidified the financial precarity in which many of them live (Petit & Tedds, 2020). The loss of income experienced by many people with disabilities due to the COVID-19 pandemic stems from systemic inequities that existed pre-pandemic. Unequal access to employment opportunities and insufficient government income supports, restrict housing options for some people with disabilities, as they are priced out of the rental market. This is particularly true for women with disabilities, people with developmental disabilities, and those that live with poverty. Further, for many participants, the discrepancy between the COVID-19 income supports they received and the supports in place to mitigate decreased income evoked feelings of being "second-class citizens": "Why is, is it considered that an able-bodied person is worth $2,000 a month, but a person with disabilities is not? We have the same expenses. We have the same, the same needs... well, actually, we have, and maybe more. You know, it's, in every case we're an afterthought" (Stienstra et al., 2021, p. 84). The symbolic message of government measures – or lack thereof – reaffirms a sense of institutional abandonment for some people with disabilities, which long existed before the pandemic.

A policy framework which starts with the lived experiences of people with disabilities would be more responsive to the increased costs caused by the pandemic and other crises, because it would center the types of systemic – and often invisible – policy exclusions which shape the relationships between poverty, employment, income support, and housing for people with disabilities. Regardless of race, age, and impairment type, most of our participants voiced a need for improved levels of income support as a facilitator to meeting their housing needs and living well. Consistent with the United Nations Partnership on the Rights of

Persons with Disabilities' call for state governments to extend income supports to all persons with disabilities (UNPRPD, 2020), establishing a national disability benefit is a crucial first step to addressing the poverty that diverse people with disabilities live in. The Liberal Government of Canada announced a Canadian Disability Benefit in the September 2020 Throne Speech, existing alongside current provincial income supports, but the legislation was delayed due to the 2021 federal election. Many disability advocates celebrate the Canadian Disability Benefit as a more systemic and inclusive measure (Plan Institute, 2020), but - similar to Canada's Disability Tax Credit - others argue that restrictive eligibility criteria exclude many marginalized people with disabilities, like sponsored immigrants and people living with a mental illness (BakerLaw, 2020). Nevertheless, a national disability benefit constitutes a tangible first step to address the inequities faced by diverse people with disabilities which increased during the pandemic (Stienstra et al., 2021), including supporting access to adequate housing.

CARE, SAFETY, AND RELATIONSHIPS

> I think the biggest changes would be around shift in, like, the support structure for, for me and for my partner. In terms of like last external support being available. And so we're kind of managing a lot more of our support needs with each other. We're doing the bulk of our care between the two of us – *a queer person discussing changes to in-home care work availability due to COVID-19*. (Stienstra et al., 2021, p. 71)

The housing situation in which people live is linked to the type of care and support they receive. Because disability and COVID-19 policies shaped where and with whom people can live, people with disabilities had to negotiate relationships with family members, friends, caregivers, and their communities to meet their care needs. People who required assistance for living tasks or with multiple disabilities indicated they lost access to formal care services due to the pandemic, due to changes in access to in-home care attendants, or they could not safely receive healthcare in person (Stienstra et al., 2021). Many other people with disabilities, especially those with mental health disabilities and those living with poverty, faced challenges to accessing the care and support that they needed (Stienstra et al., 2021). They had to craft alternatives to access care, including finding means to ensure their own care, that of their neighbors and members of their household. Most significant for the participants was the emotional care that they negotiated within and outside of their household, finding creative ways to respect their safety and that of their loved ones. In this section, we illustrate how the housing situation in which people lived shaped the choices that they made to access care. We highlight the negotiations that diverse people with disabilities made between access to care and safety, which often resulted in building care relationships with their closest ones.

Negotiating Access to Professional Care and Infection Risk

> Nobody's allowed in, and nobody's allowed out, and I'm sorry, but anybody who lives in a congregate care facility is in a very vulnerable position on care for a person with a disability, or your senior. And when nobody else is allowed in that place. And nobody out. It only makes you way more vulnerable – *Disability advocate at a national civil society organization for people with intellectual disabilities.* (Stienstra et al., 2021, p. 68)

Adequate housing is intimately bound to the availability of disability-related supports. Federal and provincial support for community care programming which allows people with disabilities to live independently has declined since the 1990s (Chouinard, 2006; Hulchanski, 2006), resulting in reduced access to supportive programming pre-COVID-19. As the pandemic took hold, housing became a key site of interest both in terms of how "shelter-in-place" and "lockdown" orders shaped and regulated the movement of care labor. The restricted access to disability-related supports was especially true for those in congregate settings including group homes, long-term care (LTC) facilities, assistive living, and other institutional settings, as well as for those who need care assistance for daily living tasks and those living with mental health disabilities (Stienstra et al., 2021). The ways in which various levels of policies (federal, provincial, municipal, and Indigenous) interacted shaped the care choices that diverse people with disabilities made.

In our study, most participants discussed a decline in the quantity and quality of care and community supports they received, including increased barriers to medical and attendant care, concerns about infection risk, and worries related to agency COVID-19 infection prevention policies (Stienstra et al., 2021). These concerns were voiced by white and racialized men, women, and non-binary people living in urban areas who required assistance for daily living tasks or attendant care at home. One white woman from Ontario with physical disabilities told us that they "live in assisted living and there are 15 other people with disabilities that live here. And the agency has not put anything in place to ensure that staff get tested on a regular basis. I asked them when they would be doing that, and they said they don't have any plans to do it in the future as of right now" (Stienstra et al., 2021, p. 67). We note that racialized and Indigenous people living in congregate settings did not express concerns over their agency's policies, which may stem from historical and ongoing exclusions from state protections, which in turn has led to low expectations about the role of government policies and programs in sustaining their needs.

COVID-19 also deeply affected the safety of those living in congregate care. Participants living in privatized congregate settings indicated losing access to care and not being heard by their agency, while publicly funded congregate settings, which had emergency plans – albeit inadequate – to ensure that residents received some attendant care throughout the pandemic. People living in residential care represented 66% of Canada's fatalities (Loreto, 2021). While we are still reckoning with the scope of the human cost of the pandemic due to the failure to implement policies protecting people residing in congregate settings, the links between poor health outcomes and neoliberal policy which privileges for-profit care is increasingly becoming clear. As an example, one recent analysis of LTC in Ontario found that for-profit LTC providers were associated with more COVID-19 outbreaks and increased numbers of resident deaths (Stall et al., 2020).

Across the country and even across agencies within the same province, there appeared to be unclear, contradictory, and confusing policy responses to protecting those who reside in congregate settings. The responses included strict lockdowns and restrictions on visitors that left some people with disabilities living in congregate settings isolated from their essential and unpaid support people (Stienstra et al., 2021). The feeling of isolation was reported by participants who identify as women or Indigenous. Advocates and scholars recognize the importance of integrating loved ones in the care provided in institutionalized settings as they hold unique knowledge and skills regarding the person in care, which often leads to this person's empowerment (Canadian Foundation for Healthcare Improvement, 2020; Parmer et al., 2021). The responses also included the uneven implementation of daily testing or screening for residents of congregate settings, which at once ensured their safety, but also caused stress for some people with disabilities who have difficulty communicating their health status (Stienstra et al., 2021). The few standardized guidelines regarding testing and screening which did exist were often unevenly applied, with the overall situation within congregate living leading one disability leader to conclude that "during this pandemic, we saw clearly that seniors and people with disabilities who actually lived in their own homes, or whatever with supports were way safer" (Stienstra et al., 2021, p. 67).

For decades, disability scholars and activists have denounced the forms of discrimination and neglect that people with disabilities experience in the name of care, such as institutionalization, sterilization, physical restraint, and isolation (Eales & Peers, 2020). Participants who identify as women and wheelchair users, and live with multiple disabilities, feared experiencing neglect and discrimination in institutionalized care settings, such as hospitals or long-term care homes (Stienstra et al., 2021). For example, a quadriplegic woman expressed a lot of worry about people with disabilities being forced into institutions due to being unable to access community care during the pandemic. As this section illustrates, policies have disproportionately negative impacts on people with disabilities living in congregate care and those who require attendant care at home, including young and older adults living in long-term care homes and people with intellectual or mental health disabilities living in group homes or institutions. This is evident in high mortality rates, unclear, inadequate, and contradictory safety policies, and strictly enforced isolation, all of which negatively affected diverse people with disabilities' well-being and health.

Fostering Care Relationships

Many participants, especially those living in congregate settings and those caring for relatives or friends, told us that they experienced heightened isolation, which compromised their feelings of safety and connectedness. Yet people with disabilities leveraged their relationships and housing situation in creative ways to obtain the care they needed. Care relationships are often reciprocal for people with disabilities, across all social groups, meaning that they often provide some type of care to those caring for them. During the pandemic, many of the participants who identified as white women or non-binary, racialized people, and people living in multigenerational home, noted an increase in their caregiving responsibilities due to decrease in care services that the members of their household received. Research has well documented the increased burden of unpaid care work on women, especially racialized and immigrant women (Dugarova, 2020). We also found that members of the LGBTQ2S+ also took on more unpaid care responsibilities. For example, a trans disabled person did injections for themself and their disabled partner, because they faced barriers accessing care.

While they had to provide more care to others and often received less professional care themselves, people with disabilities who lived with a friend or family member that they could trust and rely on reported feeling relieved from the constant mental load of managing several care services. For those without these close interpersonal connections, the lack or inadequate care they received and the isolation they lived with negatively affected their physical and emotional well-being (Stienstra et al., 2021). Yet, most participants across social groups shared how they developed a routine of checking-in on the well-being of their friends, family members, and/or neighbors, as a way to both provide and receive support from those around them. They encouraged each other to develop plans in case they become sick with COVID-19 or other illnesses, as they realized that formal care services were not equipped to ensure their care in times of crisis.

Networks of caregiving also shifted, although imperfectly, according to the emotional, physical, and financial resources that people had at a given time. In our study, women and members of the LGBTQ2S+ talked about negotiating the amount of care they provided to their closest ones compared to the care they received, depending on urgency of care and access to external care services. At times when it was unsafe for people within a household to do their groceries, they mobilized relationships with friends to get their food and other necessities. They also made compromises of their own well-being by securing more urgent care to those in need. People requiring assistance for daily living tasks, racialized people with disabilities, and people with mental health and cognitive disabilities were often not in situation where they could negotiate care responsibilities, sometimes leaving them without the necessary supports or with additional responsibilities.

Relationships with extra-human beings, such as pets and nature, were also important to participants given the constraints of their housing situation. People with disabilities living alone or with people with whom they did not feel well connected talked about their interactions with dogs or cats as mitigating the negative impacts caused by their living situation. This aligns with research that has established that people build caring relationships with animals during times of crisis (Franklin, 1999). A racialized man with a cognitive disability who had to move back with his parents due to the lack of job opportunities during the pandemic explained that his dog was the most important support for him to live well, providing emotional care and physical activity. Similarly, participants living in urban areas indicated that spending time outdoors, especially in parks and trails, was particularly important to nurture their mental, physical, and emotional well-being. They discussed being grateful for nearby parks that would allow them to connect with nature, their friends, and cultivate a sense of community by seeing people, even from a distance. Nature and parks thus allowed participants to decide who they would spend time with, as opposed to the restrictions imposed on households: it allowed people with tense relationships in the home to get some space, and to choose their interactions with friends and family members that support them.

CONCLUSION: BUILDING BACK BETTER

In this chapter, we examined how the housing situation of diverse Canadians with disabilities shaped their paths to livelihoods during the pandemic. The influence of neoliberal policies combined with lack of meaningful income supports for people with disabilities shaped access to safe, accessible, and affordable housing for diverse people with disabilities in Canada. The housing situation of Canadians with disabilities, in turn, often restricted their paths to livelihoods, meaning that it limited the choices that they had in accessing their needs and desires. These constraints were especially true for people requiring assistance for daily living tasks, those living in congregate settings, people with mental health disabilities, and racialized people. Included here is confusion stemming from tensions between securing profit, mitigating risk, and providing necessary care.

Our interviews with diverse Canadians with disabilities confirm and expand the literature on the impacts of COVID-19 on people with disabilities, showing that they faced increased and disability-specific impacts, such as loss of care, employment, decrease in income, increase in costs, and isolation (Stienstra et al., 2021). Our research also shows the creative ways in which they met their needs and nurtured their well-being. They did that by leveraging informal relationships of care, engaging in reciprocal relationships and networks of care, and connecting with others, with pets, and with nature. We found that certain groups of people faced obstacles that built from each other or led to additional obstacles, which both resulted in greater exclusion. For example, we found that people with mental health disabilities, especially those who were racialized and part of the LGBTQ2S+ community, were more likely to have lost their employment or have limited employment opportunities, which led to choosing a housing situation that created stress and additional care responsibilities, and/or restricted their access to necessary care and supports. An intersectional livelihoods approach uniquely exposes the cumulative and cascading challenges that certain groups face in accessing and advocating for supports and information and in negotiating care. The livelihoods paths of diverse people with disabilities emphasize how policies addressing specific experiences, such as disability or loss of employment, may remain inaccessible for people facing multiple and intersecting barriers.

Our research also indicates several important implications as we aim to build a more just world post-pandemic. We need a policy system that is responsive to the different situations that people have in addition to community building and people's agency (Stienstra et al., 2021). In other words, it is about creating policy mechanisms that recognize and facilitate access to the supports that help people live well. In the context of the pandemic in Canada, this means providing people with disabilities with access to the supports that they need while considering the complexity of public health restrictions, which may look like financially supporting community initiatives. To achieve a responsive policy response that addresses the cascading impacts of risk and care, it is necessary for governments to, early and often, engage with people with disabilities, disability leaders and organizations in emergency planning and beyond. By acknowledging that people with disabilities are experts in their own lives and have knowledge of the types of emergency responses which ensure accessibility and inclusion, many of the tragedies and horrors of the COVID-19 pandemic could have been lessened (Stienstra et al., 2021). Further, establishing a national disability benefit along with dismantling existing neoliberal policies will stem many of the negative impacts which relate to income insecurity and systemic inequalities experienced by diverse people with disabilities in Canada.

REFERENCES

Abilities Centre & Canadian Disability Participation Project. (2020). *Covid-19 disability survey*. https://abilitiescentre.org/Abilities/media/Documents/Covid-survey-report-Dec-18_1.pdf

Adams, F., Ot, B., & Maseko, P. (2014). Livelihoods of youths with and without disabilities in peri-urban South Africa. *South African Journal of Occupational Therapy*, *44*(3), 8. http://www.scielo.org.za/scielo.php?script=sci_arttext&pid=S2310-38332014000300005&lng=en&tlng=en

Alzheimer Society of Canada, ARCH Disability Law Centre, Canadian Association for Community Living, Canadian Mental Health Association – Toronto Branch, Council of Canadians with Disabilities, IRIS – Institute for Research and Development on Inclusion and Society, People First of Canada, Social Rights Advocacy Centre, & Wellesley Institute. (2017). Meeting Canada's obligations to affordable housing and supports for people with disabilities to live independently in the community. https://inclusioncanada.ca/wp-content/uploads/2018/05/Canada-Right-to-Housing-for-Persons-with-Disabilities-May-15-2017.pdf

BakerLaw (2020, October 9). Throne speech unveils new Canadian disability benefit. https://www.bakerlaw.ca/legal-issues/human-rights/throne-speech-unveils-new-canadian-disability-benefit/

Berrigan, P., Scott, C. W. M., & Zwicker, J. D. (2020). Employment, education, and income for Canadians with developmental disability: Analysis from the 2017 Canadian survey on disability. *Journal of Autism and Developmental Disorders*. https://doi.org/10.1007/s10803-020-04603-3

Braun, V., & Clarke, V. (2019). Reflecting on reflexive thematic analysis. *Qualitative Research in Sport, Exercise and Health*, *11*(4), 589–597. https://doi.org/10.1080/2159676X.2019.1628806

Canada Revenue Agency. (2019). *First annual report of the Disability Advisory Committee: Enabling access to disability tax measures [Annual report]*. Government of Canada. https://www.canada.ca/en/revenue-agency/corporate/about-canada-revenue-agency-cra/disability-advisory-committee/2019-full-report.html#_Toc5712826

Canadian Foundation for Healthcare Improvement. (2020). Better together: Re-integration of family caregivers as essential partners in care in a time of COVID-19. https://www.cfhi-fcass.ca/docs/default-source/itr/tools-and-resources/bt-re-integration-of-family-caregivers-as-essential-partners-covid-19-e.pdf

Cho, S., Crenshaw, K., & McCall, L. (2013). Toward a field of intersectionality studies: Theory, applications, and praxis. *Signs: Journal of Women in Culture and Society*, *38*(4), 785–810. https://doi.org/10.1086/669608

Chouinard, V. (2006). On the dialectics of differencing: Disabled women, the state and housing issues. *Gender, Place & Culture*, *13*(4), 401–417. https://doi.org/10.1080/09663690600808528

Christensen, A. D., & Jensen, S. Q. (2012). Doing intersectional analysis: Methodological implications for qualitative research. *Nora: Nordic Journal of Women's Studies*, *20*(2), 109–125. https://doi.org/10.1080/08038740.2012.673505

Clarke, V., & Braun, V. (2017). Thematic analysis. *The Journal of Positive Psychology*, *12*(3), 297–298. https://doi.org/10.1080/17439760.2016.1262613

Collins, S. B. (2004). Sustainable livelihoods: A contribution to our understanding of poverty. *Canadian Review of Social Policy; Toronto*, *54*, 1–17.

Crenshaw, K. (1991). Mapping the margins: Intersectionality, identity politics, and violence against women of color. *Stanford Law Review*, *43*(6), 1241–1299. https://doi.org/10.2307/1229039

De Haan, L. J. (2017). Livelihoods in development. *Canadian Journal of Development Studies/Revue Canadienne d'études du développement*, *38*(1), 22–38. https://doi.org/10.1080/02255189.2016.1171748

Deng, Z., Morissette, R., & Messacar, D. (2020). Running the economy remotely: Potential for working from home during and after COVID-19. Statistics Canada. https://www150.statcan.gc.ca/n1/pub/45-28-0001/2020001/article/00026-eng.htm?HPA=1

Denzin, N., & Lincoln, Y. (2018). Introduction: The discipline and practice of qualitative research. In N. Denzin, & Y. Lincoln (Eds.), *The sage handbook of qualitative research* (pp. 29–71). Sage Publications.

DisAbled Women's Network of Canada/Réseau d'actions des femmes handicapées du Canada. (2019). Plus qu'une note de bas de page: Rapport de recherche sur les femmes et les filles en situation de handicap au Canada. https://www.dawncanada.net/media/uploads/news_data/news-278/rapport_de_recherche_plus_qu'une_note_de_bas_de_page.pdf

Dugarova, E. (2020, June 16–18). Unpaid care work in times of the COVID-19 crisis: Gendered impacts, emerging evidence and promising policy responses. [Paper presentation]. United Nations Department of Economic and Social Affairs (UNDESA) division for inclusive social development's (online) expert group meeting on families in development: Assessing progress, challenges and emerging issues. Focus on modalities for IYF+30 & parenting education, New York, United States. https://www.un.org/development/desa/family/wp-content/uploads/sites/23/2020/06/UN.MegaTrends.Final_.Trask_.2020.pdf

Eales, L., & Peers, D. (2020). Care haunts, hurts, heals: The promiscuous poetics of queer crip Mad care. *Journal of Lesbian Studies*, *25*(3), 163–181. https://doi.org/10.1080/10894160.2020.1778849

Egale Canada, African-Canadian Civic Engagement Council, Innovative Research Group. (2020). Impact of COVID-19 on Canada's LGBTQI2S Community. https://egale.ca/wp-content/uploads/2020/08/COVID-2_EgaleACCECIRG-FINAL.pdf

Employment and Social Development Canada. (2021). Building understanding: The first report of the National Advisory Council on Poverty. Employment and Social Development Canada. https://www.canada.ca/en/employment-social-development/programs/poverty-reduction/national-advisory-council/reports/2020-annual.html

Franklin, A. (1999). *Animals and modern cultures: A sociology of human-animal relations in modernity*. London: Sage.

Groce, N., Kett, M., Lang, R., & Trani, J. (2011). Disability and poverty: The need for a more nuanced understanding of implications for development policy and practice. *Third World Quarterly*, *32*(8), 1493–1513. http://www.jstor.org/stable/41300297

Hanass-Hannock, J., & Mitra, S. (2016). Livelihoods and disability: The complexities of work in the Global South. In S. Grech & K. Soldatic (Eds.), *Disability in the global South: The critical handbook* (pp. 133–151). Springer International Publishing.

Handicap International (2015). Disability in humanitarian context: Views from affected people and field organisations. https://d3n8a8pro7vhmx.cloudfront.net/handicapinternational/pages/1500/

attachments/original/1449158243/Disability_in_humanitarian_context_2015_Study_Advocacy.pdf?1449158243

Hankivsky, O., Grace, D., Hunting, G., Giesbrecht, M., Fridkin, A., Rudrum, S., Ferlatte, O., & Clark, N. (2014). An intersectionality-based policy analysis framework: Critical reflections on a methodology for advancing equity. *International Journal for Equity in Health*, *13*(1), 119. https://doi.org/10.1186/s12939-014-0119-x

Hill Collins, P., & Bilge, S. (2016). *Intersectionality*. Polity Press.

den Houting, J. (2020). Stepping out of isolation: Autistic people and COVID-19. *Autism in Adulthood*, *2*(2). 103–105. https://doi.org/10.1089/aut.2020.29012.jdh

Hulchanski, D. (2006). What factors shape Canadian housing policy? The intergovernmental role in Canada's housing system. In R. Young & C. Leuprecht (Eds.), *Canada: The state of the federation 2004 : Municipal-federal-provincial relations in Canada* (pp. 210–247). Montreal: McGill-Queen's University Press.

Inclusion Canada. (2018). A right to housing for all: Ensuring a human rights approach inclusive of all persons with developmental disabilities. https://inclusioncanada.ca/wp-content/uploads/2018/07/CACLNHSsubmissionJN8-FINAL.pdf

Ingstad, B., & Eide, A. (2011). Introduction: Disability and poverty: A global challenge. In B. Ingstad & A. Eide (Eds.), *Disability and poverty: A global challenge* (pp. 1–13). Policy Press.

Kraus De Camargo, O., Ahmad, F., Pozniak, K., & Freeman, M. (2020). *COVID-19 Survey at a glance*. CanChild Survey. https://canchild.ca/system/tenon/assets/attachments/000/003/346/original/COVID-19_Survey_V3.pdf

Levine, S. (2014). How to study livelihoods: Bringing a sustainable livelihoods framework to life. Secure Livelihoods Research Consortium. https://securelivelihoods.org/wp-content/uploads/How-to-study-livelihoods-Bringing-a-sustainable-livelihoods-framework-to-life.pdf

Loreto, N. (2021). Deaths in residential care by facility. (September 13, 2021) [Dataset]. https://docs.google.com/spreadsheets/d/1M_RzojK0vwF9nAozI7aoyLpPU8EA1JEqO6rq0g1iebU/edit?usp=sharing

MacLean, C. (2020, November 16). Tenant with heart failure fears he'll be homeless as Manitoba ban on evictions, rent increases ends. CBC News. https://www.cbc.ca/news/canada/manitoba/tenants-with-disabilities-homelessness-covid-19-1.5745140

Manning, S., Stienstra, D., Baikie, G., & Hutchison, C. (2016). Experiences of women with disabilities in Canada's North [Fact sheet]. FemNorthNet. https://www.criaw-icref.ca/publications/experiences-of-women-with-disabilities-in-canadas-north/

Mitchell, D., & Karr, V. (2014). *Crises, conflict and disability: Ensuring equality*. Routledge.

Morris, S., Fawcett, G., Brisebois, L., & Hughes, J. (2018). *A demographic, employment and income profile of Canadians with disabilities aged 15 years and over, 2017*. No. 89-654-X2018002. Statistics Canada. https://www150.statcan.gc.ca/n1/en/pub/89-654-x/89-654-x2018002-eng.pdf?st=HBynR5Ph

Ndumbe-Eyoh, S., Muzumdar, P., Betker, C., & Oickle, D. (2021). 'Back to better': Amplifying health equity, and determinants of health perspectives during the COVID-19 pandemic. *Global Health Promotion*, *28*(2), 7–16. https://doi.org/10.1177/17579759211000975

Parmar, J., Anderson, S., Dobbs, B., Tian, P. G. J., Charles, L., Triscott, J., Stickney-Lee, J., Brémault-Phillips, S., Sereda, S., & Poole, L. (2021). Neglected needs of family caregivers during the COVID-19 pandemic and what they need now: A qualitative study. *Diseases*, *9*(4), 70. https://doi.org/10.3390/diseases9040070

Pearce, E. (2014). Disability inclusion: Translating policy into practice in humanitarian action. Women's Refugee Commission. https://reliefweb.int/sites/reliefweb.int/files/resources/Disability%20Inclusion_Translating%20Policy%20into%20Practice%20in%20Humanitarian%20Action.pdf

Petit, G., & Tedds, L. (2020). The effect of differences in treatment of the Canada emergency Response benefit across provincial and territorial income assistance programs. *Canadian Public Policy*, *46*(S1), S29–S43. https://doi.org/10.3138/cpp.2020-054

Pettinicchio, D., Maroto, M., Chai, L., & Lukk, M. (2021). Findings from an online survey on the mental health effects of COVID-19 on Canadians with disabilities and chronic health conditions. *Disability and Health Journal*, *14*(3). https://doi.org/10.1016/j.dhjo.2021.101085

Plan Institute. (2020, October). Canada disability benefit part 1 – Webinar 2 – What we want and need [Video]. *YouTube*. https://www.youtube.com/watch?v=DP0vWZes4Y4

Plouin, M., Adema, W., Fron, P., & Roth, P. M. (2021). *A crisis on the horizon: Ensuring affordable, accessible housing for people with disabilities.* [(OECD Social, Employment and Migration Working Papers No. 261)]. Directorate for employment, labour and social affairs committee, Organisation for Economic Co-operation and Development. https://www.oecd-ilibrary.org/social-issues-migration-health/a-crisis-on-the-horizon_306e6993-en

Rodrigue, S. (2016). Insights on Canadian society: Hidden homelessness in Canada. Statistics Canada. Retrieved from https://www150.statcan.gc.ca/n1/pub/75-006-x/2016001/article/14678-eng.htm

Srijuntrapun, P. (2018). Sustainable livelihoods framework of visually impaired people. *Asia Pacific Journal of Social Work and Development*, *28*(1), 27–38. https://doi.org/10.1080/02185385.2017.1394217

Stall, N. M., Jones, A., Brown, K. A., Rochon, P. A., & Costa, A. P. (2020). For-profit long-term care homes and the risk of COVID-19 outbreaks and resident deaths. *Canadian Medical Association Journal*, *192*(33), E946–E955. https://doi.org/10.1503/cmaj.201197

Statistics Canada (2020). Impacts of COVID-19 on persons with disabilities. https://www150.statcan.gc.ca/n1/en/daily-quotidien/200827/dq200827c-eng.pdf?st=avvw6y9j

Statistics Canada (2021). Housing vulnerabilities among Canadians with mental health-related disabilities. https://www150.statcan.gc.ca/n1/pub/11-627-m/11-627-m2021007-eng.htm

Stienstra, D., Grand'Maison, V., Pin, L., Rodenburg, E., Garwood, K., & Reinders, K. (2021). Disability inclusion analysis of lessons learned and best practices of the Government of Canada's response to the COVID-19 pandemic. University of Guelph - Live Work Well Research Centre and DisAbled Women's Association of Canada. https://liveworkwell.ca/sites/default/files/pageuploads/DisabilityInclusionAnalysisCOVID-19_Final_031621_protected.pdf

Stienstra, D., & Lee, T. M. (2019). Disabilities and livelihoods: Rethinking a conceptual framework. *Societies*, *9*(4), 67. https://doi.org/10.3390/soc9040067

Tint, A., & Weiss, J. A. (2018). A qualitative study of the service experiences of women with autism spectrum disorder. *Autism*, *22*(8), 928–937. https://doi.org/10.1177/1362361317702561

UN Partnership on the Rights of Persons with Disabilities (UNPRPD). (2020). Disability inclusive social protection response to COVID-19 crisis. http://inprf.gob.mx/inprf/archivos/2020/disability_covid-19.pdf

UNHCR. (2016). *UNHCR age, gender, and diversity accountability report 2015*. United Nations High Commissioner for Refugees. https://www.unhcr.org/protection/women/5769092c7/unhcr-age-gender-diversity-accountability-report-2015.html

Zwicker, J., & Dunn, A. (2018). Breaking down barriers to the disability tax credit. *Policy Options*. https://policyoptions.irpp.org/magazines/january-2018/breaking-down-barriers-to-the-disability-tax-credit/

Chapter 3

"A ROLLERCOASTER OF EMOTIONS": SOCIAL DISTANCING, ANXIETY, AND LONELINESS AMONG PEOPLE WITH DISABILITIES AND CHRONIC HEALTH CONDITIONS

Michelle Maroto, David Pettinicchio, Lei Chai and Andy Holmes

ABSTRACT

Purpose: *Although social distancing measures enacted during COVID-19 prevented the spread of the virus and acted as important coping mechanisms during this stressful time, they also contributed to loneliness and anxiety. The pros and cons of social distancing measures were especially relevant among people with disabilities and chronic health conditions – a high-risk group concerned about infection through contact with non-household members and visiting public places like school, healthcare providers, and work.*

Methods/Approach: *Drawing on data from a national online survey (*N = *1,027) and in-depth virtual interviews (*N = *50) with Canadians with disabilities and chronic health conditions, we examine the positive and negative effects of three types of social distancing measures – avoiding public places, transitioning to remote work or school, and avoiding contact with non-household members – on perceptions of increases in anxiety and loneliness during the pandemic.*

Findings: *We find that the relationships between engaging with social distancing measures and anxiety and loneliness could be positive or negative,*

Disability in the Time of Pandemic
Research in Social Science and Disability, Volume 13, 49–73

ISSN: 1479-3547/doi:10.1108/S1479-354720230000013004

with measures acting as both adaptive and maladaptive coping mechanisms. Although avoiding public places or non-household members and transitioning to remote work or school often resulted in increased anxiety and loneliness, respondents also described situations where these measures helped them cope with concerns about catching COVID-19.

Implications: *Our findings highlight potential implications for public health policy in allocating different coping resources among marginalized groups during times of crisis and demonstrate the importance of using a social model of stress, coping mechanisms, and mental health.*

Keywords: Disability; mental health; social distancing measures; public policy; COVID-19; mixed methods

INTRODUCTION

The COVID-19 pandemic has clearly been a stressful global life event. Stemming from the fear of infection and growing economic insecurity, many groups have reported declining mental health in relation to the added stress (Bierman & Schieman, 2020; Hub Staff Report, 2020; Statistics Canada, 2020). To combat COVID-19, social distancing measures intended to reduce social contact were governments' primary way to curb the spread of the virus and protect vulnerable groups, especially prior to the widespread distribution of vaccines. By restricting travel, closing schools and businesses, and asking individuals to reduce in-person contacts, many countries were able to limit COVID-19 cases, hospitalization, and deaths. These measures were especially important for protecting at-risk communities, including people with disabilities, people with chronic illness, older adults, and people in low-income neighborhoods, who were more vulnerable to COVID-19, especially at school, work, and in other public settings.

Despite these protective benefits, such restrictions also disrupted day-to-day living, led to economic hardship, and increased isolation by limiting social ties (Pfefferbaum & North, 2020). COVID-19 fatigue and repeated periods of lockdown have generated social unrest. Some, including anti-maskers, anti-vaxxers, and more recently, the "trucker protestors," have mobilized this unrest into organized demonstrations and occupations (Martin & Vanderslott, 2021). For others, their disability and health status made them especially vulnerable to the virus, which required that they strictly adhere to safety and social distancing measures, even when "following the rules" potentially generated other adverse effects including increased loneliness, disconnectedness, and anxiety. Being disproportionately at risk for complications from the virus and already marginalized by ableist institutions and cultures, people with disabilities and chronic health conditions experienced deteriorating mental and physical wellbeing during COVID-19 (Kavanagh et al., 2022; Turk et al., 2020) with varying outcomes among this group, particularly in relation to their relative access to resources, supports, and coping mechanisms.

For people with disabilities and chronic health conditions, social distancing measures present a complicated coping mechanism for dealing with pandemic stress. Coping strategies include "behavioral and/or cognitive attempts to manage specific situational demands which are appraised as taxing or exceeding one's ability to adapt" (Thoits, 1995, p. 60). Strategies can act as maladaptive coping mechanisms, such as when COVID-19 related restrictions like staying home and limiting social interaction result in prolonged isolation and social disconnectedness, contributing to increased fear, anger, stress, and anxiety (Choi et al., 2021; Summaka et al., 2021). However, because these strategies effectively curb viral transmission, they can also be adaptive, relieving anxiety about having to engage with non-household members, increasing feelings of safety and security, and potentially mitigating some pandemic-related stress. And so, for many, adherence to social distancing measures became an important coping strategy for managing the stress and risk involved with COVID-19.

This chapter explores how three types of social distancing measures – avoiding public places, transitioning to remote work or school, and avoiding contact with non-household members – functioned as both adaptive and maladaptive coping strategies for people with disabilities and chronic health conditions during the COVID-19 pandemic, a period of increased stress, especially for high-risk groups. Exposure to stressors and access to coping mechanisms depend on a person's positionality within the social structure (Brown, 2003; Pearlin & Bierman, 2013), meaning that certain groups like people with disabilities and chronic health conditions face different barriers but also stand to benefit in different ways from protections provided by coping mechanisms like social distancing measures. Building on this perspective, we address two central questions. How is adherence to social distancing measures associated with experiences of loneliness and anxiety among people with disabilities and chronic health conditions? Does the relationship differ based on the specific type of social distancing?

We use a mixed-methods approach to address these questions, employing a national online survey (June 2020, $N = 1{,}027$) and integrated set of in-depth virtual qualitative interviews (August–November 2020, $N = 50$) among people with disabilities and chronic health conditions. We find that social distancing measures acted as both adaptive and maladaptive coping strategies, depending on how each was implemented. Our findings speak to the impacts of crises and corresponding public health and policy responses, as well as broader understandings about how marginalized communities attempt to manage stressful events. We therefore contribute to the sociological tradition of understanding mental health disparities as a function of social status and social group membership (Link & Phelan, 1995; Pearlin, 1999; Reichard et al., 2011).

SOCIAL BARRIER-BASED UNDERSTANDINGS OF ANXIETY AND LONELINESS

Anxiety, loneliness, and other forms of psychological distress are common among people with disabilities and chronic health conditions (Brown & Turner, 2010;

Cage et al., 2018; Chan et al., 2011; Turner & Beiser, 1990; Turner et al., 2006). This is also true for specific subgroups, like individuals on the autism spectrum (Cage et al., 2018; Gillott & Standen, 2007; Park et al., 2019). Excluded from social networks, people with disabilities have weaker social ties and experience greater social isolation (Macdonald et al., 2018; Nosek & Hughes, 2003; Schafer, 2018; Shandra, 2017, 2021), which further contribute to distress (Bierman et al., 2021). This is partly due to mobility-related issues (Rosso et al., 2013; Schafer, 2018), but also because of disablist attitudes and ableist structures that stigmatize, marginalize, and exclude (Maroto & Pettinicchio, 2022; Schafer, 2018; also see Cage et al., 2018; Ciciurkaite et al., 2022; Moloney et al., 2019). Here, disablism reflects negative attitudes that support the unequal treatment of people with disabilities, but ableism is much broader, reflecting structures designed to support certain abilities (Campbell, 2009; Maroto & Pettinicchio, 2022; Wolbring, 2008).

Although the links between disability, loneliness, and anxiety are well documented, only recently have health scholars borrowed from disability studies to apply a social model or barrier-based approach to explain these links. This approach moves the focus away from individual impairment to socially constructed or environmental barriers that contribute to marginalization. In the context of mental health, social policies, ableist institutional practices, negative attitudes, and stigmatizing labels undermine social ties that act as key coping mechanisms buffering against everyday stressors that add to depression and anxiety, lowering social welfare and personal wellbeing (Brown, 2017; Cross, 2013; Oliver, 1996).

A social barrier-based framework further demonstrates how loneliness results from lack of or poor-quality social ties and the feelings it brings on (Dahlberg & McKee, 2014). As Hawkley and Cacioppo explain, loneliness is "distressing feeling that accompanies the perception that one's social needs are not being met by the quantity or especially the quality of one's social relationships" (2010, p. 218). Consequently, loneliness has increasingly been used as a proxy for social disconnectedness, which people with disabilities experience at greater rates (Emerson et al., 2021; Mithen et al., 2015).

Structural alienation and social disconnectedness are a result of disabling barriers across different spheres of life including work and school. These barriers not only contribute to loneliness but also to anxiety (MacDonald et al., 2018), a negative affect that decreases personal well-being (Emerson et al., 2020). Living alone, lack of employment, and lack of community resources all contribute to worsening loneliness and anxiety (Emerson et al., 2021). Low social connectedness contributes to anxiety because the quality of contact with others – a coping mechanism – is low or altogether absent. Already higher levels of loneliness and anxiety then leave this group more vulnerable to further negative outcomes under stressful situations, especially when coping mechanisms are lacking.

EXPOSURE TO STRESSORS AND ACCESS TO COPING MECHANISMS

Uncovering how coping mechanisms (or lack thereof) buffer stressors particular to given social groups and statuses – so-called minority stressors (Meyer, 2003) that include alienation, devaluation, and exclusion – requires a within-group focus rather than a between-group comparison because stressors are experienced differently by different groups (Brown, 2017; Nosek & Hughes, 2003). Although research on disability and mental health emphasizes disability as a "chronic stressor" leading to increased depression and anxiety (Chan et al., 2011; Zheng et al., 2021), multiple social contexts and factors like social ties, employment, marriage and household structure, access to formal and informal care, and social supports and resources provide coping mechanisms to protect people from stressors (Bierman, 2012; Schieman & Plickert, 2007). As Brown (2017) finds, coping mechanisms against depressive symptoms like supportive social relationships are less effective at buffering disability-relevant social stressors when they are diminished. Social ties therefore help mitigate the negative effects of stressors when they are available, promoting positive mental health outcomes through the provision of social, emotional, informational, and instrumental supports (see Thoits, 1995, 2011; Umberson & Karas Montez, 2010).

Crises including natural disasters, economic emergencies, and pandemics lead to increased stress throughout the population. A chief stressor during health pandemics is increased "health anxiety" which disproportionately affects vulnerable and at-risk groups (Asmundson & Taylor, 2020). But because crises represent major exogenous shocks, secondary stressors also include loss of work, financial insecurity, and breaks in social ties (Zheng et al., 2021). These secondary stressors affect already vulnerable groups disproportionately, including people with disabilities (Maroto et al., 2021). Crises also make coping resources unavailable. This is particularly true in the case of COVID-19 as social distancing, self-isolation, and lockdowns affected everything from work and school, to being with family and friends, and accessing healthcare professionals.

SOCIAL DISTANCING MEASURES: ADAPTIVE OR MALADAPTIVE COPING MECHANISMS?

Examining the circumstances that simultaneously increase stressors and undermine coping mechanisms provides an important contribution to the scholarship on group-specific stressors, access to coping mechanisms, and mental health outcomes. COVID-19 is one such circumstance. Zheng et al. (2021) found that pandemic-related secondary stressors led to depressive symptoms, and Summaka et al. (2021) showed not only increased fear, anger, annoyance, stress, and sadness, but also increases in anxiety. Pettinicchio et al. (2021) found that Canadians with disabilities and chronic health conditions reported increased anxiety, stress, despair, and loneliness. These studies reveal how health-related concerns and disruptions to social ties (i.e., stress buffers) because of social distancing and lockdown measures contribute to negative mental health outcomes, including anxiety and loneliness (Kar et al., 2020). We build on this research by examining the potential positive and negative effects of adherence to different social distancing measures.

Social distancing measures implemented by the Canadian government and others starting in March 2020 limited the spread of COVID-19 and mortality from the virus (Courtemanche et al., 2020). They have also been important for protecting people who are especially vulnerable to complications from the virus. However, although these sweeping measures provided important protection against the spread of COVID-19, they also disrupted key supports (Douglas et al., 2020). People's day-to-day living and routines – everything from meeting friends for lunch and going shopping, to getting adequate home care or visiting a mental health professional – were affected. Many people with disabilities and chronic health conditions living at home lost in-person paid health care services due to COVID-19 related restrictions (Jeste et al., 2020). With increased obstacles in accessing healthcare and social supports, they faced challenges in managing their health throughout the pandemic (Lunsky et al., 2022; Pendo, 2020). As a result of social distancing measures interrupting social ties and support systems, many individuals felt disconnected and experienced elevated mental health issues during the pandemic, a stressful time where individuals need social supports the most (Brooks et al., 2020; Scharf & Oinonen, 2020).

With already high levels of social isolation and weak social ties, social distancing and stay-at-home orders can act as maladaptive coping mechanisms, adding to feelings of loneliness and anxiety among people with disabilities and chronic health conditions. Despite the increases in social isolation, however, social and physical distancing measures still provided important protections for combatting the spread of COVID-19, especially among people with disabilities and chronic health conditions for whom the dangers of getting sick were much greater. This means that measures like limiting contact with people outside the household, working from home, and spending less time in public add to a sense of safety and assuage some pandemic-related fears. And so, these may not negatively affect mental health. Indeed, as adaptive coping mechanisms, they may improve mental health, especially among members of communities whose health is a salient feature of daily life (Pettinicchio et al., 2021). In other words, distancing and self-isolation are also adaptive coping mechanisms providing mental health benefits by limiting fears and concerns.

DATA AND METHODS

We use a mixed-methods approach to study the relationship between social distancing measures, loneliness, and anxiety among people with disabilities and chronic health conditions. We classified disability using six questions following the Canadian Survey on Disability (CSD), the World Health Organization, and the Washington Group on Disability Statistics (Morris et al., 2020; see also Pettinicchio & Maroto, 2021). Questions asked respondents if they never, sometimes, often, or always experienced difficulties seeing, hearing, walking, or doing other physical activities, or learning, remembering, or concentrating. They also asked if respondents had any emotional, psychological, or mental health conditions or any other health concern or long-term condition that has lasted or is expected to last for six months or more. We classified chronic conditions based on whether the respondent indicated the presence of the following nine conditions: asthma, cancer, chronic kidney disease, chronic respiratory or lung disease, diabetes, hypertension, heart disease, immunocompromised, or obesity.

The present study uses data from a quota-based online survey conducted from June 11 to June 22, 2020 (N = 1,027) and a set of follow-up interviews collected from August through November 2020 (N = 50). Participants were recruited by *Qualtrics*, an Internet-based survey company using paid research panels. All respondents were 18 years or older at the time of surveying, resided in a Canadian province, and reported one or more of the six listed disabilities or nine listed chronic health conditions. To ensure that we obtained a representative sample of all 10 Canadian provinces, data were collected via quota-based sampling based on 2016 Census provincial population estimates. We did not employ post-stratification weights (Bethlehem, 2010). Many of the characteristics observed in our sample (e.g., age, gender, and education) mirror those for individuals sampled in the CSD and Canadian Community Health Survey (CCHS) (Pettinicchio et al., 2021).

Supplementing our quantitative data, we conducted 50 qualitative in-depth phone interviews between August and November 2020 with a sample of respondents from our survey. In-depth interviews allowed us to further explore and seek clarity about how respondents were experiencing the pandemic by asking integrated follow-up questions not often available through surveys alone (Lamont & Swidler, 2014; Pugh, 2013). From our initial survey, 506 respondents requested to be contacted for a follow-up interview. We then selected 100 respondents to ensure a diversity of characteristics (i.e., age, gender, race) as well as different disabilities and health conditions, and then drew 50 who were ultimately interviewed. We provided respondents a $30 incentive, informed them of ethical clearance from our university review boards, and noted that all names used would be pseudonyms to protect their confidentiality.

Survey Analysis and Measures

We examine two outcome variables that measure whether a respondent self-reported any increase in *anxiety* or *loneliness* within the last 14 days (a time referring to early June 2020). These were part of a series of 10 questions that asked respondents: "Have you experienced any changes in the following feelings within the last 14 days?" Respondents were given choices of decrease, about the same, and increase. We coded variables for anxiety and loneliness as binary variables indicating an increase in these feelings.

We connect these outcomes with three predictor variables accounting for the major social distancing measures taken and their potential negative effects. They indicate whether the respondent reported *avoiding public places, avoiding in-person work or school*, and *avoiding contact with non-household members*. These variables were created from a set of questions that first asked respondents about 14 potential measures that they took to combat COVID-19 and then asked to what extent these measures affected them negatively or made things worse to capture the adaptive or maladaptive dimensions of each strategy. Combing these questions, the final variables include three categories – did not use this measure (no strategy), used the measure with no negative effects (adaptive strategy), and used the measure with at least some negative effects (maladaptive strategy).

Several control variables were included. We measure disability condition/severity as the *number of reported disabilities and health conditions*, which indicated whether the respondent reported one, two or three, four or five, or six or more disabilities or chronic health conditions. We also control for *age*, measured in years; *gender* measured as male, female, and other or non-binary; and *marital status* measured as never married, cohabiting, married, and formerly married (i.e., widowed, separated, or divorced). We include an indicator variable for the *presence of children* in the household. Education is measured as obtaining a Bachelor's degree or higher. We also control for whether the respondent was *employed*. We include an indicator for *race/ethnic minority*. Finally, *region* includes the following categories: Ontario, Québec, British Columbia, Prairie provinces, and Atlantic province. Descriptive statistics are presented in the appendix.

With binary outcome variables, we use logistic regression models to examine the association between social distancing practices and increases in anxiety and loneliness. We primarily discuss our results as predicted probabilities and average marginal effects (AMEs). Applied to our categorical focal variables, AMEs indicate the average percentage point difference in the probability of experiencing increased anxiety or loneliness associated with a discrete change in the predictor variable.

Interview Data Analysis

We combined these quantitative analyses with results from our in-depth interviews that reveal more about how social distancing, especially not going to work, contributed to loneliness and declining mental health. Interviews lasted from 12 to 60 minutes in length with an average of 34 minutes and were transcribed verbatim by a team of research assistants and coded on Dedoose – a qualitative data analysis program. We first open coded transcripts to create a preliminary coding scheme (Strauss, 1987), which was deductively based on our research questions and inductively through emergent themes from respondents (Deterding & Waters, 2021). Here, we looked for discursive claims from participants (Strauss & Corbin, 1990) before we analytically coded and identified common themes across respondents (Auerbach & Silverstein, 2003) to establish inter-coder reliability. Our in-depth interviews provide rich descriptions of our respondents' experiences of loneliness, anxiety, and social isolation during the COVID-19 pandemic.

FINDINGS

Most survey respondents engaged in at least one social distancing measure, but the usage and effects varied considerably. As shown in Fig. 1, 22% of respondents reported that they did not avoid public places, 60% reported that avoiding public places negatively affected them, and 18% reported avoiding public places with no negative effects. Most respondents reported that they were not able to transition to remote work or school, 29% reported that they were negatively affected by a remote school or work transition, and 15% reported that they were not negatively affected. Finally, 29% of respondents reported that they were still socializing with people outside their household, 52% reported that avoiding contact with individuals outside their household negatively affected them, and 18% reported that avoiding contact with non-household members did not negatively affect them. These findings indicate that social distancing measures can act as both adaptive and maladaptive coping strategies, which means that may not always contribute negatively to anxiety and loneliness.

To address the adaptive and maladaptive dimensions of social distancing behaviors, we use two sets of logistic regression models predicting increased anxiety or loneliness in Table 1 (Model Sets 1–2) and Figs. 2–4. The table includes model coefficients and average marginal effects for all focal variables. Figures present predicted probabilities of increased anxiety and loneliness associated with avoiding public places (Fig. 2), avoiding in-person work/school (Fig. 3), and avoiding contact with non-household members (Fig. 4).

Table 1 shows that engaging with different social distancing measures offered both benefits and drawbacks for loneliness and anxiety that varied with the specific measure. Avoiding public places and transitioning to remote work or school were associated with increased anxiety and loneliness, but only when they were reported as having negative effects in a maladaptive context. When not accompanied by negative effects, these measures were associated with reduced anxiety, showing that they can also be adaptive.

The pattern differed for avoiding contact with non-household members. Engaging with this type of social distancing without negative effects was associated with decreased anxiety and loneliness. It was the only measure associated with decreased loneliness. When negative effects were present, however, this measure did not significantly increase anxiety but it was associated with increased loneliness.

These varying effects were further supported by our interview data, where respondents discussed both the benefits and drawbacks of different measures. The interviews allowed us to explore patterns established within the quantitative data. Following the goals of mixed methods research, we integrate our discussion of these findings with the quantitative results below.

Avoiding Public Places

When accompanied by negative effects, avoiding public places was associated with an 11.7 percentage point increase in the probability of experiencing increased anxiety and a 16.4 percentage point increase in the probability of

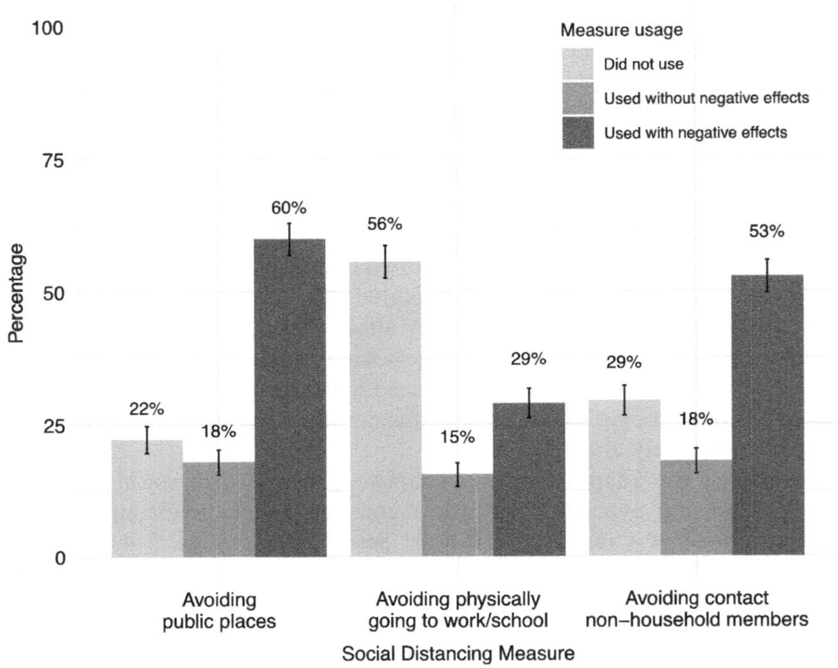

Fig. 1. Use of Social Distancing Measures. *Source:* 2020 COVID-19 Response Survey of People with Disabilities and Chronic Health Conditions. N = 1,027 adults.

loneliness (Table 1). However, when not accompanied by negative effects, this measure was associated with a 9.5 percentage point reduction in anxiety. Expanding these findings, Fig. 2 shows that 44% of respondents who reported that avoiding public places negatively affected them experienced increased anxiety compared to 33% of those who did not avoid public places and 23% who avoided public places with no negative effects. Differences were also apparent in terms of increased loneliness; 38% of respondents who avoided public places with negative effects experienced increased loneliness compared to 21% of those who did not avoid public places and 19% who avoided public places with no negative effects.

Interview respondents echoed these findings. In the words of one study participant, Lina, a 36-year-old homemaker with asthma, "if you're unwell for physical reasons and then you're told to isolate, I feel like that's hard on a person's mental health. At the same time, you can't even really go get the mental health help." Lina further discusses the implications for people with disabilities, saying, "It's hard for the average person, but for people with disabilities and seniors and for your quality of life, it's hard to sit in a room. It's hard to just sit in a house with nobody in to contact, right?" Indeed, for Margo, avoiding public

Table 1. Results From Logistic Regression Models Predicting Increased Anxiety and Loneliness.

	Model Set 1: Anxiety				Model Set 2: Loneliness			
	b	SE	AME	SE	*B*	SE	AME	SE
Intercept	0.329	(0.429)			−1.018	(0.641)		
Avoiding public places (Ref: Did not use)								
Yes, without negative effects	−0.520*	(0.244)	−0.095*	(0.044)	−0.164	(0.412)	−0.025	(0.061)
Yes, with negative effects	0.547***	(0.123)	0.117***	(0.025)	0.875***	(0.154)	0.164***	(0.024)
Pseudo R-Squared	0.101				0.099			
Intercept	0.367	(0.507)			−0.819	(0.533)		
Remote work or school (Ref: Did not use)								
Yes, without negative effects	−0.540*	(0.216)	−0.104**	(0.040)	−0.026	(0.206)	−0.005	(0.037)
Yes, with negative effects	0.633***	(0.156)	0.140***	(0.034)	0.687***	(0.175)	0.140***	(0.034)
Pseudo *R*-Squared	0.099				0.084			
Intercept	0.514	(0.485)			−0.728	(0.674)		
Avoiding contact with non-household members (Ref: Did not use)								
Yes, without negative effects	−0.668*	(0.279)	−0.129*	(0.052)	−0.485**	(0.163)	−0.079**	(0.024)
Yes, with negative effects	0.254	(0.145)	0.055	(0.031)	0.503**	(0.184)	0.099**	(0.036)
Pseudo *R*-Squared	0.092				0.088			

Notes: Logistic regression models predicting probability of a reported increase in anxiety (Column set 1) and loneliness (Column set 2) based on three sets of social distancing measures. All models include control variables: number of disabilities or chronic health conditions, age, gender, racial/ethnic minority status, marital status, presence of children, education, employment status, and province. Full model results appear in the appendix. "*b*" refers to logit model coefficients. Odds ratios can be obtained by exponentiating (*b*). AME refers to average marginal effects, which can be interpreted as a percentage point change in the probability of the outcome category associated with a unit change in the predictor variable. Standard errors are in parentheses. Standard errors account for clustering by province/region.

$^{***}p < 0.001$, $^{**}p < 0.01$, $^{*}p < 0.05$.

Source: 2020 COVID-19 Response Survey of People with Disabilities and Health Conditions, $N = 1{,}027$ adults.

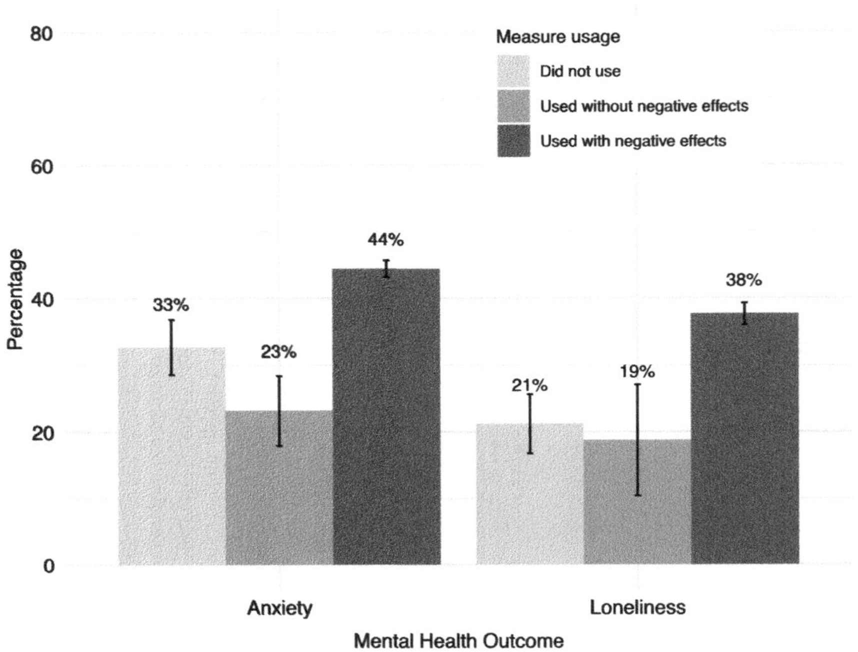

Fig. 2. Increase in Anxiety and Loneliness by Experiences Avoiding Public Places. *Notes:* Predicted probabilities (expressed as percentages) and 95% confidence intervals based on logistic regression models predicting increased anxiety and loneliness in relation to experiences avoiding public places. Models appear in Table 1. *Source:* 2020 COVID-19 Response Survey of People with Disabilities and Chronic Health Conditions. $N = 1{,}027$ adults.

places made her situation "really tough." She told us: "I don't get dressed. I wander around. Some days, I just sit and cry. That makes it really tough."

Anxieties associated with being physically confined at home were captured well by Reagan:

> There were stories from other parts of the province where there were people who ran out of food because they were older. They couldn't get to the store or they were afraid to go to the store, and they had nobody else who could help them... I think more should have been put in place to help people like that, and older people and people with a disability.

It is not only older people with disabilities and chronic health conditions who reported mental health related issues around social distancing. As Allison, a 47-year-old administrative assistant working from home with asthma and obesity told us: "So, I kind of feel like a shut-in. Because I start to hyperventilate. I do all my grocery shopping online and just have it, once at Walmart, they'll put it in the back of the car for me." Allison and many participants point to the negative

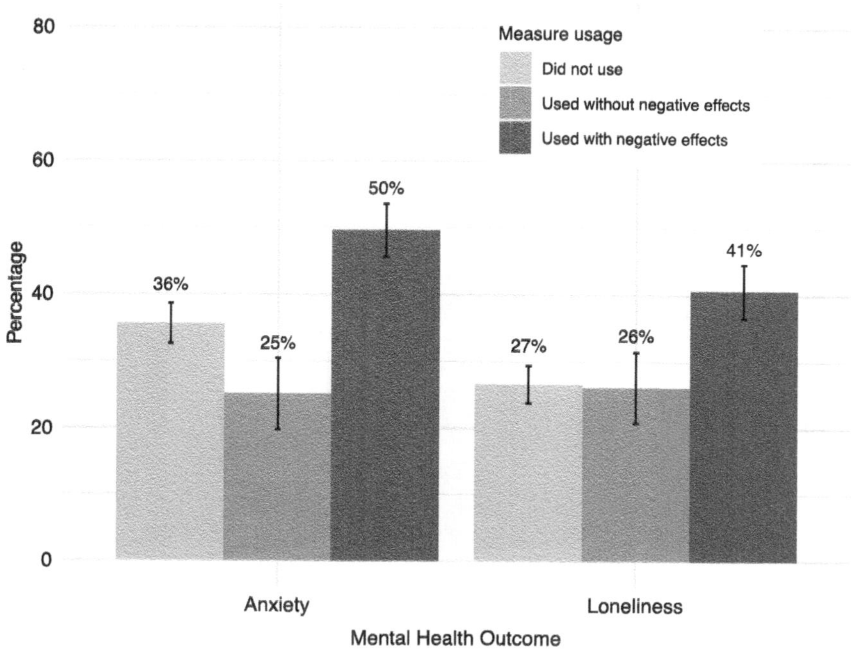

Fig. 3. Increase in Anxiety and Loneliness by Experiences Avoiding Physically Attending Work/School. *Notes:* Predicted probabilities (expressed as percentages) and 95% confidence intervals based on logistic regression models predicting increased anxiety and loneliness in relation to experiences avoiding physically attending work or school. Models appear in Table 1. *Source:* 2020 COVID-19 Response Survey of People with Disabilities and Chronic Health Conditions. N = 1,027 adults.

mental health consequences of avoiding public places and disruptions to social ties, which generated feelings of isolation, loneliness, and anxiety.

Avoiding In-Person Work or School

The associations between transitioning to remote work or school and anxiety and loneliness also depended on whether negative effects were present, demonstrating how this strategy could be both adaptive and maladaptive. Respondents who reported that avoiding going into work or school negatively affected them were 14.0 percentage points more likely to report increased anxiety and to report increased loneliness (Table 1). For example, Maryam, a 35-year-old coach with claustrophobia and obesity, explained that working from home during the pandemic "has taken a toll mentally too for me because I've always worked all my life... I have mostly done jobs that required me to be at the office." Maryam told us how the move to remote work posed challenges to her mental wellbeing: "mentally, I feel quite restless and I actually want to go out." Yet, given her

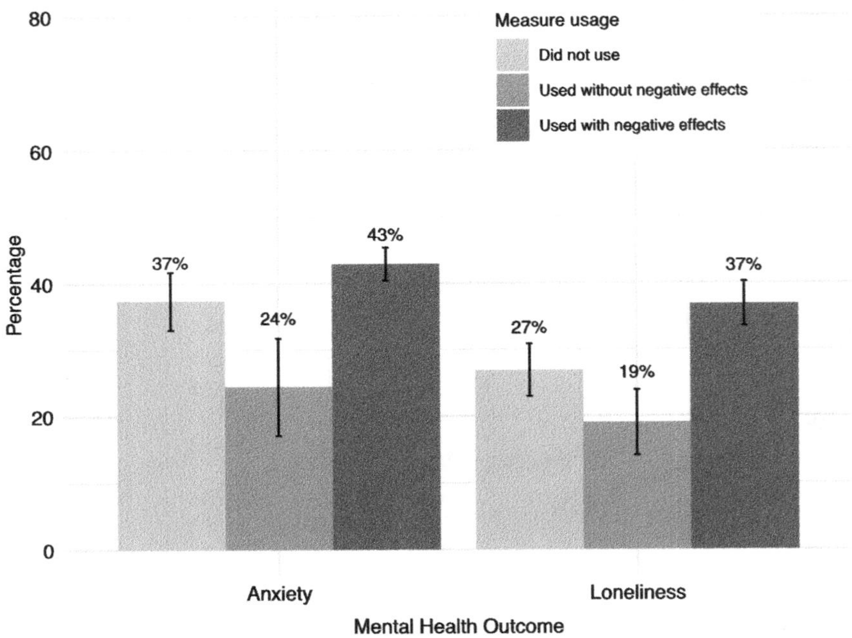

Fig. 4. Increase in Anxiety and Loneliness by Experiences Avoiding Contact with Non-household Members. *Notes:* Predicted probabilities (expressed as percentages) and 95% confidence intervals based on logistic regression models predicting increased anxiety and loneliness in relation to experiences avoiding contact with non-household members. Models appear in Table 1. *Source:* 2020 COVID-19 Response Survey of People with Disabilities and Chronic Health Conditions. $N =$ 1,027 adults.

heightened stress about being more at-risk of getting COVID, she remained "very fearful" and was "literally not even opening the house door to take a breath." Like many others, Maryam was wrestling with the effects of social disruption, on the one hand, and concerns about safety if those disruptions had not taken place, on the other.

However, those who reported that avoiding in-person work or school did not negatively affect them were 10.4 percentage points *less* likely to experience increased anxiety than respondents who were still attending work or school in-person (Table 1). According to Dillan's experience about working from home, "I transitioned to working from home and teaching from home. So, I was still getting paid, so it wasn't really an issue. In June, the teachers all went back to work for a month and just in the school building. At that point, I still hadn't been okay to go back." It appears working and attending school remotely offered benefits for some respondents but not others.

Those who were able to work or attend school from home without negative effects reported some of the lowest rates of anxiety. As shown in Fig. 3, only 25% reported increased anxiety and 26% reported increased loneliness. However, those who worked or attended school remotely and reported negative effects from this situation experienced the *highest* rates of anxiety and loneliness. Among these respondents, 50% experienced increased anxiety and 41% experienced increased loneliness.

For many respondents with disabilities and chronic health issues, the thought of working in person during the pandemic brought new challenges and anxieties. Aayan, a 31-year-old recreational therapist who was considered an essential worker, described her anxiety of having to go in to work:

> I was mandated to still come in and that is stressful because I work for a hospital in Toronto and I'm frontlined with a vulnerable population. So, I found that it did affect me even more so than I think the average person because not only was I… I already have the anxiety in general but then I had to, on top of that, go into an environment where I was at a very high risk of getting it. I would be traveling by TTC [public transit] there and back, which was also very anxiety inducing because not everyone followed the protocols.

Dora, a 76-year-old retired teacher, described her concerns about the potential distancing measures taken by the schools. She says: "I'm not even sure about taking the teaching job, because I'd be involved with kids again. I don't know how careful they're going to be… So, my son does not want me going…so I kind of dropped that job."

Avoiding in-person work or school was not always linked with increased anxiety. This makes sense because individuals with disabilities and chronic health conditions have heightened concerns about getting COVID-19 and have a higher risk of developing serious complications if they did. Respondents had to balance safety, the need to earn an income, and concerns over mental health. According to Ramona, "it's so hard because it's like I know I want to work, but then the numbers are going up, and so there's this conflict between wanting to keep myself safe, but also wanting to work." Similarly, as Maryam explained, "Eventually, I have to go out for an interview and hopefully to work as well" yet expressed some anxieties when she said, "but then there is still that uncertainty because we can [at least] control our lives within our homes at the most." For some, the opportunity to work from home meant feeling less anxious and stressed.

Avoiding Contact With Non-Household Members

Compared to the first two measures, patterns differed with avoiding contact with non-household members. Avoiding contact with non-household members without negative effects was associated with a 12.9 percentage point decrease in anxiety and a 7.9 percentage point decrease in loneliness, net of other covariates (Table 1). Negative effects with this measure, however, were associated with a 9.9 percentage point increase in loneliness but were not significantly associated with anxiety. Fig. 4 shows that 43% of people who had limited contact with non-household members with negative effects reported increased anxiety and 37% reported increased loneliness, much higher percentages than those who limited contact but did not see any negative effects. Here, it is likely that being isolated to protect one's health is seen as taking precedence over socializing with non-household members and risking infection. However, this still did often lead to greater loneliness, as many respondents described.

Some respondents, like Esther, a 60-year-old woman with hypertension, were aware of the risks of contact with others. She noted, "The one thing I'm worried about is even if I worked frontline . . .and I know they have the PPE for it, what's to say that I won't catch it? I'm afraid of that. That's what's cautioning me so terribly. Is it worth going out there to die?" However, for people like Slater, a 33-year-old man with depression, not being able to meet people in public was associated with loneliness. According to Slater: "I went on Facebook and there's people that I see are interested in me and I was going to make a date, but then I couldn't. . .So, my depression, it's on a day-to-day basis. . .It's gotten a little worse over the time. Can't go on dates, can't meet up for friends, feel pretty lonely, feel pretty depressed. It's pretty difficult."

Dora emphasized the negative effects of being isolated from family, saying, "I feel very isolated, and I'm going through emotional times right now, and I've got nobody except my son, when he's here, to share it with." For Dora, being isolated and lacking in-person interactions was similar to Ramona, a 28-year-old market researcher with vision and hearing impairments who described "not being able to hug people" alongside strictly virtual communication which she felt was isolating.

Sydney, a 71-year-old retired woman, further described the negative effects of avoiding social interactions, like socializing with friends, during the pandemic. She says: "I feel like I'd want to cry. . .And I think, well, I'm 71 and a half. This is a really crappy bunch of years at the end of my life if this keeps going." For Sydney, who described herself as a "social person," not being able to participate in her exercise group, celebrate birthdays, or have lunch with friends created significant feeling of loneliness. This was also true for Allison, who indicated: "I don't see loved ones nearly as much. We would have got together as a family for Easter and Thanksgiving. And I'm sure Christmas was also canceled. So, I'm kind of feeling disenfranchised and not connected to anybody, anymore."

Again, though, avoiding contact with people outside the household also offered vulnerable respondents certain protections. For Nicki, a 50-year-old woman with kidney failure on dialysis, avoiding contact with those outside her household gave her a sense of security, at the same time contributing to her loneliness: "No one wants to be around you. Now that there's this 10-person bubble, no one wants me in it because I have to maintain all of those 10 people and know that they don't do bad things. And no one wants to commit to that. It has completely changed my life and made it worse." While maintaining her social bubble granted Nicki safety during the pandemic, she described her isolation from her family: "You think that my own family would at least understand and make changes for me." And part of me says, "They got to live too." So, I don't know. It's a roller coaster of emotions."

Nicki's experience demonstrates both the benefits and drawbacks of social distancing for those who have underlying conditions that make them vulnerable to COVID-19. Although not socializing with people can relieve those with disabilities and chronic health conditions from worrying about contracting a harmful virus, this is at the expense of minimizing contact with loved ones.

DISCUSSION AND CONCLUSION

Our examination of social distancing measures' associations with loneliness and anxiety among people with disabilities and chronic health conditions shows how these measures can function as both adaptive and maladaptive coping mechanisms for dealing with the stress of COVID-19. People who reported that avoiding public places and transitioning to remote work or school negatively affected them were more likely to experience anxiety and loneliness. But, those who did not report negative consequences experienced decreases in anxiety, demonstrating some of the protective benefits of using these social distancing measures to cope with the stress brought on by COVID-19. Avoiding contact with non-household members was also associated with decreased anxiety and loneliness in some situations, and associated with increased loneliness in others. As respondents described in interviews, these strategies resulted in both benefits and drawbacks.

Our findings from the only mixed method study incorporating a national survey and set of interviews with Canadians with disabilities and chronic health conditions collected during the COVID-19 pandemic offer important insights regarding the benefits and drawbacks of social distancing measures. However, there are limitations associated with our sampling methods.

First, even though it was a useful strategy for contacting a marginalized community, our non-probability quota-based sample limited the generalizability of our results. Although quota sampling does not meet the requirements of probability sampling, our survey did provide representation of our population of interest by mirroring demographic characteristics as compared to the CSD and the CCHS. Second, we were unable to recruit individuals without access to the Internet, alongside people with more severe disabilities requiring assistance from caregivers. This means that these groups are likely underrepresented in our study. Third, our smaller sample sizes limited our ability to examine differences by specific disability type, which has been shown to matter for outcomes like loneliness and isolation (MacDonald et al., 2018). Future research would benefit from incorporating these differences. Finally, given that we sought to create an accessible survey, we included single question measures associated with recent self-reported anxiety and loneliness by instructing respondents to recall their health only during the last two weeks. More expansive measures could reveal broader differences. However, our follow-up interviews also allowed respondents to expand on their experiences, providing more detail about their mental health during the pandemic.

Our study advances the growing need for public health studies of vulnerable populations during pandemics (McLaren & Dutton, 2020) by exploring an important but understudied research area involving the mental health effects of social distancing (Scharf & Oinonen, 2020). We show that social distancing measures do not necessarily contribute to greater mental health disparities among people with disabilities and chronic health conditions. For instance, those who were able to use the strategies of avoiding public places and contact with non-household adaptively did not experience increased anxiety and loneliness. In fact, those who adaptively transitioned to remote work or school were among the least likely to experience increased anxiety.

Although some studies emphasize the negative effects of social distancing on mental health (Brooks et al., 2020; Scharf & Oinonen, 2020), our findings suggest that adherence to social distancing measures is not always tied to worsening mental health. Pointing to important scope conditions, one explanation we put forth is that individuals with disabilities and chronic health conditions who are at greater risk and disproportionately worried about contracting a deadly virus (Kavanagh et al., 2022; Lunsky et al., 2022) nevertheless understand the benefits of social distancing as a way to avoid these risks. As a result, avoiding socialization with nonfamily members, such as friends and coworkers, is deemed more beneficial than putting oneself or others at risk of contagion. For many but not all, virtual alternatives to keep in touch and maintain social ties partially filled the gaps caused by social distancing measures. In the words of one of our participants, Glenn, a 46-year-old retail manager from Alberta, who spoke on adapting to living in a pandemic, "it's a brand-new world" of socialization.

REFERENCES

Asmundson, G. J., & Taylor, S. (2020). How health anxiety influences responses to viral outbreaks like COVID-19: What all decision-makers, health authorities, and health care professionals need to know. *Journal of Anxiety Disorders*, *71*, 1–2. https://dx.doi.org/10.1016/j.janxdis.2020.102211

Auerbach, C. F., & Silverstein, L. B. (2003). *Qualitative data: An introduction to coding and analysis*. New York University Press.

Bethlehem, J. (2010). Selection bias in web surveys. *International Statistical Review*, *78*(2), 161–188. https://doi.org/10.1111/j.1751-5823.2010.00112.x

Bierman, A. (2012). Functional limitations and psychological distress: Marital status as moderator. *Society and Mental Health*, *2*(1), 35–52. https://doi.org/10.1177/2156869312442884

Bierman, A., & Schieman, S. (2020). Social estrangement and psychological distress before and during the COVID-19 pandemic: Patterns of change in Canadian workers. *Journal of Health and Social Behavior*, *61*(4), 398–417. https://doi.org/10.1177/0022146520970190

Bierman, A., Upenieks, L., & Schieman, S. (2021). Socially distant? Social network confidants, loneliness, and health during the COVID-19 pandemic. *Social Currents*, *8*(4), 299–313. https://doi.org/10.1177/23294965211011591

Brooks, S. K., Webster, R. K., Smith, L. E., Woodland, L., Wessely, S., Greenberg, N., & Rubin, G. J. (2020). The psychological impact of quarantine and how to reduce it: Rapid review of the evidence. *The Lancet*, *395*(10227), 912–920. https://doi.org/10.1016/S0140-6736(20)30460-8

Brown, T. N. (2003). Critical race theory speaks to the sociology of mental health: Mental health problems produced by racial stratification. *Journal of Health and Social Behavior*, *44*(3), 292–301. https://www.jstor.org/stable/1519780

Brown, R. L. (2017). Functional limitation and depressive symptomatology: Considering perceived stigma and discrimination within a stress and coping framework. *Stigma and Health*, *2*(2), 98–109. https://doi.org/10.1037/sah0000042

Brown, R. L., & Turner, R. J. (2010). Physical disability and depression: Clarifying racial/ethnic contrasts. *Journal of Aging and Health*, *22*(7), 977–1000. https://doi.org/10.1177/0898264309360573

Cage, E., Di Monaco, J., & Newell, V. (2018). Experiences of autism acceptance and mental health in autistic adults. *Journal of Autism and Developmental Disorders*, *48*(2), 473–484.

Campbell, F. K. (2009). *Contours of ableism: The production of disability and abledness*. Palgrave MacMillan.

Chan, N., Anstey, K. J., Windsor, T. D., & Luszcz, M. A. (2011). Disability and depressive symptoms in later life: The stress-buffering role of informal and formal support. *Gerontology*, *57*(2), 180–189. https://doi.org/10.1159/000314158

Choi, J. W., Han, E., Lee, S. G., Shin, J., & Kim, T. H. (2021). Risk of COVID-19 and major adverse clinical outcomes among people with disabilities in South Korea. *Disability and Health Journal*, *14*(4), 101127. https://doi.org/10.1016/j.dhjo.2021.101127

Ciciurkaite, G., Marquez-Velarde, G., & Brown, R. L. (2022). Stressors associated with the COVID-19 pandemic, disability, and mental health: Considerations from the Intermountain West. *Stress and Health*, *38*(2), 304–317. https://doi.org/10.1002/smi.3091

Courtemanche, C., Garuccio, J., Le, A., Pinkston, J., & Yelowitz, A. (2020). Strong social distancing measures in the United States reduced the covid-19 growth rate: Study evaluates the impact of social distancing measures on the growth rate of confirmed COVID-19 cases across the United States. *Health Affairs*, *39*(7), 1237–1246. https://doi.org/10.1377/hlthaff.2020.00608

Cross, M. (2013). Demonised, impoverished and now forced into isolation: The fate of disabled people under austerity. *Disability & Society*, *28*(5), 719–723. https://doi.org/10.1080/09687599.2013.808087

Dahlberg, L., & McKee, K. J. (2014). Correlates of social and emotional loneliness in older people: Evidence from an English community study. *Aging & Mental Health*, *18*(4), 504–514. https://doi.org/10.1080/13607863.2013.856863

Deterding, N. M., & Waters, M. C. (2021). Flexible coding of in-depth interviews: A twenty-first century approach. *Sociological Methods & Research*, *50*(2), 708–739. https://doi.org/10.1177/0049124118799377

Douglas, M., Katikireddi, S. V., Taulbut, M., McKee, M., & McCartney, G. (2020). Mitigating the wider health effects of COVID-19 pandemic response. *BMJ*, *369*, m1577. https://doi.org/10.1136/bmj.m1557

Emerson, E., Fortune, N., Aitken, Z., Hatton, C., Stancliffe, R., & Llewellyn, G. (2020). The wellbeing of working-age adults with and without disability in the UK: Associations with age, gender, ethnicity, partnership status, educational attainment and employment status. *Disability and Health Journal*, *13*(3), 1–7. 100889. https://doi.org/10.1016/j.dhjo.2020.100889

Emerson, E., Fortune, N., Llewellyn, G., & Stancliffe, R. (2021). Loneliness, social support, social isolation and wellbeing among working age adults with and without disability: Cross-sectional study. *Disability and Health Journal*, *14*(1), 1–7. 100965 https://doi.org/10.1016/j.dhjo.2020.100965

Gillott, A., & Standen, P. J. (2007). Levels of anxiety and sources of stress in adults with autism. *Journal of Intellectual Disabilities*, *11*(4), 359–370. https://doi.org/10.1177/1744629507083585

Hawkley, L. C., & Cacioppo, J. T. (2010). Loneliness matters: A theoretical and empirical review of consequences and mechanisms. *Annals of Behavioral Medicine*, *40*(2), 218–227. https://doi.org/10.1007/s12160-010-9210-8

Hub Staff Report, John Hopkins University. (2020). COVID-19 poses unique challenges for people with disabilities. https://hub.jhu.edu/2020/04/23/how- covid-19-affects-people-with-disabilities

Jeste, S., Hyde, C., Distefano, C., Halladay, A., Ray, S., Porath, M., Wilson, R. B., & Thurm, A. (2020). Changes in access to educational and healthcare services for individuals with intellectual and developmental disabilities during COVID-19 restrictions. *Journal of Intellectual Disability Research*, *64*(11), 825–833. https://doi.org/10.1111/jir.12776

Kar, S. K., Yasir Arafat, S. M., Kabir, R., Sharma, P., & Saxena, S. K. (2020). Coping with mental health challenges during COVID-19, *Coronavirus disease 2019 (COVID-19)* (pp. 199–213). Springer.

Kavanagh, A., Hatton, C., Stancliffe, R. J., Aitken, Z., King, T., Hastings, R., Totsika, V., Llewellyn, G., & Emerson, E. (2022). Health and healthcare for people with disabilities in the UK during the COVID-19 pandemic. *Disability and Health Journal*, *15*(1), 101171. https://doi.org/10.1016/j.dhjo.2021.101171

Lamont, M., & Swidler, A. (2014). Methodological pluralism and the possibilities and limits of interviewing. *Qualitative Sociology*, *37*(1), 153–171. https://doi.org/10.1007/s11133-014-9274-z

Link, B. G., & Phelan, J. (1995). Social conditions as fundamental causes of disease. *Journal of Health and Social Behavior*, 80–94.

Lunsky, Y., Durbin, A., Balogh, R., Lin, E., Palma, L., & Plumptre, L. (2022). COVID-19 positivity rates, hospitalizations and mortality of adults with and without intellectual and developmental disabilities in Ontario, Canada. *Disability and Health Journal*, *15*(1), 101174.

Macdonald, S. J., Deacon, L., Nixon, J., Akintola, A., Gillingham, A., Kent, J., Ellis, G., Mathews, D., Ismail, A., Sullivan, S., Dore, S., & Highmore, L. (2018). 'The invisible enemy': Disability, loneliness and isolation. *Disability & Society*, *33*(7), 1138–1159. https://doi.org/10.1080/09687599.2018.1476224

Maroto, M., & Pettinicchio, D. (2022). Relational inequality and the structures that disadvantage. In R. L. Brown, M. Maroto, & D. Pettinicchio (Eds.), *The Oxford handbook of the sociology of disability*. Oxford University Press.

Maroto, M. L., Pettinicchio, D., & Lukk, M. (2021). Working differently or not at all: COVID-19's effects on employment among people with disabilities and chronic health conditions. *Sociological Perspectives*, *64*(5), 876–897. https://doi.org/10.1177/07311214211012018

Martin, S., & Vanderslott, S. (2021). Any idea how fast 'It's just a mask!' can turn into 'It's just a vaccine!': From mask mandates to vaccine mandates during the COVID-19 pandemic. *Vaccine*. (in press). https://doi.org/10.1016/j.vaccine.2021.10.031

McLaren, L., & Dutton, D. J. (2020). The social determinants of pandemic impact: An opportunity to rethink what we mean by "public health spending". *Canadian Journal of Public Health*, *111*(4), 451–453. https://doi.org/10.17269/s41997-020-00395-2

Meyer, I. H. (2003). Prejudice, social stress, and mental health in lesbian, gay and bisexual populations: Conceptual issues and research evidence. *Psychological Bulletin*, *129*, 674–697. https://doi.org/10.1037/0033-2909.129.5.674

Mithen, J., Aitken, Z., Ziersch, A., & Kavanagh, A. M. (2015). Inequalities in social capital and health between people with and without disabilities. *Social Science & Medicine*, *126*, 26–35. https://doi.org/10.1016/j.socscimed.2014.12.009

Moloney, M. E., Brown, R. L., Ciciurkaite, G., & Foley, S. M. (2019). "Going the extra mile": Disclosure, accommodation, and stigma management among working women with disabilities. *Deviant Behavior*, *40*(8), 942–956. https://doi.org/10.1080/01639625.2018.1445445

Morris, S., Fawcett, G., Brisebois, L., & Hughes, J. A. (2020). *Demographic, employment and income profile of Canadians with disabilities aged 15 years and over, 2017*. Statistics Canada Catalogue No. 89-654-X201800; 2020. https://www150.statcan. gc.ca/n1/pub/89-654-x/89-654-x2018002-eng.htm

Nosek, M. A., & Hughes, R. B. (2003). Psychosocial issues of women with physical disabilities: The continuing gender debate. *Rehabilitation Counseling Bulletin*, *46*(4), 224–233. https://doi.org/10.1177/003435520304600403

Oliver, M. (1996). *Understanding disability from theory to practice*. Palgrave.

Park, S. H., Song, Y. J. C., Demetriou, E. A., Pepper, K. L., Norton, A., Thomas, E. E., Hickie, I. B., Hermens, D. F., Glozier, N., & Guastella, A. J. (2019). Disability, functioning, and quality of life among treatment-seeking young autistic adults and its relation to depression, anxiety, and stress. *Autism*, *23*(7), 1675–1686. https://doi.org/10.1177/1362361318823925

Pearlin, L. I. (1999). The stress process revisited: Reflections on concepts and their interrelationships. In C. S. Aneshensel, J. C. Phelan, & A. Bierman (Eds.), *Handbook of the sociology of mental health* (pp. 395–415). Kluwer Academic/Plenum Publishers.

Pearlin, L. I., & Bierman, A. (2013). Current issues and future directions in research into the stress process. In C. S. Aneshensel, J. C. Phelan, & A. Bierman (Eds.), *Handbook of the sociology of mental health* (pp. 325–340). Springer.

Pendo, E. (2020). COVID-19 and disability-based discrimination in healthcare. https://www.americanbar.org/groups/diversity/disabilityrights/resources/covid19-disability-discrimination/

Pettinicchio, D., & Maroto, M. (2021). Who counts? Measuring disability cross-nationally in Census data. *Journal of Survey Statistics and Methodology*, *9*(2), 257–284. https://doi.org/10.1093/jssam/smaa046

Pettinicchio, D., Maroto, M., Chai, L., & Lukk, M. (2021). Findings from an online survey on the mental health effects of COVID-19 on Canadians with disabilities and chronic health conditions. *Disability and Health Journal*, *14*, 1–11. 101085. https://doi.org/10.1016/j.dhjo.2021.101085

Pettinicchio, D., Maroto, M., & Lukk, M. (2021). Perceptions of Canadian federal policy responses to COVID-19 among people with disabilities and chronic health conditions. *Canadian Public Policy*, *47*(2), 231–251. https://doi.org/10.3138/cpp.2021-012

Pfefferbaum, B., & North, C. S. (2020). Mental health and the COVID-19 pandemic. *New England Journal of Medicine*, *383*(6), 510–512. https://doi.org/10.1056/NEJMp2008017

Pugh, A. J. (2013). What good are interviews for thinking about culture? Demystifying interpretive analysis. *American Journal of Cultural Sociology*, *1*(1), 42–68. https://doi.org/10.1057/ajcs.2012.4

Reichard, A., Stolzle, H., & Fox, M. H. (2011). Health disparities among adults with physical disabilities or cognitive limitations compared to individuals with no disabilities in the United States. *Disability and Health Journal*, *4*(2), 59–67. https://doi.org/10.1016/j.dhjo.2010.05.003

Rosso, A. L., Taylor, J. A., Tabb, L. P., & Michael, Y. L. (2013). Mobility, disability, and social engagement in older adults. *Journal of Aging and Health*, *25*(4), 617–637. https://doi.org/10.1177/0898264313482489

Schafer, M. H. (2018). (Where) is functional decline isolating? Disordered environments and the onset of disability. *Journal of Health and Social Behavior*, *59*(1), 38–55. https://doi.org/10.1177/0898264313482489

Scharf, D., & Oinonen, K. (2020). Ontario's response to COVID-19 shows that mental health providers must be integrated into provincial public health insurance systems. *Canadian Journal of Public Health*, *111*(4), 473–476. https://doi.org/10.17269/s41997-020-00397-0

Schieman, S., & Plickert, G. (2007). Functional limitations and changes in levels of depression among older adults: A multiple-hierarchy stratification perspective. *Journals of Gerontology Series B: Psychological Sciences and Social Sciences*, *62*(1), S36–S42. https://doi.org/10.1093/geronb/62.1.S36

Shandra, C. L. (2017). Disability and social participation: The case of formal and informal volunteering. *Social Science Research*, *68*, 195–213. https://doi.org/10.1016/j.ssresearch.2017.02.006

Shandra, C. L. (2021). Disability and patterns of leisure participation across the life course. *The Journals of Gerontology: Series B*, *76*(4), 801–809. https://doi.org/10.1093/geronb/gbaa065

Statistics Canada (2020). *Impacts on mental health*. Statistics Canada Catalogue No. 11-631-X. https://www150.statcan.gc.ca/n1/pub/11-631-x/2020004/s3-eng.htm

Strauss, A. L. (1987). *Qualitative analysis for social scientists*. Cambridge University Press.

Strauss, A. L., & Corbin, J. M. (1990). *Basics of qualitative research: Grounded theory procedures and techniques*. Sage.

Summaka, M., Zein, H., Naim, I., & Fneish, S. (2021). Assessing the psychological impact of COVID-19 outbreak and its related factors on Lebanese individuals with physical disabilities. *Disability and Health Journal*, *14*(3), 1–7. 101073. https://doi.org/10.1016/j.dhjo.2021.101073

Thoits, P. A. (1995). Stress, coping, and social support processes: Where are we? What next? *Journal of Health and Social Behavior, Extra Issue*, 53–79. https://doi.org/10.2307/2626957

Thoits, P. A. (2011). Mechanisms linking social ties and support to physical and mental health. *Journal of Health and Social Behavior*, *52*(2), 145–161. https://doi.org/10.2307/2626957

Turk, M. A., Landes, S. D., Formica, M. K., & Goss, K. D. (2020). Intellectual and developmental disability and COVID-19 case-fatality trends: TriNetX analysis. *Disability and Health Journal*, *13*(3), 1–4. 100942. https://doi.org/10.2307/2626957

Turner, R. J., & Beiser, M. (1990). Major depression and depressive symptomatology among the physically disabled: Assessing the role of chronic stress. *The Journal of Nervous and Mental Disease*, *178*(6), 343–350. https://doi.org/10.1097/00005053-199006000-00001

Turner, R. J., Lloyd, D. A., & Taylor, J. (2006). Physical disability and mental health: An epidemiology of psychiatric and substance disorders. *Rehabilitation Psychology*, *51*(3), 214–223. https://doi.org/10.1037/0090-5550.51.3.214

Umberson, D., & Karas Montez, J. (2010). Social relationships and health: A flashpoint for health policy. *Journal of Health and Social Behavior*, *51*(Suppl. 1), S54–S66. https://doi.org/10.1177/0022146510383501

Wolbring, G. (2008). The politics of ableism. *Development*, *51*(2), 252–258. https://doi.org/10.1057/dev.2008.17

Zheng, J., Morstead, T., Sin, N., Klaiber, P., Umberson, D., Kamble, S., & DeLongis, A. (2021). Psychological distress in North America during COVID-19: The role of pandemic-related stressors. *Social Science & Medicine*, *270*, 1–8. 113687. https://doi.org/10.1016/j.socscimed.2021.113687

APPENDIX A. DESCRIPTIVE STATISTICS FOR MODEL VARIABLES

		Percentage or Mean		
			95% Confidence Interval	
	Sample Frequency	Estimate	Lower	Higher
Increased anxiety	392	0.382	0.352	0.411
Increased loneliness	316	0.308	0.279	0.336
Avoiding public places				
No	228	0.222	0.198	0.249
Yes, without negative effects	184	0.179	0.157	0.204
Yes, with negative effects	615	0.599	0.568	0.628
Avoiding physically going into work or school				
No	571	0.556	0.525	0.586
Yes, without negative effects	159	0.155	0.134	0.178
Yes, with negative effects	297	0.289	0.262	0.318
Avoiding contact with non-household members				
No	302	0.294	0.267	0.323
Yes, without negative effects	184	0.179	0.157	0.204
Yes, with negative effects	541	0.527	0.496	0.557
Number of disabilities or conditions				
One	109	0.106	0.089	0.127
Two or three	359	0.350	0.321	0.379
Four or five	333	0.324	0.296	0.354
Six or more	226	0.220	0.196	0.246
Age (mean)				
Gender				
Male	472	0.460	0.429	0.490
Female	544	0.530	0.499	0.560
Non-binary or other	11	0.011	0.006	0.019
Member of a racialized minority group	183	0.178	0.156	0.203
Marital status				
Never married	324	0.315	0.288	0.345
Cohabiting	138	0.134	0.115	0.157
Married	406	0.395	0.366	0.426
Formerly married	159	0.155	0.134	0.178
Presence of children	246	0.240	0.214	0.267

(Continued)

	Sample Frequency	Percentage or Mean		
			95% Confidence Interval	
		Estimate	Lower	Higher
Ba or higher	360	0.351	0.321	0.380
Employed	490	0.477	0.447	0.508
Province (reduced variable)				
Ontario	399	0.389	0.359	0.419
Quebec	230	0.224	0.199	0.251
British Columbia	134	0.130	0.111	0.153
Prairie provinces (AB, MA, SK)	199	0.194	0.171	0.219
Atlantic provinces (NB, NL, NS, PEI)	65	0.063	0.050	0.080

Notes: Estimates refer to sample data.
Source: 2020 COVID-19 Response Survey of People with Disabilities and Health Conditions, $N = 1{,}027$ adults.

APPENDIX B. RESULTS FROM LOGISTIC REGRESSION MODELS PREDICTING INCREASED ANXIETY

	Model 1		Model 2		Model 3	
	B	SE	*B*	SE	*B*	SE
Intercept	0.329	(0.429)	0.367	(0.507)	0.514	(0.485)
Avoiding public places (Ref: Did not use)						
Yes, without negative effects	−0.520*	(0.244)				
Yes, with negative effects	0.547***	(0.123)				
Remote work or school (Ref: Did not use)						
Yes, without negative effects			−0.540*	(0.216)		
Yes, with negative effects			0.633***	(0.156)		
Avoiding contact with non-household members (Ref: Did not use)						
Yes, without negative effects					−0.668*	(0.279)
Yes, with negative effects					0.254	(0.145)
Number of reported disabilities and health conditions (Ref: One)						
Two or three	0.588	(0.370)	0.570	(0.356)	0.565	(0.349)
Four or five	0.899	(0.479)	0.945	(0.489)	0.895	(0.474)
Six or more	1.265***	(0.320)	1.243***	(0.318)	1.214***	(0.320)
Age	−0.040***	(0.004)	−0.038***	(0.003)	−0.039***	(0.004)
Gender (Ref: Male)						
Female	0.126	(0.100)	0.101	(0.142)	0.121	(0.102)
Other or non-binary	0.097	(0.417)	0.048	(0.567)	0.083	(0.458)
Marital status (Ref: Never married)						
Cohabiting	0.266	(0.207)	0.261	(0.165)	0.219	(0.188)
Married	0.210	(0.178)	0.208	(0.137)	0.151	(0.165)
Formerly married	0.404	(0.321)	0.453	(0.234)	0.399	(0.297)

(Continued)

	Model 1		Model 2		Model 3	
	B	SE	*B*	SE	*B*	SE
Any children	−0.048	(0.309)	−0.069	(0.292)	−0.017	(0.324)
BA or higher	−0.013	(0.080)	0.001	(0.078)	0.016	(0.064)
Employed	−0.329**	(0.107)	−0.325**	(0.102)	−0.344***	(0.094)
Member of a racialized minority group	−0.197	(0.144)	−0.231	(0.158)	−0.164	(0.154)
Province (Ref: Ontario)						
Quebec	−0.045	(0.041)	0.027	(0.051)	0.021	(0.052)
British Columbia	0.267***	(0.041)	0.376***	(0.026)	0.296***	(0.030)
Prairie provinces	−0.195***	(0.021)	−0.195***	(0.028)	−0.195***	(0.026)
Atlantic provinces	0.322***	(0.053)	0.256***	(0.036)	0.289***	(0.062)
Pseudo *R*-Squared	0.101		0.099		0.092	

Notes: Logistic regression models predicting probability of reported increase in anxiety. Continuous variables are mean centered. "*b*" refers to logit model coefficients. Odds ratios can be obtained by exponentiating (*b*). Standard errors are in parentheses. Standard errors account for clustering by province/region.

***$p < 0.001$, **$p < 0.01$, *$p < 0.05$.

Source: 2020 COVID-19 Response Survey of People with Disabilities and Health Conditions, $N = 1{,}027$ adults.

APPENDIX C. RESULTS FROM LOGISTIC REGRESSION MODELS PREDICTING INCREASED LONELINESS

	Model 1		Model 2		Model 3	
	b	SE	B	SE	*B*	SE
Intercept	−1.018	(0.641)	−0.819	(0.533)	−0.728	(0.674)
Avoiding public places (Ref: Did not use)						
Yes, without negative effects	−0.164	(0.412)				
Yes, with negative effects	0.875***	(0.154)				
Remote work or school (Ref: Did not use)						
Yes, without negative effects			−0.026	(0.206)		
Yes, with negative effects			0.687***	(0.175)		
Avoiding contact with non-household members (Ref: Did not use)						
Yes, without negative effects					−0.485**	(0.163)
Yes, with negative effects					0.503**	(0.184)
Number of reported disabilities and health conditions (Ref: One)						
Two or three	0.743	(0.387)	0.700*	(0.324)	0.701*	(0.344)
Four or five	0.956***	(0.227)	0.968***	(0.231)	0.952***	(0.246)
Six or more	1.024***	(0.169)	1.000***	(0.146)	0.984***	(0.166)

(Continued)

	Model 1		Model 2		Model 3	
	b	SE	B	SE	*B*	SE
Age	−0.022*	(0.011)	−0.019*	(0.009)	−0.021*	(0.010)
Gender (Ref: Male)						
Female	0.037	(0.089)	0.025	(0.092)	0.055	(0.096)
Other or non-binary	0.177	(0.692)	0.103	(0.737)	0.185	(0.709)
Marital status (Ref: Never married)						
Cohabiting	−0.565***	(0.132)	−0.601***	(0.118)	−0.632***	(0.141)
Married	−0.597***	(0.166)	−0.585***	(0.134)	−0.652***	(0.163)
Formerly married	0.433	(0.407)	0.473	(0.306)	0.413	(0.403)
Any children	−0.060	(0.349)	−0.054	(0.340)	−0.028	(0.364)
BA or higher	−0.046	(0.154)	−0.045	(0.133)	−0.001	(0.130)
Employed	0.068	(0.137)	0.086	(0.160)	0.046	(0.143)
Member of a racialized minority group	0.070	(0.170)	0.069	(0.167)	0.088	(0.175)
Province (Ref: Ontario)						
Quebec	0.413***	(0.033)	0.452***	(0.033)	0.474***	(0.052)
British Columbia	−0.175***	(0.029)	−0.079***	(0.023)	−0.142***	(0.032)
Prairie provinces	0.044	(0.028)	0.012	(0.022)	0.015	(0.032)
Atlantic provinces	−0.121***	(0.032)	−0.166**	(0.058)	−0.134*	(0.063)
Pseudo *R*-Squared	0.099		0.084		0.088	

Notes: Logistic regression models predicting probability of reported increase in loneliness. "*b*" refers to logit model coefficients. Odds ratios can be obtained by exponentiating (*b*). Standard errors are in parentheses. Standard errors account for clustering by province/region.
***$p < 0.001$, **$p < 0.01$, *$p < 0.05$.
Source: 2020 COVID-19 Response Survey of People with Disabilities and Health Conditions, $N = 1{,}027$ adults.

Chapter 4

BARRIERS IN THE ACCESS TO HEALTHCARE FACILITIES DURING COVID-19 FOR PEOPLE WITH DISABILITIES IN MUMBAI'S INFORMAL SETTLEMENTS

Srishti Jaitely and Navjit Gaurav

ABSTRACT

Purpose: *In India, people with disabilities (PWDs) have emerged as one of the most vulnerable populations during COVID-19, particularly those living in informal settlements. Although the government has made efforts to ensure healthcare access for all, these efforts seem inadequate considering that PWDs' needs vary greatly depending on type and degree of disability. The purpose of the study is to identify barriers in healthcare access for PWDs in Mumbai's informal settlements during COVID-19.*

Methods: *A qualitative approach employed multiple case study methods. Eight PWDs were selected as cases from the informal settlements of M-East Ward, Mumbai. The data was gathered using observation and interaction with the PWDs. Data were analyzed for emergent themes to explore the presence, meaning, and relationships of barriers faced by PWDs accentuated by pandemic.*

Findings: *Findings indicate a complex and compounded interplay of structural, administrative, psycho-social, and technological factors which created numerous challenges for PWDs to access healthcare provisions during pandemic. These factors include socioeconomic challenges, the built*

Disability in the Time of Pandemic
Research in Social Science and Disability, Volume 13, 75–94

Published under exclusive licence by Emerald Publishing Limited
ISSN: 1479-3547/doi:10.1108/S1479-354720230000013005

environment inaccessibility, limited transportation facilities, and lack of trained healthcare personnel to support PWDs.

Implications: *This research adds to an understanding of the barriers faced by PWDs and provides insights for formulating contextualized policies to ensure accessible health services for PWDs when needed. Findings point out ways in which understanding the barriers would help to identify the gaps in the resource system, and to mobilize required resources in the relevant healthcare departments.*

Keywords: Barriers; access to healthcare; people with disability; COVID-19; informal settlements; India

INTRODUCTION

COVID-19 has impacted people globally in different ways (Buheji et al., 2020), based on where and how they are positioned in the socio-economic policies (Bashir et al., 2020) and practices that have been adopted to ensure better healthcare facilities for all (Kumar et al., 2020). However, people living in informal settlements are facing significant challenges in accessing healthcare (Wilkinson, 2020), among them, people with disabilities (hereinafter referred to as PWDs) are disproportionately affected (Auerbach & Thachil, 2021). In India, settlements with insecure housing tenure tend to be the ones with poverty and low health status (Ganguly, 2019), making people further vulnerable to multiple disabling conditions due to lost social bond and insecurity leading emotional isolation and psychological stress (Mopari et al., 2019). These multiple vulnerability factors have also made it challenging for PWDs to access health care services during COVID-19 (Raju et al., 2021). In such situations where Mumbai overall have limited resources and infrastructure (Naydenova et al., 2017), it is difficult for PWDs living further in low resource informal settlements to access healthcare facilities. Meanwhile, PWDs are vulnerable to communicable diseases due to their physical, sensory, and cognitive limitations as they have limited understanding about such infections (Jesus et al., 2020). PWDs are also at an increased risk of comorbidities with COVID-19 (Senjam & Singh, 2020), calling out for an urgent need to improve localized healthcare access during the pandemic for them.

During the COVID-19 pandemic, isolation, disconnect, disrupted routines, and diminished health services have greatly impacted the lives and mental well-being of PWDs (Jesus et al., 2020). The phenomenon of safe distancing and isolation made space an important aspect in the COVID era (Raju et al., 2021). Spaces around us are designed in a way that is more than often not accessible for PWDs and there are different ways PWDs negotiate with various spaces in their day-to-day life (Subbaraman & Murthy, 2015). In simplest terms, disability can be understood as a state which is caused by the interaction of social, occupational, physical, and psychological conditions (Falvo & Holland, 2017). Apart from the healthcare impact, PWDs were more vulnerable to socioeconomic challenges such as job loss (Raju et al., 2021), increased social discrimination (Koschorke et al., 2014), limited access to good quality food (Prasad et al., 2021), lack of information about the epidemic, and behavioral challenges (Parsons & Johal, 2020). These challenges create a wide range of inequalities that overlap into a complex form of social exclusion.

PROBLEM STATEMENT

COVID-19 had a cascading impact on the lives of people living in low-resource settings. Mumbai, the densely populated city of India has witnessed significant challenges to manage healthcare services and provide adequate healthcare access to the people amidst COVID-19 (Bhattacharjee & Sattar, 2021). Studies highlights that Mumbai's private health system collapsed due to the exponential pressure from the rapid rise in COVID-19 cases (Raju et al., 2021). To mitigate this rapid rise in cases a collaboration was formed between the municipality and local low-cost private-health practitioners (Bai et al., 2020). This collaborative effort eventually managed to control the spread of the coronavirus in the Dharavi settlement (Kumar et al., 2020).

Prior studies highlight how the social, political, and structural inequalities that are common features in Mumbai's informal settlements, create barriers for PWDs and women while they access healthcare and other basic facilities (Aravind et al., 2021; Bajpai & Wadhwa, 2020; Subbaraman & Murthy, 2015). In short, being disabled exposes individuals to many vulnerabilities that others do not face. There is a need to understand PWDs' disability-specific requirements, daily living activities and take appropriate and timely measures to ensure their protection and safety during COVID-19 (Devendeck & Sonne, 2021). There has been limited understanding from a PWDs' perspective about the barriers in healthcare access during COVID-19. It is imperative to explore PWDs' experiences, to develop strategies to mitigate the further consequences of COVID-19 on their wellbeing. Hence, there is an immediate need to explore the barriers faced by PWDs while accessing healthcare, with a purpose to advocate for support that is disability inclusive, and community driven.

LITERATURE REVIEW

After the onset of COVID-19 in India, the central and state governments took a series of policy measures designed to address emerging issues such as rising cases of infection, shortages of essential goods such as medicines, ration kits, and hospitals equipment, and widespread loss of jobs and livelihoods (Sengupta & Jha, 2020). People in informal settlements witnessed targeted measures like delivery of ration kits at doorsteps by local organizations and Anganwadi centers, creating awareness about vaccination, maintaining physical distancing, and practicing handwashing and sanitization to prevent the spread of COVID-19 (Bajpai & Wadhwa, 2020; Prasad et al., 2021). However, continuous and careful handwashing to prevent COVID-19 is not always an option for people due to their living conditions such as lack of access to water, sanitation, and healthcare inside informal settlements (Raju et al., 2021).

Similarly, limited access to healthcare systems inhibits their health-seeking behavior (Parsons & Johal, 2020) and individuals with disabilities in India found themselves impaired to seek redressal for their health conditions (Aravind et al., 2021). Research has also long shown that negative health outcomes can be aggravated by stigma and discrimination due to certain health conditions, such as physical and mental disability (Koschorke et al., 2014; Subbaraman & Murthy, 2015). Furthermore, the response of the Indian government toward improving the disparaging effects of the pandemic on PWDs was perceived to be inadequate considering PWDs' needs vary greatly depending on type and degree of disability (Aravind et al., 2021). It is important to explore the barriers faced by people with different disabilities living in Mumbai's informal settlements while accessing healthcare services during COVID-19.

RESEARCH QUESTIONS

This study explored the following questions:

- What are the barriers faced by people with disabilities in accessing healthcare services amidst COVID-19?
- How do these barriers influence the psycho-social wellbeing of people with disabilities in low-resource communities?

METHODOLOGY

Study Context

The M-East Ward, one of the 24 administrative divisions of Mumbai and home to over 807,720 (Census of India, 2011) residents, is also one of the poorest areas in the city. The population density of the ward is 24,852 people per square kilometer (Census of India, 2011). The ward is marked by high rates of vulnerability, poverty, everyday violence, and precarity (TISS, 2015). The ward located on the peripheries of the city is a convenient option to set foot in the city for individuals and families who migrate in search of livelihood, predominantly in the informal sector.

Migrants from various parts of the country move into the ward in huge numbers. The migrants have limited social capital and belong to historically marginalized sections (Dalits, minority groups), which makes it difficult for them to survive in this city. Human development index is the lowest in the city, with an infant mortality rate of around 66.47 per thousand live births, 1,490 children under the age of 6 are out of school, and more than half of children malnourished (Municipal Corporation of Greater Mumbai, 2009). A disability report published by Apnalaya (Kumar & Mehta, 2019) indicates that 1.3% of the M-East Ward is disabled. Compared to official data (0.3%), these numbers indicate an under-reporting of disabled cases in the M-East Ward. Reports indicate growing rates of disability, creating an intersection of various geriatric and disability-related concerns.

Study Design

A qualitative study, based on multiple-cases design (Stake, 2013; Yin, 2014), was conducted in the informal settlements of Mumbai's M-East Ward. Our approach is grounded in the quest to explore how PWDs access healthcare, and the barriers that arise while accessing healthcare across different healthcare settings during COVID-19 (Fabregues & Fetters, 2019; Jachyra et al., 2015). The healthcare settings within and nearby the informal settlements were war rooms, quarantine centers, and primary healthcare centers. For our observations, we chose a multiple-case study method as it allowed us to observe the particularities of each case inside these different healthcare settings (Bortoleto et al., 2020; Thomas, 2011). An interpretive naturalist's perspective (Thomson, 1981) was adopted to preserve the 'naturalness' of the environment by considering the unique study context of M-East Ward (Harrison et al., 2017).

Participants

Our study participants were PWDs living in the informal settlements of Mumbai's M-East Ward. Eight PWDs were selected as cases, we adopted non-probabilistic procedures and employed convenient sampling (Sedgwick, 2013). The reason for choosing convenient sampling was to allow researchers to be flexible, and select participants from proximity (QuestionPro, 2021) while making field visits across healthcare settings. To ensure case diversity, this research considered the variations among the PWDs in terms of their demographics like impairments, age, gender, employment, and marital status. The variation in the sample was opted to capture PWDs' varied experiences with the barriers amidst COVID-19.

Data Collection

The primary researcher (SJ) is a community mental health professional working for more than 2 years (before and during COVID) with the Transforming M-East Ward project in the informal settlements of Mumbai's M-East Ward.[1] SJ collected data by observing multiple participants ideal for case study (Yin, 2014). Using participant observation (Spradley, 2016), SJ observed people, including healthcare workers, family caregivers, and PWDs, coming to the war rooms, quarantine centers, and other healthcare settings.[2] The purpose of observing participants across different set-ups was to develop a deeper understanding of the barriers faced by PWDs in accessing healthcare services in different settings so, a comprehensive action plan could be prepared.

For this study, several criteria were applied to observation. SJ is experienced in counseling and trained in working with the clients and observation methodology.

The procedures used in the observations were the same for all cases. To create an environment of empathy, as recommended by Wacquant (2006), and to build rapport in the participatory observation process (Jachyra et al., 2015), the researcher employed the following strategy: she did not participate in any clinical activities, instead slowly building informal interactions with PWDs over time, especially with those who spontaneously approached her during their healthcare visits. Field notes and observation notes were taken during and after observation and were written in the researcher's field diary.

The interactions and observations took place for one year. She observed and interacted with the PWDs weekly while they were trying to access quarantine facilities in nearby quarantine centers, the procedure of getting a bed inside the quarantine center, accessing food and sanitation facilities inside the quarantine center, accessing the center's physical built environment. SJ interacted with PWDs and with their caregivers (family members) to understand their disability-related need, she further observed PWDs while they went to the war rooms seeking help, and while they accessed hospitals, community healthcare services for treatment and support during COVID-19. Additionally, SJ also maintained notes from the interaction with PWDs and caregivers and wrote them in the field diaries along with any key insights from the interaction.

Data Analysis

The field diaries were transcribed and translated into English. The field notes and data from the interaction with the PWDs and caregivers were translated by NG and then memo-ed based on the transcripts to complement observational notes. Memos are crucial to the analysis and discussion of data (Bortoleto et al., 2020), and they offered supportive sources of evidence to corroborate the research findings and improve the data credibility during analysis (Phillippi & Lauderdale, 2018).

The data was organized in Atlas Ti for analysis by NG. The data included notes on eight case studies, interactions memos, observation notes, and field notes. Analysis was done considering the thematic categories using content analysis (Stake, 1995, 2013). Both researchers are experienced in the content analysis method, and they analyzed data by developing thematic categories (Krippendorff, 2004) and interpreted into those categories, using a critical hermeneutics lens (Bourdieu & Wacquant, 1992). A critical hermeneutic lens allowed interpretations by understanding the factors that influences participants' experience. The data were analyzed based on the emergent themes to explore the presence, meaning, and relationships of barriers faced by PWDs in accessing healthcare services.

To conduct analysis data were collaboratively read multiple times by both the researchers, each time developing and applying codes and seeking to reduce the systematic codes into categories. Thematic categories were created from recurring patterns and codes (e.g., structural, psycho-social, and technological) (Denzin & Lincoln, 2011). After the first three observation notes both the researcher sat together to discuss the coding pattern and emergent themes. This peer debriefing

(Henry, 2015; Spall, 1998) helped in maintaining coherency in the analysis process. Themes developed from observational data were contrasted with the field notes and interaction memos, whose convergences and divergences contributed to consolidating thematic categories (Anguera et al., 2017). We developed four thematic categories highlighting the barriers faced by PWDs in accessing healthcare services amidst COVID-19.

Ethical Consideration

Informed verbal consent was obtained from the participants before documenting their experiences and their participation was voluntary. Considering the engagement with their narrative could be traumatic and understanding scarcity and need for mental health care, a free M-iCall helpline was provided to each case. M-iCall, an M-East ward specific psychosocial helpline service, was developed under the Community-Led Action Learning and Partnership (CLAP) project to address the scarcity and need for mental health care. The helpline successfully provided free client-centered counseling services to callers with a client empowerment and education model. A prerecorded message was played before each call informing callers that the call recording will be used for training and research purposes while maintaining closer confidentiality. Verbal consent was also obtained to use their case stories.

RESULTS

This study involved eight PWDs, and there was variation among the participants concerning the types of disability, participants' age, gender, having disability certificate, employment, and marital status. The average age of the participants was 32 years and there were 5 men and 3 women (Table 1).

Findings from the eight case studies indicate a complex and compounded interplay of structural, administrative, psycho-social, and technological factors which created numerous challenges for PWDs to access healthcare provisions during COVID-19.

Structural

A person's quality of life is affected by the availability of physical space for mobility and accessibility. The M-East Ward has over 85% of people living in informal settlements with inadequate access to basic amenities like water, electricity, and sanitation. Many of these informal settlements are also prone to frequent environmental disasters. The ward has 380 toilet blocks, but only 13 of those are disabled-friendly. Only 56% of the area has access to water. There are 15 healthcare posts, 11 dispensaries, and one secondary care hospital that offers basic health care services to more than 1 million population (TISS, 2015). The nearest tertiary care hospital is 12 km away, which is challenging for a PWD to access.

Table 1. Participants' Demographic Characteristics.

Type of Disability	Age	Gender	Marital Status	Have Disability certificate[b]	Can Read and Speak Marathi[a]	Employment Status	Caste
Intellectual disability	21	Female	Unmarried	Yes	Yes	Unemployed	OBC
Autism	16	Female	Unmarried	No	Yes	Student	OBC
Physical disability	83	Male	Married	Yes	Yes	Retired	OBC
Physical disability	13	Female	Unmarried	No	Yes	School dropout	SC
Physical disability	15	Male	Unmarried	Yes	No	School dropout	SC
Cerebral palsy	19	Male	Unmarried	No	Yes	School dropout	OBC
Acquired physical disability due to accident	42	Male	Married	No	Yes	Employed (Autorickshaw driver)	SC
Visual impairment	54	Male	Unmarried	No	Yes	Unemployed	SC

Note: OBC = Other backward classes, SC = Scheduled caste.
[a]Marathi is the local language spoken in Mumbai.
[b]Disability certificate (DC) is a document provided by the government hospitals in India to any person with a disability who has impairment ≥ 40%, and DC enable them to access various social security entitlements and supports.

The built environment limitations included no provision for PWDs toilet, usable ramps, signboard, and instruction sheets in an accessible format making hospitals, quarantine, isolation, and vaccination centers inaccessible for PWDs (refer Table 2). Some participants reported the transport responsibility was often on the PWDs and their families during lockdown. The ambulances did not have facilities to accommodate the PWDs' special needs. One of the participants mentioned

> My mother had to request neighbours to help move me in the ambulance. She told authorities I cannot move by myself, still there was no one to help us or an accessible ambulance to take me to Isolation Center. – Man with cerebral palsy, 19 years

Participants reported that isolation and quarantine centers were set up overnight to house people and high-risk contacts. These centers were originally constructed and designed as low-cost housing options to accommodate people who have been relocated from various informal settlements across M-East Ward. However, they had little to no provisions for persons with visual impairment, and so they found it difficult to navigate these healthcare settings. There were also no provisions for people with neurodevelopmental needs, to help them manage their own needs and their stress levels (refer Table 2). One of the participants reported

> Building [quarantine center] did not have any provisions to help people like us. I was dependent on others for using common building services regularly, which was very frustrating. – Man with visual impairment, 54 years

Table 2. Disability-Specific Challenges.

S.no.	Pseudonyms	Types of Disability	Case Context	Challenges
1	PWID	Intellectual disability	A 21-year-old girl with intellectual disability, who is dependent on her mother for her needs and decision making.	• Severe intellectual disability made the PWID dependent on others for their basic hygiene and survival needs. • Challenge in understanding of COVID-19 protocols and precautions.
2	PWA	Autism	A 16-year-old girl with Autism, whose caregiver was tested COVID positive.	• The COVID-19 protocols and restrictions led to various environmental changes, i.e., being confined to specific spaces, sharing space with others. Due to neurodivergent sensory needs, adaptation to changed environments was challenging, for PWA. • Discontinuity in autism specific therapy support. Intervention was limited to talk therapy, with no access to intervention-specific equipment and occupational therapies.
3	PWPD1	Physical disability	A PWPD who lived with his wife for years and now were separated because of COVID. They had created a sense of co-dependency on each other.	• Mobility issue due to non-user-friendly built environment of healthcare settings and ambulance services.
4	PWPD2	Physical disability	The case indicated the plight of a young girl suffering from chronic illness and physical disability	• No support in the hospital, PWDs had to move on their own from their bed to washroom services.
5	PWPD3	Physical disability	A 15-year-old boy with physical disability, school dropout and living with family with limited social support.	• Inaccessible washrooms at the quarantine and isolation centers. • Separation from partner and long-term caregivers. • Discontinued supportive and responsive healthcare support posing threat to life and financial burden on family.
6	PWCP	Cerebral palsy	A 19-year-old male, who spent a decade in his one-room house with his mother and 8 siblings.	It was impossible to transport him without ignoring the physical distancing norms.
7	PWAPD	Acquired physical disability due to accident	A 42-year-old rickshaw driver and sole earner of the family met an accident and lost a leg.	A medical trust helped him manage prosthetic leg costs. However, after the trust diverted support grant toward

Table 2. (Continued)

S.no.	Pseudonyms	Types of Disability	Case Context	Challenges
				COVID-19, he had to use a walking stick.
8	PWVI	Visual impairment	A 54-year-old man with congenital blindness living in a disability shelter home faced barriers to accessing treatment and moving out of the isolation ward.	• Information shared in form of scanned documents for public health directives were not readable through screen reader. • COVIN app, for booking online vaccination slot was not PWVI friendly without a screen reader. • Mobility stick was not thoroughly sanitized, after the stay of the person is over in the isolation center.

With the most focus being laid on COVID-19 care, PWDs faced challenges in accessing rehabilitation support-based care, as they were unable to visit hospitals. There were limited services, and funds leading to longer waiting periods and gaps in ongoing treatments. One of the caregivers we interacted with mentioned

> My daughter was supported by trust which would provide financial support for her therapy, but they have stopped since COVID. Madam, the trust understands our need, but they have no money for us. (Mother of a girl with physical disability, 13 years)

The residential placement of PWDs led to further discrimination as they did not have COVID-19 equipped health care hospitals nearby their informal settlements. Participants also reported treatment being denied to them based on their residential location as the area is infamous for high crime rates and violence. One of the respondents mentioned

> In hospital when they hear we are from Govandi [one of the areas in M-East Ward], they look at us with suspicion. – Woman with intellectual disability, 21 years

PWDs reported that residential addresses were not compatible with software's map and with nearest landmarks being a few hundred kilometers away it was challenging to avail doorstep deliveries.

Administrative

The pandemic was a novel challenge for all with no awareness on how to deal and manage the situation. There was a lack of policy provisions for PWDs who have been infected with COVID-19. One of the participants reported

> I know under the pension scheme [Indira Gandhi National Disability Scheme] I deserve money, but I have not received any money from the government. – Man with visual impairment, 54 years

Several participants reported that at the administrative level, policymakers' perception toward the occupants of informal settlements is more of a liability, rather than a participatory approach. PWDs with lived experiences are not included in policy formulations, making the process non-collaborative and top-down in nature. One of the caregivers we interacted with mentioned

> Both my father and I have tested positive. My sister, who has autism, is dependent on us. Please give us some time to make some care arrangements for her. – Sister of a girl with Autism, 16 years

Having no disability certificate also restricted individuals to access social security entitlements. One of the participants stated

> I have been trying for disability certificate for 2 years before COVID, but no help. Even when they could see my leg cut, I was made to make multiple visits to hospitals. Some pension would have helped my family during lockdown. – Man with acquired physical disability, 42 years

All the participants reported limitations regarding the number of specialized care centers and trained health care professionals for PWDs, that led to incidents such as denial of treatments, ignoring the immediate emergency care need of PWDs, and no provision of beds (refer Table 2). One of the caregivers mentioned

> If I leave my sister in an isolation ward, she would not be able to express what she needs. We need to leave her with someone who understands what she wants and is aware of her routine, otherwise, my sister can be very irritable. – Sister of a girl with Autism, 16 years

Participants reported a lack of training of healthcare personnel regarding how to support people with different disabilities also made their journey of treatment distressing. The process of caregiving and receiving is often viewed as a functional relationship where they are a personal and intimate bond for various PWDs, developed over several years. One of the caregivers mentioned

> My mother does all work for my sister. After Aai(mother) tested positive my aunt helped to take care of my sister, but now even my sister has tested positive. Can you help us in providing same hospital room for them. . .we have been requesting you for 2 days? – Brother of a woman with intellectual disability, 21 years

Besides training on how to respond to PWDs' specific needs, caregivers stated that the healthcare professionals need to be empathetic with PWDs to facilitate developing a safe space for them to express their needs and requirements. Across disabilities, women faced challenges related to water, sanitation, and hygiene (WASH) services. One of the participants shared menstrual hygiene products not being provided in hygiene kits, others reported that considering lockdown, sanitary napkins should be provided to women in institutional and home isolation.

Psychosocial

Across stages of prevention, treatment, and rehabilitation, PWDs faced unique challenges due to their disability specific need. This included difficulty to follow prevention protocol like keeping a safe social distance, from their caregiver affecting their emotional bond. One of the participants mentioned

> My wife is not with me in the hospital, so I have to always call someone for even basic works. I do not feel good about it. We have been disabled but we have never been dependent on anyone else. We always had each other. This is a very difficult time for both of us. I at least have other people in hospital, but my wife is completely alone at home. – Men with physical disability, 83 years

Caregivers reported that PWDs found it more challenging to access testing services as they were unable to afford private testing services and were heavily dependent on government-run testing camps and centers. Due to unavailability of support, it was challenging for them to reach testing sites. In cases where PWDs required hospitalization, it was challenging to find services that suited their disability-specific needs (refer Table 2). Participants reported that hospitals refused to admit them as it would require hospital to provide special assistance. One of the participants reported

> I suffer from TB and when I told them, they asked me to wait. People without other severe conditions were getting hospital admissions before me. Are they saying TB patients like me do not deserve treatment? – Man with visual impairment, 54 years

Post COVID-19, rehabilitation care is an integral part of complete recovery. Participants reported that they feel physically and emotionally fatigued stemming from their experience of isolation and uncertainty. One of the participants reported

> Every PWD should be provided with someone to talk to and share their anxieties in the initial days. That was the most challenging time for me. – Man with visual impairment, 54 years

The narrative of loss has been attached to post COVID-19 times, various PWDs shared that it has been a constant theme of their life. Participants reported that these narratives build a sense of shame, discouraging them from seeking treatment. The psychological trauma of living in a new world and the need to adapt quickly was evident. People shared that often they were blamed for not following preventive measures, leading to the spread of the virus.

There was a constant uncertainty concerning COVID-19 guidelines, the availability of health services, and treatment options for those with diverse disabilities. Several participants reported that the lockdown led to reduced opportunities for independence and becomes a situation of a sudden shift from social support to no care situation. Caregivers of people with intellectual disabilities reported how activities of daily living form an integral part of their participants' life and post COVID-19 care often leads to disruptions in those spaces. It was challenging for caregivers to help the PWDs understand the change in routines (refer Table 2). Caregivers reported the lost sense of familiarity creates anxiety in PWDs, often leading to harmful behavior as they share unique ecosystem bonded by understanding of mutual response, needs, and anxieties. Caregivers reported that these are personalized system, and it takes some time for other systems to establish, adapt and become stable. In such cases where caregivers tested positive, it was extremely challenging for them as well as PWDs to find alternative support systems.

An alternate observation was, PWDs who were left to take care of themselves for the first time in their lives explored new ways for self-care. They faced challenges and high levels of frustration in the initial phase, although when left on their own they learned to manage their own affairs, which helped to build their self-confidence and esteem, something they would have never explored had they not been cornered in isolation due to COVID-19, turning out to be a blessing in disguise for them to manage their health conditions more positively. One of the participants mentioned

> I see this as the experience where I have stayed all alone, in a confined space. This was the first time in my life where I was being responsible for my own needs and taking care of myself. It was a bit isolating initially, but gradually I started to understand nothing will change. I am now more confident about taking care of my needs when I move out of this building [quarantine center]. – Man with visual impairment, 54 years

In the case of accessing vaccination, a person with a physical disability found it challenging to travel to vaccine centers to get vaccinated.

> The government vaccination center is far. I have to change buses to reach the center and if I do not get a vaccination even after going there, it will be waste of time. Sarkar(government) knows our condition, they should provide us vaccination at home. – Boy with physical disability, 15 years

A person with visual impairment reported that the door-to-door vaccination drive was targeting only bedridden population, hence excluding any other forms of disability. To avail vaccination facility PWD should have a disability certificate and availability of a doctor for 30 minutes post-vaccination, which is a challenge in the informal settlement. Many PWDs opt-out of the vaccination process after facing these hurdles for getting a dose of vaccine. A participant reported

> I have been told, if I am blind, I cannot get a vaccination at home. They are only provided if you are bedridden. My condition is no better. I have been infected once, and I want to take the vaccine, but I won't be able to travel to the center to get the vaccine. – Man with visual impairment, 54 years

An alternate observation was participants' hesitancy and low trust toward the vaccination due to lack of clear messaging and communication around the impact of vaccination on their ongoing health condition. In case of side effects, there was no set of instructions or provisions for PWDs in the local language (Marathi), which would be accessible to them and their caregivers in case of emergency.

Technological

The ability to access and use technology also emerged as a major barrier in accessing healthcare during COVID-19 times. Several participants and caregivers reported that the process of bed management and COVID-19 test report circulation was done through a helpline and WhatsApp respectively. Those with neurodevelopmental and neurocognitive needs were unable to access the service as it was challenging for them to use the mobile phones and follow automated call instruction. The modes of communication were reported challenging to be used by people with visual impairment (refer Table 2). One of the participants stated

> I would have taken the vaccination, but I could not because the vaccination booking apps have not been screen reader enabled. – Man with visual impairment, 54 years

Talking about the technological barrier he further added

> After I tested positive, it was very difficult for me to understand where to go, as all helpline numbers and guidelines about hospitalization were not screen reader friendly. I was dependent on calling others and pleading with them to provide me with information. – Man with visual impairment, 54 years

A person with visual impairment reported that the process of accessing vaccinations for COVID-19 has been made digital, making it challenging to register for vaccination slots. The applications were not compatible with screen-reader and text-to-voice support leading to PWDs being dependent on others for their registrations (refer Table 2).

DISCUSSION

There has been work already done by Indian organizations on the impact of COVID on various groups of PWDs highlighting challenges, availability of support, resources and need to contextualize care (Aravind et al., 2021; Auerbach & Thachil, 2021; Bajpai & Wadhwa, 2020; Bhattacharjee & Sattar, 2021; Kumar et al., 2020). This study is unique because while there is much disability rights activism in India, very little of it surrounds or deals with the experiences of poor, lower caste, and migrant PWDs or those living in low-resource informal settlements such as M-East Ward.

Studies have highlighted that individual come across various psychological situations (Aravind et al., 2021; Mopari et al., 2019). Often when we face challenges, we experience distress, and the distressing psychological situations can be a new challenge. Similarly in our study, participants have shared different forms of psychologically distressing situations including a new psychological challenge due to COVID-19, distress as they were unable to access and reach the healthcare support. We suggest while addressing the issues of PWDs, their distressing situation should be understood by involving them in the rehabilitation process.

Understanding these challenges can help health care professionals to design better treatment and rehabilitation services. The psychosocial approach explores the intersection and interaction of social, cultural, and environmental influences on the mind and behavior of people living in the informal settlements (Ganguly, 2019). Here the social component is one's ability to use social supports, and ability to adapt to various situations amidst COVID-19 (Auerbach & Thachil, 2021; Bhattacharjee & Sattar, 2021). PWDs' face challenges due to the inaccessibility of the built environment; structured initial support and redesigning components of the built environment based on their feedback can create healthier structures (Ganguly, 2019; Kumar et al., 2020). Building an understanding of the distressing situations and core challenges and exploring their expression for different disabilities may help to build friendlier rehabilitation services for PWDs similar to Bhattacharjee and Sattar (2021). Psychological the poor design of systems often left participants feeling further trapped in the never-ending maze, which can also have an overall negative impact on their lives (Aravind et al., 2021). A better understanding the needs and desires of PWDs can help design their rehabilitation activities with higher chances of positive response to the intervention and facilitate learned optimism. We recommend including PWDs in co-creation of ideas to design their rehabilitation activities to positively impact their empowerment.

Social support requires resources and conducive conditions. The interventions of care should be designed keeping in mind the long-lasting psychological impact of PWDs' interaction with the health system (see Table 3).

The experience of working with health care systems including policy recommendations, implementation has helped to understand the possible gaps that creates challenges for PWDs to access dignified health care services. The interventions should be designed considering its implementation at promotion, prevention, treatment, and rehabilitation phase. Possible interventions that can be implemented to ensure last-mile connectivity are as follows:

- Consulting PWDs on their needs and ideal service systems while respecting and acknowledging PWDs voices and choices.
- Designing accessible awareness material and toolkits for caregivers on how to take care of PWDs who tested positive and are in home isolation.
- Devising contingency plan and preparing essential item kit for PWDs while in quarantine.
- Vulnerability-based analysis of PWDs data by concerned government departments for need-based distribution of resources and disability-specific care. This can be achieved by creating a reliable NGO network that work with PWDs and connecting them to individuals in need. Resource directories for different services can be made available to various stakeholders and connecting them with local helpline services.
- Ensuring accessible rehabilitation and post treatment support to facilitate speedy recovery.
- Ensuring home delivery of essential services (food, water, sanitary pads, medicines) and special provisions for PWDs in ration shops to avoid long queues and discomfort.

Table 3. Disability-Specific Recommendations.

S.no.	Pseudonyms	Types of Disability	Recommendations
1	PWID	Intellectual disability	Creating easy to understand IEC material in various modalities, inclusive of different intellectual needs of people.
2	PWA	Autism	• Designing activities, in collaboration with PWA to establish routine and helping them adapt to changed routines. • Accommodations to make digital learning more inclusive for PWA. • Creating spaces for various groups to interact and share experiences. These exercises are therapeutic as to reduce the feeling of isolation.
3	PWPD1	Physical disability	• Beds of PWPDs should be near washrooms, which are accessible and usable. • Facility of accessible bell system. • Accessible quarantine centers, healthcare settings with provisions of accessible washrooms. • Provision for accessible transport facilities to travel from community to the healthcare settings. • Trained health care staff, about how to manage the distress of PWPD. • Arranging online facilities which help them connect with their family members regularly. • Providing targeted and long-term therapeutic support.
4	PWPD2	Physical disability	
5	PWPD3	Physical disability	
6	PWCP	Cerebral palsy	• Provision of local language communication board. • Hygiene kit to have CP user friendly material. • Positioning of furniture in the room to enable easy access to door and calling devices. • Putting safety bars and handles in room and washrooms for safe mobility.
7	PWAPD	Acquired physical disability due to accident	• Accessible quarantine centers, healthcare settings with provisions of accessible washrooms. • Provision for accessible transport facilities to travel from community to the healthcare settings
8	PWVI	Visual impairment	• Door to door visits for helping to book the slots for vaccination. • Booking slots on behalf of a PWVI through a helpline. • Accessible quarantine and isolation center.

- Providing safety gears and preventive practices to enhance low spread of virus in case of physical contact with PWDs.
- Empowering communities, local actors whose capacities can be utilized and developed as citizen helpers.
- Promoting collaboration with community-based organizations (CBOs) with high quality and people-centered public health care. This approach can help to sensitize people about case-specific needs of PWDs.

- Promoting models of localized care for PWDS, for example, Community Care Centers to house high risk and COVID-19 positive individuals in their community and in proximity to caregivers. These centers can further be connected to work in collaboration with community kitchens and psycho-social helpline.

STUDY LIMITATIONS

We have been able to interact and observe PWDs who were visiting the healthcare settings. Community interaction was not intense, only narrative that were brought to the healthcare settings were facilitated through online calls. Given that we were majorly connecting over phone, no participation was observed from individuals with speech impairment. A more aggressive on field engagement would have helped us engage with such disabilities as well. Further engaging deeply with the caregivers (family members and friends) would have provided comprehensive understanding to the challenges faced by PWDs. Our interaction was limited to only a few of the caregivers.

CONCLUSION

We have documented how systems interact in complex in low resource urban settings like Mumbai's M-East Ward, make healthcare services inaccessible for PWDs during COVID-19. We argue that inaccessible preparedness and response planning in informal settlements does not consider or include PWDs diverse needs. This creates barriers to their participation in services and care. An understanding of the barriers can aid in formulating context-relevant policies incorporating the lived experience of PWDs. Health services should be available, accessible, and usable to PWDs in informal settlements. Healthcare systems, where the element of care is at the core of it, need to develop a better understanding of what makes it holistic and accessible care. This entails learning about accessible infrastructure, particularly within informal settlements and healthcare settings, designing population-specific training programs for healthcare professionals. Understanding the barriers would help to understand the gaps in the resource system, helping to mobilize required resources in the relevant healthcare departments.

ACKNOWLEDGMENTS

We extend our deep gratitude to the research participants of M-East Ward, Mumbai for providing us insights about the barriers they faced in accessing healthcare provisions amidst COVID-19. We would like to thank the CLAP (COPING with COVID via COMMUNITY-LED ACTION, LEARNING) and Transforming M-Ward Project for supporting us with this research.

NOTES

1. Transforming M-East Ward project by Tata Institute of Social Sciences, Mumbai involves various action-research project in the fields of education, healthcare, nutrition, livelihood in M-East ward.

2. WAR Room is 24/7 COVID-19 patient management, decentralized helpline run by Brihanmumbai Municipal Corporation.

REFERENCES

Anguera, M. T., Camerino, O., Castañer, M., Sánchez-Algarra, P., & Onwuegbuzie, A. J. (2017). The specificity of observational studies in physical activity and sports sciences: Moving forward in mixed methods research and proposals for achieving quantitative and qualitative symmetry. *Frontiers in Psychology*, *8*, 2196. https://doi.org/10.3389/fpsyg.2017.02196

Aravind, R., Kolhe, V., & Kumar, D. (2021). Social spending during COVID-19: Impact on disability institutions and persons with disabilities in India. *IAHRW International Journal of Social Sciences Review*, *9*(4), 338–346.

Auerbach, A. M., & Thachil, T. (2021). How does COVID-19 affect urban slums? Evidence from settlement leaders in India. *World Development*, *140*, 105304.

Bai, X., Nagendra, H., Shi, P., & Liu, H. (2020). *Cities: Build networks and share plans to emerge stronger from COVID-19*. Springer Nature Limited. https://www.nature.com/articles/d41586-020-02459-2

Bajpai, N., & Wadhwa, M. (2020). *COVID-19 in India: Issues, challenges and lessons*. Center for Sustainable Development. Earth institute, Columbia university. ICT India working paper. file:///C:/Users/user/Downloads/ICT_India_Working_Paper_34.pdf

Bashir, M. F., Benjiang, M. A., & Shahzad, L. (2020). A brief review of socio-economic and environmental impact of COVID-19. *Air Quality, Atmosphere & Health*, *13*(12), 1403–1409.

Bhattacharjee, S., & Sattar, S. (2021). COVID-19 pandemic and the poor in the urban spaces of India with special reference to Mumbai. *Equality, Diversity and Inclusion: An International Journal*. https://doi.org/10.1108/EDI-07-2020-0196

Bortoleto, M. A. C., Ontañón Barragán, T., Cardani, L. T., Funk, A., Melo, C. C., & Santos Rodrigues, G. (2020, December). Gender participation and preference: A multiple-case study on teaching Circus at PE in Brazilians schools. *Frontiers in education* (Vol. 5, p. 260). Frontiers.

Bourdieu, P., & Wacquant, L. J. D. (1992). *An invitation to reflexive sociology*. University of Chicago Press.

Buheji, M., da Costa Cunha, K., Beka, G., Mavric, B., De Souza, Y. L., da Costa Silva, S. S., Hanafi, M., & Yein, T. C. (2020). The extent of COVID-19 pandemic socio-economic impact on global poverty. A global integrative multidisciplinary review. *American Journal of Economics*, *10*(4), 213–224.

Census of India (2011). Census of India website: Office of the Registrar General & Census Commissioner, India. Gov.in website. https://censusindia.gov.in/2011Census/pes/pes_highlights.html. Accessed on September 30, 2021.

Denzin, N. K., & Lincoln, Y. S. (2011). *The SAGE handbook of qualitative research* (4th ed.). Sage Publications.

Duvendack, M., & Sonne, L. (2021). Responding to the multifaceted COVID-19 crisis: The case of Mumbai, India. *Progress in Development Studies*. https://doi.org/10.1177/14649934211030449

Fabregues, S., & Fetters, M. D. (2019). Fundamentals of case study research in family medicine and community health. *Family Medicine and Community Health*, *7*(2).

Falvo, D., & Holland, B. E. (2017). *Medical and psychosocial aspects of chronic illness and disability* (6th ed.). Jones & Bartlett Learning.

Ganguly, N. (2019). *Slums of India*. MJP Publisher.

Harrison, H., Birks, M., Franklin, R., & Mills, J. (2017, January). Case study research: Foundations and methodological orientations. *Forum Qualitative Sozialforschung/Forum: Qualitative Social Research*, *18*(1).

Henry, P. (2015). Rigor in qualitative research: Promoting quality in social science research. *Research Journal of Recent Sciences*, 2502. ISSN, 2277.

Jachyra, P., Atkinson, M., & Washiya, Y. (2015). 'Who are you, and what are you doing here': Methodological considerations in ethnographic Health and Physical Education research. *Ethnography and Education*, *10*, 242–261. https://doi.org/10.1080/17457823.2015.1018290

Jesus, T. S., Kamalakannan, S., Bhattacharjya, S., Bogdanova, Y., Arango-Lasprilla, J. C., Bentley, J., Gibson, B. E., & Papadimitriou, C. (2020). People with disabilities and other forms of vulnerability to the COVID-19 pandemic: Study protocol for a scoping review and thematic analysis. *Archives of Rehabilitation Research and Clinical Translation*, *2*(4), 100079.

Koschorke, M., Padmavati, R., Kumar, S., Cohen, A., Weiss, H. A., Chatterjee, S., ... Patel, V. (2014). Experiences of stigma and discrimination of people with schizophrenia in India. *Social Science & Medicine*, *123*, 149–159. https://doi.org/10.1016/j.socscimed.2014.10.035

Krippendorff, K. (2004). *Content analysis: An introduction to its methodology* (2nd ed.). Sage.

Kumar, A., & Mehta, A. (2019). *Disability in M-East ward: A study prevalence, access and barriers*. Apanalaya Studies, Series II.

Kumar, A., Pareek, V., Narayan, R. K., Kant, K., & Kapoor, C. (2020). Covid-19 in India: Dharavi's success story. *BMJ*, *370*. https://doi.org/10.1136/bmj.m3264

Mopari, R., Garg, B., Puliyel, J., & Varughese, S. (2019). Measuring disability in an urban slum community in India using the Washington Group questionnaire. *Disability and Health Journal*, *12*(2), 263–268.

Municipal Corporation of Greater Mumbai. (2009). *Human development report Mumbai 2009*. MCGM, Mumbai.

Naydenova, E., Raghu, A., Ernst, J., Sahariah, S. A., Gandhi, M., & Murphy, G. (2017). Healthcare choices in Mumbai slums: A cross-sectional study. *Wellcome Open Research*, *2*.

Parsons, J. A., & Johal, H. K. (2020). Best interests versus resource allocation: Could COVID-19 cloud decision-making for the cognitively impaired? *Journal of Medical Ethics*, *46*(7), 447–450.

Phillippi, J., & Lauderdale, J. (2018). A guide to field notes for qualitative research context and conversation. *Qualitative Health Research*, *28*(3), 381–388. https://doi.org/10.1177104973231 7697102

Prasad, U., Sarwal, R., Gopal, K. M., & Paul, V. K. (2021). *Mitigation and management of COVID-19: Practices from India's state & union territories*. National Institution for Transforming India (NITI) Aayog. https://doi.org/10.7910/DVN/7MHJEM

QuestionPro. (2021, October 02). Convenience sampling: Definition, applications, advantages, method, and examples. https://www.questionpro.com/blog/convenience-sampling/

Raju, E., Dutta, A., & Ayeb-Karlsson, S. (2021). COVID-19 in India: Who are we leaving behind? *Progress in Disaster Science*, *10*, 100163. https://doi.org/10.1016/j.pdisas.2021.100163

Sedgwick, P. (2013). Convenience sampling. *BMJ*, 347.

Sengupta, S., & Jha, M. K. (2020). Social policy, COVID-19 and impoverished migrants: Challenges and prospects in locked down India. *The International Journal of Community and Social Development*, *2*(2), 152–172.

Senjam, S. S., & Singh, A. (2020). Addressing the health needs of people with disabilities in India. *Indian Journal of Public Health*, *64*(1), 79.

Spall, S. (1998). Peer debriefing in qualitative research: Emerging operational models. *Qualitative Inquiry*, *4*(2), 280–292.

Spradley, J. P. (2016). *Participant observation*. Waveland Press.

Stake, R. E. (1995). *The art of case study research*. Sage Publications.

Stake, R. E. (2013). *Multiple case study analysis*. Guilford Press.

Subbaraman, R., & Murthy, S. L. (2015). The right to water in the slums of Mumbai, India. *Bulletin of the World Health Organization*, *93*, 815–816. https://doi.org/10.2471/BLT.15.155473

Thomas, G. (2011). A typology for the case study in social science following a review of definition, discourse, and structure. *Qualitative Inquiry*, *17*, 511–521. https://doi.org/10.1177/ 1077800411409884

Thomson, J. B. (1981). *Critical hermeneutics: A study in the thought of Paul Ricoeur and Jurgen Habermas*. Cambridge University Press. https://doi.org/10.1017/CBO9780511609176

TISS. (2015). *Socio-economic conditions and vulnerabilities: A Report of the Baseline Survey of M(East) Ward, Mumbai*. Tata Institute of Social Sciences. http://urk.tiss.edu/images/pdf/M-Ward-Report.pdf. Accessed on July 21, 2021.

Wacquant, L. (2006). *Body and Soul: Notebooks of an Apprentice Boxer*. Oxford University Press.

Wilkinson, A. (2020). Local response in health emergencies: Key considerations for addressing the COVID-19 pandemic in informal urban settlements. *Environment and Urbanization*, *32*(2), 503–522.

Yin, R. K. (2014). *Case Study Research Design and Methods* (p. 282). Sage. Canadian Journal of Program Evaluation, 30(1).

Chapter 5

EXCESSIVE CHILDHOODS, SELF-RELIANT CITIZENS: DISCURSIVE CONSTRUCTIONS OF CARE FOR DISABLED CHILDREN IN INDIA DURING THE COVID-19 PANDEMIC

Kim Fernandes and Tanushree Sarkar

ABSTRACT

Purpose: *In this chapter, we examine how the media in India constructed the lives, needs, and desires of disabled children in India during the tumultuous pandemic.*

Methods/Approach: *Through critical discourse analysis, we address how children's bodies and needs have been explicitly discursively constructed as "excessive," while implicitly drawing upon neoliberal, ableist logics of loss and productivity.*

Findings: *We foreground how the framing of COVID-19 as a disaster in the Indian context obscures state neglect, suggesting that inequality has been the result of the pandemic rather than the limits of state care under neoliberal ableism. Despite the recognition of gaps in the care received by disabled children, neoliberal, entrepreneurial solutions have emerged as a new, widely touted form of care during the pandemic.*

Implication/Value: *Through our analysis, we highlight how disabled children have been neglected by the state and constructed as burdensome and vulnerable. We argue that this occurs when disabled children's bodyminds do not conform to an ideal of the self-reliant, independent citizen under the logics of*

Disability in the Time of Pandemic
Research in Social Science and Disability, Volume 13, 95–112

ISSN: 1479-3547/doi:10.1108/S1479-354720230000013006

neoliberal ableism. Our work demonstrates how children with disabilities are discursively rendered absent from conceptualizations of normate citizenship, unless seen as contributing to current or future aspirations for state productivity and growth.

Keywords: Disability; neoliberal ableism; children; COVID-19; India; media

INTRODUCTION

On March 24, 2020, at 8 p.m., Indian Prime Minister Narendra Modi announced a 21-day nationwide lockdown to prevent the spread of COVID-19 (Hindustan Times, 2020). This announcement, which came without prior warning and allowed less than 4 hours' notice to a nation of 1.3 billion people, was extended in phases until May 31, 2020 (Times of India, 2020). Both sudden and severe, the lockdown required all citizens across the country to remain inside their homes for a total period of six weeks, ending access to any form of public transport, disrupting ongoing healthcare services, and completely halting food and medicine supply chains across the country. Well after the end of the lockdown, concerns about food insecurity, the lack of access to medical care, and insufficient financial support for those affected by the pandemic continue to persist nationwide. Attending to these concerns, in this paper, we ask: How do these persistent concerns demonstrate an interface between ableism and neoliberalism (Chaudhry, 2018; Kumar et al., 2012)? Further, what might an analysis of media constructions of disabled children's childhoods reveal about the contours of citizenship and belonging under neoliberal ableism?

Such questions can be answered by exploring how in India, the pandemic has widely been framed as both a disaster and an opportunity. We begin by asserting that the framing of COVID-19 as disaster within the Indian context does the work of obscuring the expansiveness of state neglect, instead discursively suggesting that many current experiences of inequality under COVID-19 have been the result only of the pandemic rather than the limits of state care under neoliberal ableism (Goodley, 2014; Goodley & Lawthom, 2019). Additionally, focusing on COVID-19 singularly as disaster gestures away from the ways in which state care, when neglectful, can have disastrous consequences.

We also assert that the framing of the pandemic as an opportunity relies on deploying children as a site for thinking about a post-pandemic future. We see this framing as occurring through two primary notions about the ways in which children with disabilities inhabit their bodies. First, in presenting the pandemic as an opportunity and sidelining the tremendous impact that this moment has had on so many children, these accounts assume that disability is something that can be overcome by trying hard enough, thereby also placing the onus of "overcoming" systemic ableism on disabled people. This framing denies that disability can be a source of identity and pride, and a basis for forming close communities (Kafer, 2013). Secondly, it also places disabled lives under close scrutiny in ways that abled children are often not subject to. The framing of the pandemic as an opportunity urges disabled people to move past what are perceived to be their inhibitions to rise to normative (Schalk, 2016) expectations of productivity and worth.

We bring perspectives from disabled children's childhood studies to bear on media representations of state care during the pandemic, arguing that care for children's needs has been described by the media and provided by the state through two primary lenses – first, physical care for the needs of bodies that are seen as "excessive" and therefore requiring exceptional kinds of care. This framing, we argue, obscures the role of the state in creating the pandemic as a disaster, and shifts away from acknowledging the exceptional nature of the pandemic as a time in the lives of young children.

To counter this, we center the voices and needs of disabled children in India, particularly during the pandemic. To do so, we draw upon analytical perspectives that emerge from disabled children's childhood studies. This disciplinary lens pushes back against the exclusion embedded in conventional approaches to both disability and childhood.

BACKGROUND

The pandemic in India has been characterized by an unresponsive and repressive state, bigotry and discrimination against Muslims, and increased class and caste-based inequities and atrocities (Harriss, 2020; Mukherji, 2020; Rahman, 2020). There is no doubt that these oppressive behaviors were concerning well in advance of the pandemic. However, the state policy of self-reliant India (*Aatmanirbhar Bharat*) indicates a particular form of state neglect constructed through the pandemic. *Aatmanirbhar Bharat* fueled discursive constructions of independent, entrepreneurial citizens, empowered by the state to weather the pandemic. Yet, this rhetoric existed in absence of material and psycho-social care that allowed citizens, particularly those with disabilities, to survive social distancing and the economic consequences of the pandemic (Rahman, 2020). Thus, while the Prime Minister galvanized self-reliant citizens to bang plates to appreciate frontline "corona warriors," healthcare workers and doctors in many parts of the country did not have access to personal protective equipment (PPE) or regular pay (Dore, 2020).

School closures in response to the pandemic have meant a shift toward online and distance learning and disruption in school-based nutrition programs. These closures have impacted the lives of children in a variety of ways, including through a nationwide increase in child labor and child trafficking, rising school dropouts, especially for children belonging to minoritized communities, and food insecurity (Alvi & Gupta, 2020). Parents, already struggling with the financial upheaval and domestic chores exacerbated by the pandemic, were now required to homeschool children and provide reliable access to the internet (Alvi & Gupta, 2020). Although questions were raised about the accessibility of online and distance learning platforms for children with disabilities (Mahapatra & Sharma, 2021), educational funding was absent from the state's economic response to the pandemic (Alvi & Gupta, 2020). The closure of special schools, or segregated schools for disabled children, cut off disabled children from access to special educators and physical therapists. With residential special schools shut, disabled children were required to return home.

The media served as both a site of reportage of the state's neglect, particularly toward migrant labor (Harriss, 2020), and a space for state-supported anti-Muslim rhetoric (Sarkar, 2020). Nevertheless, the state sought to control how the media reported the state's response to the pandemic, with criminal charges registered against several journalists for their reporting on the deleterious impacts of the lockdown (Mukherji, 2020). The depleting freedom of the Indian press under the current government (Mukherji, 2020) also serves as important context to understand how state care has been discussed in media reporting on disability and disabled children during the pandemic.

LITERATURE REVIEW

Prior to the pandemic, children were widely written about as the future of the nation and a significant source of potential for economic growth in India (Behura, 2020; India Today, 2020a; Kumbhakar, 2019). However, these framings impose particular understandings of what constitutes a "good" childhood marked by "potential," and there is no doubt that these conceptualizations of normativity are closely intertwined with neoliberal ableist logics (Thomas, 2021). Such broad constructions of what constitutes a "good" childhood are inevitably ones that rely on a specific imagining of the child as on their way to becoming an adult. Many such normative framings of childhood discuss the lives of disabled children as relating to experiences of stigma, neglect, or abuse, and for their presumed inability to participate in linear developmental trajectories. In doing so, these framings therefore also obscure the rich, varied childhoods that disabled children are already experiencing.

Amidst these normative framings, disabled children are often described as inhabiting atypical childhoods, a construction that further obscures and denigrates their lived realities (Curran, 2013; Singh & Ghai, 2009).[1] In addition to the perception of disabled children's needs as excessive (Goodley & Runswick-Cole, 2013), their childhoods often fall under the shadow of imagined trajectories toward adulthood which are premised on assumptions about individual economic productivity. Attention to disabled children's everyday experiences within a wide range of scholarship that falls outside of the fields of disability studies and disabled children's childhood studies is often clouded by worries about the future prospects that disabled children will have as adults in an ableist society. In this way, disabled children's childhoods are marked as different from an able-bodied norm, although little attention is given to the presence of systemic ableism in these everyday experiences of difference.

These framings of disabled childhood reflect prior literature in critical disability studies, which critiques dominant conceptualizations of disability. For example, positioning disability as a tragedy marks disabled bodies as less than desirable (Kafer, 2013), marking both their present and future as stigmatized and subsequently open to "domination and social contempt" (Ferrante & Joly, 2016,

p. 156). When disability is framed as a tragedy, as Kafer (2013) points out, it becomes something to instinctively avoid – disabled futures are then continually produced as undesirable and stigmatized, rather than as both possible and imminently livable. Disabled presents (and often the starkness of disabled futures) are countered in the popular imagination through a prolonged emphasis on the disabled person's abilities, thereby portraying disabled bodies as worthy of normativity only if they were to be read as supercrip (Schalk, 2016).

Prior literature also shows that in the absence of state care, disabled children come to be constructed as burdensome, vulnerable, and tragic. "The framing of disabled children as burdens is intertwined with the way that their caregivers have framed their needs; as Karen Soldatic and Helen Meekosha (2012) note, 'carers' demands for support to facilitate [the] ... informal care [of disabled children] within the household have been won through the discursive positioning of disabled people as a burden" (p. 249). Soldatic and Meekosha (2012) argue that positioning disabled adults and children as burdensome to carers and the state is a feature of neoliberal ableism – to responsibilize care within the household while reducing institutional support (Thomas, 2021).

Even prior to the pandemic, the responsibility of care for disabled children was put onto families and kin (Addlakha, 2020). Parents are expected to do it all themselves, often imagined and cast as self-reliant citizens (Goodley, 2014) and held responsible for availing educational rights for their children. This framing reinforces what Robert McRuer (2006) has referred to as a "compulsory able-bodiedness" that is sustained by neoliberal ableism, which promotes a "do-it-yourself" citizenship. Vandana Chaudhry's (2018) attention to the ways in which this emphasis on individualized empowerment is a function of neoliberal governance points to the impact of responsibilization on the shaping of individual subjectivities.

Finally, Dan Goodley and Katherine Runswick-Cole (2013) theorized that the "leaking, lacking and excessive" bodies of children, which has provided a particularly compelling perspective to understand the disabled child's experiences of embodiment. It allows for an active acknowledgment of the ways in which expectations of normalcy shape the lives (and projected developmental trajectories) of disabled children, thereby often only discussing them in relation to their normate peers. Disabled children's childhood studies, therefore, begins by approaching disabled children not as "having problems or being problems, but as having childhoods" (Curran & Runswick-cole, 2014, p. 1617). This framing not only acknowledges the movement away from deficit framings of disability but also enables a re-thinking of normative notions of what might constitute childhood.

ANALYTICAL FRAMEWORK

Given the prior literature, the framing of disability as tragedy remains important to analyze precisely because it works both to reduce complex embodied experiences to questions of normative ability in the present moment and because it prevents other generative futures and possibilities for disabled people.

This chapter discusses the ways in which disabled children have been discursively constructed as vulnerable and as tragedies during the pandemic. To do so, we use Erinn Gilson's intersectional understanding of vulnerability, wherein Gilson argues that "corporeal vulnerability is accompanied by political, economic, social, and legal forms of vulnerability" (Gilson, 2016, p. 49). In particular, as Gilson demonstrates, when bodies are seen as oppressed, their vulnerability invites both neglect and exploitation (2016). While this framing of vulnerability has been immensely useful for us in making meaning of media representations of disabled children in India during the pandemic, we also draw upon Tiina Vaittinen's (2015) argument that vulnerable bodies are not just markers of frailty or reminders of the social role of embodiment but are also powerful political tools when understanding issues of state care and neglect. Amidst framings of the pandemic as a crisis, our work, therefore, draws closely upon Vaittinen's (2015) argument that vulnerable bodies represent political power within the political economy of care-relations and institutions.

We examine the needs of disabled children within the COVID-19 pandemic, where existing forms of care have failed because the very relations of care that require bodily proximity (Vaittinen, 2015) can no longer hold in the context of prolonged lockdowns and social distancing. Here, we build on the work of Tillie Curran, who argues that the childhoods of disabled children are "rarely understood as childhoods" (Curran, 2013, p. 126), and have instead been discussed primarily for their location within or relation to broader kin networks. Drawing upon disabled children's childhood studies, therefore, allows for an analytical focus on what disabled children need and want, rather than what they are often required to do to be seen as productive, worthy citizens.

Taking this approach allows us to engage with how neoliberal ableism contributes to the erosion of institutional support for families (Goodley, 2014; Thomas, 2021), our analysis shows that newspaper articles constructed an expectation from parents to "to try and work out a structure to keep their kids going" and provided advice from experts (Borthakur, 2020) on how to engage their "special children." The parental care of disabled children in the absence of the state is both valorized and denigrated, making care a moral responsibility (Trnka & Trundle, 2014). The responsibilization of care during the pandemic has not only operated by requiring individuals to be "self-reliant" but by privatizing relations of care onto families and kin (Soldatic & Meekosha, 2012; Trnka & Trundle, 2014).

In the next section, we discuss how media portrayals, often steeped in the normalcy narrative (Ahlvik-Harju, 2016), represent specific shifts in the relations of care and neglect between the state and disabled children (Vaittinen, 2015). Drawing on Vaittainen's (2015) crucial question, "Why do some bodies trigger care and others neglect?" our paper discusses the ways in which neoliberal ableist logics construct particular bodies as recipients of care. Media articles on disability serve as a lens through which to understand how disabled bodies are perceived by the state as both recipients of care and sites of neglect during the pandemic. We therefore begin by asking where and how normalcy appears in media representations of disability.

METHODOLOGY

We adopt critical discourse analysis (CDA) to examine the discursive strategies employed by the media in their construction of disability (Carvalho, 2008) and bring forth material realities and function of these discursive strategies in the production and reproduction of power (Richardson, 2007). Using CDA allows us to not only examine representations of disability but also how these representations interact with broader structures and discourses (Fairclough, 2001). In particular, discourse analysis can help make "explicit the discourses that produce disability as an oppressive category" (Grue, 2011). CDA adopts a moral and political stance that emphasizes how discourse produces and reproduces power from the perspectives of the oppressed (Grue, 2011). By examining how disabled children and adults were represented in the media, we question discourses around the pandemic as an opportunity to reimagine more inclusive and accessible futures for disabled people in India. Our paper addresses how the media represents disabled children and adults and the work these representations do during the pandemic.

Newspapers and media serve as a key mode of power – they reflect, represent, and reinforce societal inequalities and maintain dominant ideologies (Fraser & Llewellyn, 2015; Priyanti, 2018). Previous studies using CDA to examine disability representation in newspapers have highlighted the role of the media in maintaining ableist ideas of disability (Priyanti, 2018) that view disabled people as lacking agency (Fraser & Llewellyn, 2015). Further, Grue (2011) argues that using discourse analysis can explicate discourses that disability studies seeks to highlight, such as the construction of boundaries between normality and deviance.

Articles were identified using combinations of keywords such as "disability," "special needs," "school," "education," and "children" in November 2020. We focused on newspaper articles published between March and October 2020. In October 2020, the central government released guidelines for re-opening schools. These guidelines prioritized online learning and did not include special schools (Ministry of Home Affairs (Government of India), 2020). This timeframe of mandated school closure provides insights into newspaper discourses around education and disability during the pandemic, in no small part because school is often seen as a central site through which children are developed into productive citizens. As we note throughout the rest of this chapter, across articles, somewhat peculiarly – but not uncommonly – the concerns of people with disabilities were centered without centering their voices and lived experiences. This further resulted in the production of a fairly singular imagining of what the pandemic has been like for a heterogenous, diverse group of people, albeit one rooted in making explicit these concerns to those who were otherwise presumed to be unfamiliar with these realities.

Further, we focused on English language print and online newspapers, which are circulated across 31 million readers in India (Malvania, 2019). English language newspapers are published and read predominantly by urban elites, allowing us to engage with the configurations and ruptures of power brought forth by the Indian experience of the pandemic. Of several thousands of popular newspaper articles over the first few months of the pandemic in India, relatively very few discussed the lives of disabled people. Further, those articles that did discuss disabled people's experiences of the pandemic followed certain key themes, often repeating content and perspectives. In several cases, where a number of articles across media outlets reported similar content, we drew upon those the first instance of the published article for a more detailed analysis. This led us to develop a corpus of 67 newspaper articles.

We familiarized ourselves with the corpus through multiple readings. Our initial analysis examined language use in the articles, including narrative forms, choice and meaning of words, syntax, and use of metaphors and rhetorical tropes (Richardson, 2007). Following this description of the text, we proceeded to develop interpretations and explanations to examine the relationship between the text and context using Fairclough's (2001) guiding questions on intertextual references, discourse types, ideologies, and how power relations operate at different levels and their effects. We produced linked memos to ensure themes and discourses identified represented the data. Following this, we wrote informal analytic memos to think through patterns of discourse that were identified. Using notes from conversations, we then engaged in explicating and coding (Saldana, 2015) discursive resources present in the article. The series of documents produced served as the basis for producing a narrative with interpretations and explanations of the discourses around vulnerability, tragedy, care, and neoliberal ableism in the articles (Ziskin, 2019).

FINDINGS

Disability as Tragedy and the Responsibilization of Care for Disabled Children

The dominant framing of disabled people during the pandemic constructs disability as a superlative tragedy based on an inherent corporeal weakness. Disabled people are constructed as vulnerable, particularly by the state, because of their "physical, sensory, and cognitive limitations" (Bellamkonda, 2020). Further, their vulnerability is constituted by their inability to contribute as productive citizens (Erevelles, 2011). Articles use this frame to draw on the ways in which the "plight [of disabled people] has been ignored" (Tambe, 2020) and continued to urge readers to "imagine the plight" (Chandani, 2020) of disabled communities, in one instance arguing that "disabled people are not only the most deprived human beings in the world. . .they are also the most neglected" (Roy & Mehrotra, 2020). Such phrases produce the disabled person as devoid of any agency, employing an overwhelmingly ableist approach that assumes that they are to be pitied for their very evident perceived shortcomings. This framing attempts to evoke an emotional response from the able-bodied citizenry about the ill-treatment of disabled people by the state by individualizing tragedy to elicit pity. However, this narrative largely erases the structural ableism underlying the challenges faced by disabled people during the pandemic (Kafer, 2013).

This framing is almost exclusively reserved for disabled children, who are predominantly constructed as what Dan Goodley and Katherine Runswick-Cole have described as "leaking, lacking, and excessive bodies" (Goodley & Runswick-Cole, 2013). This is exemplified in the quote below from the director of a special school in an article in the Indian Express,

> Children may face "severe behavioural issues" that may crop up due to "pent up frustration, lack of occupation, change in routine and above all in case of children with relatively lower cognitive level, the inability to comprehend the reason for this sudden change in their lives." (Narayanan, 2020)

Disabled children are thus represented as excessive bodies that react to their environments – as an inherent lack (Goodley & Runswick-Cole, 2013) to be marked with difference that demands expert forms of care. Further, the concerns of disabled children are constructed as a fairly singular imagining of what the pandemic has been like for a heterogeneous, diverse group of children. A small handful of articles addressed specific kinds of disabilities, such as autism, rather than children with disabilities as a group, but often had significantly misleading portrayals that resulted from approaching all disabled children as monolithic – as an example, one article noted that "children with special needs . . . are affected because their memory and retention power is not similar to others" (India TV, 2020). Thus, most articles on disabled children's experiences of the pandemic do not provide significant details on how these experiences could differ by disability. This broad grouping additionally relies heavily on a language of incapacity without an acknowledgment of how ableist systems contribute heavily to processes of disablement.

Through the experience of the pandemic, civil society organizations (CSOs) working with parents of children with disabilities recommended shifting the responsibility of education to parents, "This heavy reliance on parents, in fact, is one of the recommendations put forth by Swabhiman's survey" (Kabilan, 2020). That is, the forms of care that families were required to provide due to the pandemic were viewed as an opportunity to responsibilize care onto them. This was also true for educational provisions for children without disabilities. An educational non-government organization (NGO) known for conducting annual surveys that reveal poor learning outcomes of children across the country recommended that "schools find ways to build on that home support going forward" (The Hindu, 2020).

As another example, a disability rights activist, quoted in their criticism of the state's policy of *Aatma Nirbhar Bharat* (self-reliant India), pointed out that disabled adults "who don't raise their voices or who are not heard, fall through the cracks if they are not self-reliant" (Bhatnagar, 2020). However, instead of attending to the neoliberal ableism built into state policies, newspaper articles largely tasked their imagined (normate) audience with a responsibility to help and care for disabled citizens. As an example, an article that discussed the experiences of children with disabilities as "bearing the brunt" of online education noted the many systemic difficulties that made online education inaccessible for disabled children, but ended with the following sentence: "Well, they say that opportunities come in the guise of adversities and perhaps the pandemic is a time for the government, schools and governing bodies of education to wake up and create the right tools to change the narrative" (Kabilan, 2020). Similarly, the article noted that the neglect of disabled adults and children was the moral failure of volunteers who are not "coming forward to extend their services" because of their fears of contracting the virus (Kabilan, 2020).

Across articles, parents are celebrated for taking on the "herculean tasks" of caring for disabled children. At the same time, parents are chastised for being "plain selfish" as they failed to educate their children. Schools argued that parents were shirking off responsibility after "admitting the child to a special school" (Tankha, 2020). In the case of poorer families, the construction of discourse around familial involvement differed slightly – here, families were largely described as unable to support homeschooling, viewed as a luxury for parents from lower-income backgrounds. Overall, the articles seek to place the responsibility of caring for disabled children squarely on parents and families at a time when many families are struggling to cope with the material hardships brought on by the absence of social security nets during the pandemic (Mahapatra & Sharma, 2021).

Neoliberal Ableism, Entrepreneurial Care, and the Production of Self-Reliant Citizens

Disabled children in India have borne the brunt of educational inequities and ableist schooling regimes well before the pandemic. During the pandemic, the "online experience" (India Today, 2020b) for all school-going children has been described as a key site through which to ensure "that students continue their learning and engagement." However, in contrast, one article titled, "India's Online Classrooms are Outdated for Disabled Kids" argued that the solution to including disabled children and ensuring that their education was on par with their normate peers was to ensure that digital classrooms had the latest technologies (Pandey, 2020). While there is no doubt that technological advances have proved immensely useful for the needs of disabled people, this framing of outdated technology as the reason for exclusion writes out more systemic factors that enable ableist logics of neglect. In particular, by placing its hopes within the realm of technology, the article pays no attention to active pedagogies of care and inclusion. It also leaves out the difficulties that many disabled children, particularly those from low-income families, face when attempting to gain access to the Internet and to devices that will enable them to continue learning online.

Although the provision of ed-tech as care operates with the further assumption that it will open up pathways for disabled children and their families that were previously unavailable, early studies that have emerged on the effectiveness of online children do not take into consideration the needs of children with disabilities.

Disabled children face a unique set of challenges relating to the ability to afford access that have largely been rendered invisible by media reports. One example of these challenges is seen in an India Spend article that details an Oxfam report on early experiences with digital schooling in India since the lockdown. Despite the many ways in which marginalized parents and families discuss the limited impacts of digital schooling on their children, this report includes no discussion of how disabled children and their families have been failed by digital schooling (Malik, 2020). Another example of how ability and access intersect in media discourse is in the following anecdote from another article: "Disha was born deaf in Nagaland. Before the lockdown, she would go to school one for special kids and play with her peers – but all that has changed now. Even if she wanted, the family cannot afford a computer or a tablet, neither can they afford data to help her study online" (Borthakur, 2020). This example assumes that Disha's needs and her family's material capabilities are lacking because they do not meet neoliberal standards for continued productivity amidst the many upheavals brought about by the pandemic.

As is often the case with technosolutionist products (cf. Pischetola, 2021), the assumptions about the possibilities of technology and the futures that they gesture to do not hold up when matched against the realities of access on the ground. Speaking of online education during the pandemic, one article noted, "much of these programmes are done on the assumption that children with disabilities have access to online programmes and sessions. The reality is that they do not" (Borthakur, 2020). Another article referred to the difficulties with access through the lens of infrastructure, arguing: "it is really important that we build the infrastructure for online education" (India Today, 2020b), although the article, like several others, did not name the shifting "we" or note what this infrastructure might look like. As a further suggestion, the article offered, "the best thing to do is offer ed-tech companies and CSOs [civil society organizations] an opportunity to reach a wider audience" (India Today, 2020b). This construction of a wider audience as the solution to difficulties of access remains at odds with numerous accounts indicating the inaccessibility of education for millions of children in India during the pandemic. Most importantly, it also relocates structural gaps in providing access to technology from the state and private providers to disabled children and their families, discursively portraying the latter as responsible for their social location and access needs during this time.

Notably, despite the diverse experiences of disabled children during the pandemic, their needs are primarily discussed through the lens of their families' experiences. For instance, a piece on the hardships that families of disabled children face offered the following detail: "families have been deprived of two things…able bodies, and financial sustainability" (Suchitra, 2020). Rooted in ableist logics, this depiction of the family as being "deprived" of ability locates the experience of being disabled in the individual, assuming ability as normalcy in a manner that frames able-bodiedness as a (largely physical) state of being that families are owed by their children.

As has been the case in many other countries around the world, the experiences of children in India during the pandemic have also been interpreted, discussed, and responded to primarily through the lens of the loss of learning. This loss has been widely discussed publicly, with several references to the vast numbers of children who are physically out of school at this point (Al Jazeera, 2020; Live Mint, 2020; Pathak, 2020). The focus on the disruption of schooling as the primary disruption experienced by children during the pandemic obscures other central concerns relating to emotional well-being, household dynamics, access to food, and physical safety. Further, the focus on the loss of learning resulting from out of school time, particularly in India, has positioned the school as the central – if not often the only – site of learning, thereby assuming that all children and their parents have experienced the pandemic through this unitary lens (Fernandes & Garg, 2020). Therefore, although time at school can often constitute an important part of a child's everyday life, it is apparent from the above narratives that the goal of this time was to fashion children into productive citizens.

Neoliberal logics of loss are particularly apparent in discussions about the school as a primary site through which learning takes place. One article, titled, "COVID-19 shut schools, but teachers make sure learning is not stopping," argues for the role of teachers as "real impact creators in the current crisis" (Senapaty & Falt, 2020). This portrayal is at odds with several conversations where teachers have expressed their unpreparedness to deal with the pandemic (Pitroda, 2020; Viney, 2020) and does not acknowledge how teachers require much more support than they are currently receiving both from the state and school administration. The loss associated with school closure is framed primarily in economic terms, emphasized for the potential it might have to disrupt the growth of the Indian economy both now and in the future. By extension, young bodies – disabled or otherwise – are only seen for how they exacerbate anxieties around narratives of loss. As a result, learning is imagined primarily through continued access to school, and the onus is placed on the child – and their family – to ensure that they do not hinder the promise of economic growth. Such a framing prioritizes a particularly adult-centric notion of what learning should look like and does not center the preferences of children. Although the school is also often a central site for childhood friendships and socialization, as a result of underlying neoliberal ableist logics, there is far less media discussion of how these social bonds have been interrupted during the pandemic.

Conversely, in moments when children are unable to attend school, their physical absence from school is framed as a "lack of learning activity" (The Hindu, 2020). Here, marginalized student populations are seen as "suffering" for their own inability to attend school when online, another framing that does not pay attention to the systemic, infrastructural support necessary for students to be able to continue learning online. Further, depicting children who are unable to attend classes online – and by extension assumed to not be learning – as suffering assumes that learning activities are only possible when initiated and carried out by an adult.

CONCLUSION

Our findings show two dominant themes that appeared across newspaper articles from March 2020–October 2020 in mainstream English newspapers in India. The first theme was the depiction of the lives of disabled children as unending tragedies and the shifting responsibilization for their care. The second theme was the emergence of entrepreneurial care under the neoliberal, ableist state, as a result of which K-12 education (both prior to and during the pandemic) was perceived largely as a vehicle through which future-oriented, self-reliant adult citizens would be developed.

In analyzing the application of neoliberal ableist logics to the lives of disabled children in India during the pandemic, we provide a critique of dominant discursive constructions within media portrayals of non-normate children as vulnerable and as tragedies. Drawing upon perspectives from disabled children's childhood studies, we argue that these portrayals of children further enable them to be described as continual recipients of care, even when their voices, preferences, and needs are not centered in the provision of this care. This was demonstrated in newspaper coverage by leaving out their voices or opinions on what was happening. We also trouble the conventional understandings of state care and neglect, noting that disabled children the portrayal of disabled children as needing exceptional amounts of care during the pandemic obscures the proportions of state neglect. Importantly, we point to how disabled children have been oppressively discussed as bodies in need of all manner of fixing, even though the responsibility for the care and labor of fixing often paradoxically falls on disabled children and their families.

Within media representations, disabled children are cast as recipients of care. Their non-normativity and the medical care that they have required are emphasized, and the threat of education disruption by the pandemic heightens these panics. Our data showed that the widespread movement from in-person classroom education to online education relied on an undying faith in the ability of online education, or technologies, to solve that manufactured crisis. Thus emerged the framing of the pandemic as an "opportunity in adversity" (India Today, 2020b) for teaching and learning. Newspaper coverage sidestepped conversations about the limits of online education (particularly as it relates to access) in marginalized contexts. Instead, media representations of technology as a technical solution, or current and future leveler, promoted the proliferation of entrepreneurial solutions to the limits of school education as a form of care provision.

This faith in technology simply existing ignores systemic questions of access; instead, it locates the responsibility for accessing them with disabled children and their families. Through an entrepreneurial refashioning of care, education technologies (ed-tech) have been presented as the solution to various system concerns that have emerged during the pandemic. We demonstrate how engagement with online learning centers children primarily for their ability to contribute in economically productive ways in the future, which in turn denies them the possibility of fully inhabiting the present.

Despite various discussions that recognize the significant gaps in the care that disabled children receive, our data highlight how entrepreneurial solutions have emerged as a new, widely touted form of care during the pandemic, often enthusiastically discussed for their potential to re-frame difficulties that disabled children face with non-pandemic schooling. This enthusiasm for the potential of technology to generate more productive citizens fails to consider the many ways in which online education has proved to be inaccessible to disabled children. That is, technologies were positioned as potentially "solving" the schooling problem when they in fact did not. The positioning of technology as a solution to larger systemic problems (Lindtner et al., 2016) simultaneously obscures the support needs that disabled children and their families have expressed during the pandemic.

At the same time, as neoliberal logics of tragedy and loss around disability circulate, disabled children are commonly discursively rendered absent from conceptualizations of normate citizenship unless they are directly seen as contributing to current or future aspirations for state productivity and growth. Meanwhile, families are asked (and blamed) if they aren't able to overcome their children's perceived differences. Neoliberal ableist logics play a significant role in the superimposition of this trajectory of presumed normalcy (and its intersections with able-bodiedness) on the lives of disabled children. As this paper has demonstrated, the discursive casting of disabled children as tragic and sad, the responsibilization of families for their care, and the misplaced faith in technology as a solution to larger systemic problems have been prominent features of media coverage of disabled children's experiences of the pandemic in India.

NOTE

1. In a nod to existing debates around the use of person-first versus identity-first language, as disabled scholars, we use identity-first language or person-first and identity-first language interchangeably depending on the context. For us, identity-first language signals autonomy, power, and a description of disability that is not based in euphemistic or negative connotations of disability, but rather one that views disability as diversity and a part of the social justice agenda (Andrews et al., 2019). Toward this decision, we also draw upon the work of Dr Morton Ann Gernsbacher (2017), who systematically traces the use of person-first language in scholarly writing and has examined over 5 million books, 25 million abstracts, and 150 million articles to make the case that (depending on the journal) person-first language is used 100–700 times more often to refer to people with disabilities than people without disabilities, implying that person-first language is significant when talking about disabled people, since all others are assumed to be "normal." Further, as Emily Ladau (2015) points out, person-first language "buys into the stigma it claims to be fighting." This is an important argument we seek to make in this paper as well. Contextualized more broadly, our citational decisions are also in line with updated guidance from the American Psychological Association (APA, 2015; APA Style, 2021).

REFERENCES

Addlakha, R. (2020). Kinship destabilized!:disability and the micropolitics of care in Urban India. *Current Anthropology*, *61*(S21), S46–S54. https://doi.org/10.1086/705390

Ahlvik-Harju, C. (2016). Disturbing bodies – Reimagining comforting narratives of embodiment through feminist disability studies. *Scandinavian Journal of Disability Research*, *18*(3), 222–233. https://doi.org/10.1080/15017419.2015.1063545

Al Jazeera. (2020, August 15). Why are so many Indian children losing out on schooling? *Al Jazeera*. https://www.aljazeera.com/program/the-stream/2020/8/15/why-are-so-many-indian-children-losing-out-on-schooling/

Alvi, M., & Gupta, M. (2020). Learning in times of lockdown: How Covid-19 is affecting education and food security in India. *Food Security*, *12*(4), 793–796. https://doi.org/10.1007/s12571-020-01065-4

American Psychological Association (APA). (2015). Choosing words for talking about disability. https://www.apa.org/pi/disability/resources/choosing-words

American Psychological Association Style (APA Style). (2021). *Disability*. https://apastyle.apa.org/style-grammar-guidelines/bias-free-language/disability

Andrews, E. E., Forber-Pratt, A. J., Mona, L. R., Lund, E. M., Pilarski, C. R., & Balter, R. (2019). #SaytheWord: A disability culture commentary on the erasure of disability. *Rehabilitation Psychology*, *64*(2), 111–118. https://doi.org/10.1037/rep0000258

Behura, S. (2020, April 19). Economic shocks to hit children. *The New Indian Express*. https://www.newindianexpress.com/magazine/voices/2020/apr/19/economic-shocks-to-hit-children-2131071.html

Bellamkonda, S. (2020, June 26). Covid-19 has further marginalised people with disabilities. *The Times of India*. https://timesofindia.indiatimes.com/blogs/developing-contemporary-india/covid-19-has-further-marginalised-people-with-disabilities/

Bhatnagar, G. V. (2020, May 15). Without the right tools, students with disabilities struggle in online classes: Activists. *The Wire*. https://thewire.in/rights/students-with-disabilities-online-classes

Borthakur, P. (2020, September 30). How children are coping with disabilities amid COVID-19 pandemic. *East Mojo*. https://www.eastmojo.com/in-depth/2020/09/30/how-children-are-coping-with-disabilities-amid-covid-19-pandemic

Carvalho, A. (2008). Media(ted) discourse and society: Rethinking the framework of critical discourse analysis. *Journalism Studies*, *9*(2), 161–177. https://doi.org/10.1080/14616700701848162

Chandani, A. (2020, April 2). How can deaf Indians call up COVID-19 helplines? Modi govt must take these steps immediately. *The Print*. https://theprint.in/opinion/deaf-indians-covid-19-modi-govt-must-take-these-steps/393514/

Chaudhry, V. (2018). Neoliberal crises of social work in the global South: Ethnography of individualizing disability and empowerment practice in India. *International Social Work*, *62*(3), 1117–1130.

Curran, T. (2013). Disabled children's childhood studies: Alternative relations and forms of authority? BT – Disabled children's childhood studies: Critical approaches in a global context. In T. Curran & K. Runswick-Cole (Eds.), *Disabled children's childhood studies* (pp. 121–135). Palgrave Macmillan UK. https://doi.org/10.1057/9781137008220_10

Curran, T., & Runswick-cole, K. (2014). Disabled children's childhood studies: A distinct approach? *Disability & Society*, *29*(10), 1617–1630.

Dore, B. (2020). Covid-19: Collateral damage of lockdown in India. *The BMJ*, *369*(April), 1–2. https://doi.org/10.1136/bmj.m1711

Erevelles, N. (2011). *Disability and difference in global contexts: Enabling a transformative body politic*. Palgrave Macmillan.

Fairclough, N. (2001). *Language and power*. Pearson Education.

Fernandes, K., & Garg, R. (2020). Anxiety and the politics of child well-being during COVID-19. *NEOS*, *12*(2). https://acyig.americananthro.org/neos/neos_current_issue/anxiety-and-the-politics-of-child-well-being-during-covid-19/%0A%0A

Ferrante, C., & Joly, E. (2016). Begging and disability: A paradigmatic way to earn one's living. In S. Grech & K. Soldatic (Eds.), *Disability in the Global South: The critical handbook* (pp. 151–166). Springer.

Fraser, V., & Llewellyn, G. (2015). Good, bad or absent: Discourses of parents with disabilities in Australian news media. *Journal of Applied Research in Intellectual Disabilities*, *28*(4), 319–329. https://doi.org/10.1111/jar.12142

Gernsbacher, M. A. (2017). Editorial perspective: The use of person-first language in scholarly writing may accentuate stigma. *Journal of Child Psychology and Psychiatry*, *58*(7), 859–861. https://doi.org/10.1111/jcpp.12706

Gilson, E. (2016). The perils and privileges of vulnerability: Intersectionality, relationality, and the injustices of the U.S. Prison Nation. *Philosophia*, *6*(1), 43–59. https://doi.org/10.1353/phi.2016.0011

Goodley, D. (2014). *Dis/ability studies: Theorising disablism and ableism*. Routledge.

Goodley, D., & Lawthom, R. (2019). Critical disability studies, Brexit and Trump: A time of neoliberal–Ableism. *Rethinking History*, *23*(2), 233–251. https://doi.org/10.1080/13642529.2019.1607476

Goodley, D., & Runswick-Cole, K. (2013). The body as disability and possibility: Theorizing the "leaking, lacking and excessive" bodies of disabled children. *Scandinavian Journal of Disability Research*, *15*(1), 1–19. https://doi.org/10.1080/15017419.2011.640410

Grue, J. (2011). Discourse analysis and disability: Some topics and issues. *Discourse & Society*, *22*(5), 532–546. https://doi.org/10.1177/0957926511405572

Harriss, J. (2020). "Responding to an epidemic requires a compassionate state": How has the Indian state been doing in the time of Covid-19? *Journal of Asian Studies*, *79*(3), 609–620. https://doi.org/10.1017/S0021911820002314

Hindustan Times. (2020, March 24). PM Modi announces all-India lockdown over Covid-19, will be in place for 21 days. *Hindustan Times*. https://www.hindustantimes.com/india-news/pm-modi-to-address-nation-on-coronavirus-shortly/story-aR7ugx57A8sRiXX5MHAcpL.html

India Today. (2020a, August 24). How to make your children empowered citizens of future India with the right preschool education. *India Today*. https://www.indiatoday.in/education-today/featurephilia/story/how-to-make-your-children-empowered-citizens-of-future-india-with-the-right-preschool-education-1591180-2019-08-24

India Today. (2020b, September 7). Covid-19 impact: Will education for persons with disabilities change, as more universities go online? *India Today*. https://www.indiatoday.in/education-today/featurephilia/story/covid-19-impact-will-education-for-persons-with-disabilities-change-as-more-universities-go-online-1719363-2020-09-07

India TV. (2020, April 3). Coronavirus pandemic's impact on education of children with special needs. *India TV*. https://www.indiatvnews.com/health/coronavirus-pandemic-impact-education-children-with-special-needs-604207

Kabilan, K. (2020, October 10). Remote realities: Children with disabilities bear the brunt of online education during the pandemic. *The New Indian Express*. https://www.newindianexpress.com/cities/chennai/2020/oct/10/remote-realities-children-with-disabilities-bear-thebrunt-of-online-education-during-pandemic-2208179.html

Kafer, A. (2013). *Feminist*. Indiana University Press.

Kumar, A., Sonpal, D., & Hiranandani, V. (2012). Trapped between ableism and neoliberalism: Critical reflections on disability and employment in India. *Disability Studies Quarterly*, *32*(3). https://dsq-sds.org/article/view/3235/3109

Kumbhakar, D. (2019, May 22). Children: The supreme assets of our nation. *The Sentinel*. https://www.sentinelassam.com/melange/children-the-supreme-assets-of-our-nation/

Ladau, E. (2015, July 20). Why person-first language doesn't always put the person first. *Think Inclusive*. https://www.thinkinclusive.us/post/why-person-first-language-doesnt-always-put-the-person-first

Lindtner, S., Bardzell, S., & Bardzell, J. (2016). Reconstituting the utopian vision of making: HCI after technosolutionism. In *Proceedings of the 2016 CHI Conference on Human Factors in Computing Systems*, CHI'16, New York, NY, USA (pp. 1390–1402). Association for Computing Machinery.

Live Mint. (2020, October 12). School closure may cost over $400 Bn to India, cause learning losses: World Bank. *Live Mint*. https://www.livemint.com/education/news/school-closure-may-cost-over-400-bn-to-india-cause-learning-losses-world-bank-11602497233954.html

Mahapatra, A., & Sharma, P. (2021). Education in times of COVID-19 pandemic: Academic stress and its psychosocial impact on children and adolescents in India. *International Journal of Social Psychiatry*, *67*(4), 397–399. https://doi.org/10.1177/0020764020961801

Malik, A. (2020, September 15). Over 80% parents in 5 states say digital schooling failed during lockdown: Study. *India Spend*. https://www.indiaspend.com/over-80-parents-in-5-states-say-digital-schooling-failed-during-lockdown-study/

Malvania, U. (2019, April 27). Print readership in India jumps 4.4% to 425 million in two years: Report. *Business Standard*. https://www.business-standard.com/article/current-affairs/print-readership-in-india-jumps-4-4-to-425-million-in-two-years-report-119042700079_1.html. Accessed on March 10, 2022.

McRuer, R. (2006). *Crip theory: Cultural signs of queerness and disability*. New York University Press.

Ministry of Home Affairs (Government of India). (2020). Guidelines for Re-opening (No. 40-3/2020-DM-I(A)). https://www.mha.gov.in/sites/default/files/MHAOrderDt_30092020.pdf

Mukherji, R. (2020). Covid vs. Democracy: India's illiberal remedy. *Journal of Democracy*, *31*(4), 91–105. https://doi.org/10.1353/jod.2020.0058

Narayanan, J. (2020, September 22). Pandemic and a lockdown: Persons with disabilities grapple with more challenges. *The Indian Express*. https://indianexpress.com/article/lifestyle/life-style/persons-with-disabilities-day-to-day-challenges-coronavirus-covid-19-lockdown-pandemic-handwashing-social-isolation-distancing-6383363/

Pandey, P. (2020, July 19). India's online classrooms are outdated for disabled kids. Covid just made it worse. *The Print*. https://theprint.in/opinion/indias-online-classrooms-are-outdated-for-disabled-kids-covid-just-made-it-worse/463438/

Pathak, A. (2020, May 23). The pandemic and the absurdity of 'Online Teaching'. *Mainstream Weekly*, *LVIII*, 23. http://mainstreamweekly.net/article9405.html

Pischetola, M. (2021). Re-Imagining digital technology in education through critical and neo-materialist insights. *Digital Education Review*, *40*, 154–171.

Pitroda, S. (2020, November 24). Digital India is not prepared for digital education. *The Indian Express*. https://indianexpress.com/article/opinion/columns/digital-education-online-classes-learning-coronavirus-national-education-policy-6580744/

Priyanti, N. (2018). Representations of people with disabilities in an Indonesian newspaper: A critical discourse analysis. *Disability Studies Quarterly*, *38*(4), 1–2. https://doi.org/10.18061/dsq.v38i4.5818

Rahman, S. Y. (2020). 'Social distancing' during COVID-19: The metaphors and politics of pandemic response in India. *Health Sociology Review*, 131–139. https://doi.org/10.1080/14461242.2020.1790404

Richardson, J. E. (2007). *Analysing newspapers: An approach from critical discourse analysis*. Palgrave Macmillan.

Roy, B., & Mehrotra, S. (2020, April 3). COVID-19: Implications for the disabled. *The Hindu Business Line*. https://www.thehindubusinessline.com/opinion/covid-19-implications-for-the-disabled/article31250730.ece

Saldana, J. (2015). *The coding manual for qualitative researchers* (3rd ed.). Sage Publications Ltd.

Sarkar, S. (2020). Religious discrimination is hindering the covid-19 response. *BMJ*, *369*, m2280. https://doi.org/10.1136/bmj.m2280

Schalk, S. (2016). Reevaluating the supercrip. *Journal of Literary & Cultural Disability Studies*, *10*(1), 71–86. https://doi.org/10.3828/jlcds.2016.5

Senapaty, H., & Falt, E. (2020, October 5). COVID shut schools, but teachers making sure learning is not stopped. *The Print*. https://theprint.in/opinion/covid-shut-schools-but-teachers-making-sure-learning-is-not-stopped/516334/

Singh, V., & Ghai, A. (2009). Notions of self: Lived realities of children with disabilities. *Disability & Society*, *24*(2), 129–145. https://doi.org/10.1080/09687590802652363

Soldatic, K., & Meekosha, H. (2012). Moving the boundaries of feminist social work education with disabled people in the neoliberal era. *Social Work Education*, *31*(2), 246–252. https://doi.org/10.1080/02615479.2012.644975

Suchitra (2020, June 15). Coronavirus lockdown: In the pandemic, the disabled remain an invisible minority. *The Hindu*. https://www.thehindu.com/news/national/coronavirus-lockdown-in-the-pandemic-the-disabled-remain-an-invisible-minority/article31828510.ece

Tambe, N. (2020, April 2). World autism day 2020: Autism under a lockdown in India. *Asiaville*. https://www.asiavillenews.com/article/autism-and-coronavirus-world-autism-day-2020-37985

Tankha, R. S. (2020, May 14). Children with special educational needs need extra care amid COVID-19 lockdown. *The New Indian Express*. https://www.newindianexpress.com/lifestyle/health/2020/may/14/children-with-special-educational-needs-need-extra-care-amid-covid-19-lockdown-2143190.html

The Hindu. (2020, October 28). Nearly 20% of rural school children had no textbooks due to COVID-19 impact, finds ASER survey. *The Hindu*. https://www.thehindu.com/news/national/coronavirus-20-of-rural-school-children-had-no-textbooks-due-to-covid-19-impact-finds-aser-survey/article32966299.ece

Thomas, G. M. (2021). Dis-mantling stigma: Parenting disabled children in an age of 'neoliberal-ableism'. *Sociological Review*, *69*(2), 451–467. https://doi.org/10.1177/0038026120963481

Times of India (2020, May 1). Coronavirus lockdown extended by 2 more weeks: Activities that will continue to remain shut across the country. *Times of India*. https://timesofindia.indiatimes.com/india/coronavirus-lockdown-extended-by-2-more-weeks/articleshow/75492140.cms

Trnka, S., & Trundle, C. (2014). Competing responsibilities: Moving beyond neoliberal responsibilisation. *Anthropological Forum*, *24*(2), 136–153. https://doi.org/10.1080/00664677.2013.879051

Vaittinen, T. (2015). The power of the vulnerable body: A new political understanding of care. *International Feminist Journal of Politics*, *17*(1), 100–118. https://doi.org/10.1080/14616742.2013.876301

Viney, K. (2020, May 22). Teaching in the time of a pandemic. *The Hindu*. https://www.thehindu.com/education/teaching-in-the-time-of-a-pandemic/article32533237.ece

Ziskin, M. B. (2019). Critical discourse analysis and critical qualitative inquiry: Data analysis strategies for enhanced understanding of inference and meaning. *International Journal of Qualitative Studies in Education*, *32*(6), 606–631. https://doi.org/10.1080/09518398.2019.1609118

Chapter 6

SOCIAL AND HEALTH EXPERIENCES OF DISABLED PEOPLE WITH COMPLEX MEDICAL CONDITIONS DURING THE COVID-19 PANDEMIC

Joana Milan Lorandi and Pamela Block

ABSTRACT

Purpose: *This chapter explores the experiences of people with complex conditions before and during the COVID-19 pandemic, their fears for imagined futures when the pandemic first appeared, their reflections on their experiences and present status, as well as plans for a post-pandemic future.*

Methods/Approach: *This research is based on semi-structured interviews conducted by phone, Zoom, or in-person with six participants, each interviewed twice – before and during the pandemic – who either have complex medical conditions or are mothers of a child with complex medical conditions, in the United States. Half the interviews were conducted before the pandemic and the other half during the pandemic.*

Findings: *The data illuminate the understanding of our participants of the COVID-19 pandemic as a disability issue, which should be analyzed with the focus of disability as an intersectional social category and that disabled people felt at higher risk due to ableism in health policies and getting their health needs met. The results demonstrated the tremendous impact of the pandemic on the lives of our participants with complex medical conditions, whether in their work, care, physical and mental health, and social relationships.*

Implication/Value: *This study points to the importance of policymakers incorporating strategies to reduce ableism in health care provision, rationing,*

Disability in the Time of Pandemic
Research in Social Science and Disability, Volume 13, 113–131

Published under exclusive licence by Emerald Publishing Limited
ISSN: 1479-3547/doi:10.1108/S1479-354720230000013007

and other forms of decision-making. Services need to be designed keeping in mind the challenges of disabled people and their need for care. In addition, adequate education, and employment opportunities for disabled people must be ensured, while continuing to expand access options to disabled people that were available throughout the lockdown.

Keywords: Disability; complex medical conditions; pandemic; disability studies; COVID-19; ableism; feminist theories

INTRODUCTION

The global COVID-19 virus has moved rapidly around the world, infecting millions. Strict mitigation efforts such as social distancing, home quarantine, face masks, vigilant hand washing, and avoiding crowds have been instituted in most countries and have impacted all groups in society. However, the vulnerabilities of certain groups of people have been worsened due to the pandemic. Many disabled people have experienced the pandemic with a unique dread due to concerns about health care rationing by ableist health professionals, reduced or lack of access to needed appointments, procedures, medicine and supplies, which could be life-threatening, and the potential for preventable illness and death of friends, family, and themselves (Block et al., 2021).

This chapter is an outgrowth of author Block's research project: "Aging Out of Children's Hospitals and Health Systems" about the experiences and activism of those who resided in or were supported by US Children's Hospitals and Health Systems in the twentieth and twenty-first centuries (Block & Diallo, 2020). The participants include people or mothers of people with complex medical conditions in the United States, between the ages of 29 and 63.[1] A mother and daughter (both of whom are disabled) chose to interview together, leading to a total of 10 interviews with six participants. Our participants shared their pandemic experiences, which we will compare to their pre-pandemic interviews. This process enabled us to understand how pandemic conditions impacted the participants' lives and how specific forms of disability expertise not only allowed them to survive but provided advantages in navigating the pandemic even as disability realities may also have accentuated vulnerabilities. Thus, we will be discussing their experiences of the pandemic, their fears when the pandemic first appeared, their reflections on their experiences, as well as plans for a post-pandemic future. We will explore how our participants' lives changed, their experiences with health systems, disability access, pandemic-related health policies. The interviews conducted during the pandemic used the same structure as that used for pre-pandemic interviews, focusing on life occupations including school, work, interpersonal relationships, and mental health. The study is relevant as research on the impact of the pandemic on disabled people is still scarce, and the opportunity to systematically compare participant experiences before and during the pandemic is unique. This study also intends to systematize contributions aimed at the construction of anti-ableist practices to promote the well-being of this population.

Our study resonates with other research and scholarship on similar themes including stressors and declining mental health status of disabled people during the pandemic through heightened concerns over contracting the virus, increases in economic insecurity, and growing social isolation (Ciciurkaite et al., 2021; Ferreira & Lopes, 2021; Pettinicchio et al., 2021). Researchers also report the exacerbation along lines of poverty, race, and gender as well as disability of social and health inequalities, discrimination, barriers to government relief and health services (Das et al., 2021; Rohwerder et al., 2021; Wickenden et al., 2021). Block et al. (2021) note that the individualization of the responsibility to "stay safe," observed around the world, has disadvantaged disabled people among other vulnerable populations across the globe. Reinforcing that vulnerability, rather than being a characteristic of individuals, is structural and multifactorial.

Disability, Vulnerability, and Social Inequalities

Theories grounded in Brazilian Feminist Disability Studies (Diniz et al., 2009; Fietz, 2019; Mello & Nuernberg, 2012) note that notions of care, dependency and interdependence are presented as transversal to all relationships and important for the construction of more potent frameworks for ensuring rights and justice for disabled people. This approach enacts a more social understanding of disability that contrasts with internationally prevalent biomedical or rehabilitation understandings (Gesser et al., 2019; Tomasini, 2019). This study aims to examine disability using feminist, disability, care, and sociocultural theories to articulate the psychological and social impacts of disability experience for people in our study before and during the pandemic. However, the pandemic was not experienced in the same way by all individuals, with the particularities of each person's interaction with society being central to survival in crises. Thus, containment, mitigation, and suppression plans must be as inclusive as possible or risk reinforcing existing barriers (Berger et al., 2020).

According to the World Health Organization (2020), disabled people are at greater risk of contracting COVID-19. The pandemic has produced disabled bodies, while also producing social experiences that have been framed by the category of disability, whether in the orientation to health protocols, in the individualization of care, or in social isolation. Ableism can naturalize processes of exclusion in different social contexts, which can have life or death consequences in a pandemic. Kochhar (2020) argues that we cannot keep up the fight against the pandemic based on a capitalist and ableist logic because these logics caused our current reality: vulnerable people dying much more than privileged ones.

Disability justice activists such as Mingus (2022) and Piepzna-Samarasinha (2018) as well as sociologists Fine and Glendinning (2005) point out that understanding dependence and interdependence as inherent to the human condition and care as relational can expand the participation and agency of people with disabilities. Indeed, Mingus (2022) identifies this as a survival strategy during the pandemic. This study analyzes the interaction of people with disabilities and their support networks during the pandemic, understanding that care and interdependence are essential to ensure the quality of life and survival of people with disabilities, especially those who depend on the support of other people to have a livable life.

METHODS

This study is qualitative and exploratory, focusing on the changes driven by the COVID-19 pandemic, experiences, or perceptions of health rationing in crises, and the relationship between intersectional inequalities and disability. We will use the lens of feminist, disability, and sociocultural theory to examine this phenomenon, to articulate the experiences of disabled people during the pandemic, and to explore the psychological and sociocultural impacts produced.

The data for this analysis come from 10 semi-structured online interviews with six participants, all with complex medical conditions or mothers of children with complex medical conditions, in the United States both before the pandemic in 2018 and during the pandemic in Spring 2021.[2] In the case of the mother/daughter duo who were interviewed together, both of them were disabled so the mother was interviewed both as a disabled person and as a mother of a disabled person (Table 1).

Interviews provide us with an understanding the lived experiences of other people and the meanings they make of those experiences, allowing for active and collaborative constructions of meaning (Seidman, 2006). The semi structured interview allows the interviewee to discuss topics without sticking to a rigid series of pre-formulated questions (Minayo, 2010). Averaging an hour and a half, the pre-pandemic interview focused on the experience of health care of these children (or adults reflecting on their childhood experiences, reflections on their bodies, disability experiences, work and schooling, accessibility, access to the health care system, and relationships). The second interview focused on change's participants experienced due to the pandemic. The pre-pandemic interviews contained questions such as "What was your relationship and experiences interacting with your/your child's doctors?" "Who are the significant people in your family that help you/your child?" The post-pandemic interviews contained questions such as:

Table 1. Sociodemographic Participants Characteristics.

Pseudonym	Disabled Person	Mother of Disabled Person	Age at Time of Second Interview	Race/ Ethnicity	Gender
Emily	X		30 years	White	Female
Sylvester	X		63 years	Black	Male
Ellen	X	X	60 years	White	Female
Denise		X	57 years	White	Female
Marta	X		29 years	White	Female
Willa		X	45 years	White	Female

"Did you have any economic issues caused by the pandemic? Additional costs? Job loss, salary cuts, and furloughs" and "What was your experience accessing the health care systems during the pandemic? Were there difficulties?"

The interviews were done virtually or in person by Dr Block or her research assistants, recorded with the consent of the participants, either through a consent form approved through either Stony Brook University or Western University research ethics procedures.[3] Participants were recruited through a children's hospital in the Northeastern United States, the Post-Polio Health Network, or via Facebook posts. Potential participants received letters or viewed social media posts describing the project, and they contacted coauthor Block if they wished to participate. This was a cross-disability sample and we did not solicit diagnosis information. All participants experienced weeks or months of hospitalization in their childhood requiring 24/7 skilled nursing and technologies for survival. For some this need was short-lived, but for others the need is a life constant for survival.

In 2021, all project participants were invited via email or phone to discuss their experiences of the pandemic, scheduled for convenience and performed on Zoom. The recordings were stored in the project's Western University One-drive to protect the privacy of the participants. After re-affirming consent, the participants answered the interviewer's (coauthor Lorandi's) questions (Table 2).[4]

The data analysis of the interviews was performed using thematic content analysis (Bardin, 2010). The recurrence of issues or experiences mentioned in the interviews was used as a criterion for identifying themes. These indicators were related to the research objectives and allowed the construction of different categories. The verbatim transcripts of the interviews were categorized from a focused reading to segment the data, focusing on areas of convergence and divergence of the results in order to connect threads and patterns among the excerpts within those categories (Seidman, 2006). The thematic analysis identified four main topics: (1) changes in daily life experiences, (2) impact on access to health care, (3) barriers, and possibilities for accessibility, and (4) expectations for a post-pandemic world.

Table 2. Characteristics of How the Interviews Were Conducted.

Name	Interviewed Pre Pandemic	Method of Communication	Interviewed Post-Pandemic	Method of Communication
Emily	X	In person	X	Virtually
Sylvester	X	Phone	X	Virtually
Ellen	X	In person	X	Virtually
Denise	X	Phone	X	Virtually
Marta	X	Phone	X	Virtually
Willa	X	In person	X	Virtually

RESULTS

The 2021 interviews unveil the impact that the pandemic had on the research participants, and revealed the interconnectedness of the process and the contextual production of disability. Different as they may be, the influences of the pandemic on participants' experience of complex medical conditions are all linked to sociocultural relations associated with larger economic and political forces. The interviews illustrate how the social construction of barriers mirrors how individualistic and meritocratic approaches influence the possibilities for access. During the pandemic, the challenge of making activities remote impacted the perception of access alternatives in various contexts. In the virtual work environment, for example, it was possible to reduce or eliminate locomotive, attitudinal, and architectural barriers to allow for the full participation of disabled people.

Mental Health and Coping Strategies

As a disability group, the people with complex medical conditions interviewed in this research require frequent medical care and often, depending on the characteristics of their diagnoses, require daily support to carry out their basic needs. Relevant topics brought up in the pre-pandemic interviews, included the construction of their identities and life experiences as disabled people. The Pandemic was not the first experience for them in being isolated, excluded, and treated differently. However, all the respondents described the effects of the pandemic on their mental health as challenging or negative due to social isolation, mentioning symptoms such as anxiety, depression, fatigue, and binge eating. Ellen and Emily Ladau are mother and daughter. Both are disabled and they opted to be interviewed together under their own names. Emily Ladau (2021) is an author and disability activist. Ellen explains that at the beginning of the pandemic, she felt:

> Definite concern, anxiety, umm definitely watching the news a lot then because everything new and newsworthy. And learning how to protect myself and my family. Following all the safety protocols as far as masking and definitely decreased outings to only essential things like the pharmacy and the grocery store. And increased ordering on amazon.

Willa is her daughter's primary caregiver. They live in a rural area and her daughter was not able to engage in as many school, work, or community activities as they might wish because of the barriers to accessing many programs in the place where they live. Willa's pandemic coping strategies included accessing reliable sources of information, reducing the amount of news, keeping social relationships online, and continuing to work. Willa says it is, "better in terms of not only was it very scary at first, but then people were kind of panicking about what was going to happen. And I'd try to find more information that came out and I think it was more..., it was easier to [feel in] control."

Sylvester is a black man born in Canada but currently living in the US. He had polio as a newborn, losing fine motor control and experiencing impaired mobility in one of his legs causing a great deal of pain throughout his life until it was amputated. He has a BA in human resources and an MA in mediation and arbitration. During the pandemic, he contracted COVID-19. A polio survivor surviving his second major pandemic, Sylvester discussed how important the contact and support of his children was during this time:

> Like they call me every day so no matter what I got, I got three awesome girls and one awesome son. I've been really, really blessed. You know, I meet people who say "that's gotta suck to have one leg." I'm like, "no, that's nothing dude I got. I got children that are out of this world. From give me polio any day than having children that ain't these." You know and like I said they call me every day; all I have to do is say hey and they're here you know. I mean they're in Florida and Colorado Springs, which is thousands of miles away. And they'll do anything for me.

Marta (pseudonym) is a journalist and poet. Since childhood she has been in and out of hospitals for surgery and research; her condition was rare, and the doctors studied it. Marta discusses how separation from people she cared about due to the pandemic caused her anxiety:

> Normally my way of coping for my concern for you is to keep you near me. And when you're worried about everyone in your life and you're not allowed to have them near you, there's this constant nervousness of "are they okay, where are they?" They could be in some sort of trouble, and I can't do nothing about it. Anxiety wheels in the back of the brain just spinning.

Marta coped with this situation by:

> (...) finding a way to make my way useful because I know that if this is a crisis for me, it's a ten times worse crisis for a lot of other people. And the thing that I can do is keep working so that whatever happens next, the work goes on...when the world picks up again, I want to be able to say "here's a book I made that you can read" or "finishing my master's degree" because I want to be contributing something.

Denise, mother to Erick, aged 23 in 2021, described how her family lived in fear of her son contracting COVID-19, applying stricter safety measures than they had used prior to the pandemic. She and another participant lost loved ones during the pandemic and had increased difficulties in coping with the deaths due to social isolation. She explains that his disorder is gradual, although it was sudden and very global when it first started at 13 months.

Work and Study Changes

In this section, we explore how participants work and school lives changed due to the pandemic. In addition, we discuss grief, isolation, and the uncertainties wrought by larger economic and technological forces. The theme of disability was interconnected in the participants' professional trajectory, as Sylvester reports about his professional journey:

> I used to repair musical instruments after I got out of high school, well after I got out of college I kind of took things a little bit more seriously. My dad used to repair musical instruments, and he taught me how to do It, and I did that for about 20 years and then post-polio syndrome kind of gave me a bit of a problem. And so, I had to kind of quit from that and said Well maybe I can be an HR manager. So, I got my bachelor's degree in HR, and I was working at Sears at that time as an HR manager. But they had me walking around a lot and I went like well, this isn't gonna work.

As post-polio syndrome resulted in Sylvester needing to switch careers, it provided him with experience in adapting his work as his body and life required it. Despite his ability to adapt, Sylvester acknowledges feelings of loss that accompanied his increasing loss of motor function.

> I pretty much lost that, that bothers me sometimes. Sometimes I go to pick something up and it goes right out of my hand. You know those things bother you, you know, because I'm kind of an old fashion kind of guy, that wanted to support his family, and I'm not really able to do that much anymore. So, um I'm more of a people person than anything, yeah, I can't do any of that stuff anymore.

During the COVID-19 pandemic Sylvester was able to continue working remotely in his job in mediation and arbitration.

The ease with which participants adapted their communication and social relations strategies to the public health measures implemented during the pandemic varied dramatically. Digital media for social participation and "bed-space activism" has been used for a long time by disabled people, especially those with complex medical conditions requiring them to practice social distancing (Piepzna-Samarasinha, 2018). For some of our participants such as Emily and Marta, the increased use of technologies imposed by the pandemic was not new. Marta states: "we always sort of did it that way because my co-editor and I, we're both disabled so we were online for accessibility reasons before we were online for Covid reasons." Similarly, Emily states that: "I'm a communications consultant. So, I do a lot of writing, editing, social media management, website management, things like that. All with a focus on disability. So, that is something that I've pretty much always been doing virtually anyway so it wasn't a big change."

On the other hand, for those who were new to working or studying online reported limitations such as lack of engagement in activities, and fatigue regarding the use of technologies. Denise reports about her son that "he's not engaged by some of the big advocacy meetings and some of the Zoom's because he can't interact with anybody now, and he'll still sometimes find some things boring if he's just kind of sitting there and he's not able to move around the room or see people."

Denise's commentary evokes the importance of creativity in adapting pandemic-era activities to the digital reality for her son. This ability is needed to ensure accessible entertainment, study, and work solutions: "So it was just a matter of trying to think outside the box now and figure out how to, how to, keep him engaged in other ways." However, she experienced guilt and frustration in her attempts to adapt her son's routine to the virtual context: "So he was really like out and about on the go and everything. And, you know, I just I just felt awful. So, I decided to try to replicate something for him by Zoom."

Changes in the Communications and Social Relations

As a result of the public health measures implemented during the COVID-19 pandemic, many participants' ways of communicating and relating to one another changed significantly. Participants discussed the centrality of technology in communication and the maintenance of social relationships, mentioning the increased use of video conferencing platforms and social networks during the pandemic. In the interviews before the pandemic both Sylvester and Marta emphasized that they were very outgoing people who enjoyed being with friends and family. During the pandemic the effects of social isolation were significant and though connecting virtually proved useful, it did not supply all the needs of our participants' social relationships. As Marta discusses this loss. "I think for us it was not seeing people at times when we normally would. Like my household is normally very communal. People come in and out, we like, we have a lot of friends in and out. I used to throw dinner parties very frequently."

In contrast, Denise discussed her more isolated reality before the pandemic, because of the need for care of her son Erick: "And because Erick's health problems have created situations for us where, sort of, over time, we're kind of shut-in and locked out." Participation in FaceBook groups and engagement activism on behalf of children with complex medical conditions helped her to feel less isolated. Similarly, Willa reports that, as she lives in a rural area, social media networks have been essential to connect with other mothers of children with the same diagnosis as her daughter:

> Well, we live in a very rural area. So, there's not a big population period and there is certainly not a big population of special needs parents. So, it's just a way to connect and you know it's just a great source of information...My daughter has been able to keep in touch. She can't use it herself but I can get it to show her pictures of people she went to school with and things like that. So, it gives her an opportunity to see them and see their kids and stuff like that. So, it's a great resource for us. It keeps us from being isolated, I think.

For Denise and Erick, remote conversations were important with disability community:

> ...video and audio technology have really stepped in. You know, to kind of plug the gaps, you know, make life better for them...I've heard other disability activists talk about this, too, and seen articles. I mean, people with disabilities have been talking or meeting, right, to do work remotely and do other things remotely. And are not they're not always able to get out all the time because their health issues and to go to meetings in person and travel and things like that. And so so ironically, I think there are ways in which Erick feels just as engaged in his community as he did in the past. It's just it's just differently.

The importance of family and friends emerge as a significant theme in both pre-pandemic and pandemic interviews. As Ellen said in her pre-pandemic interview: "families were a definite support. More my side, just because I feel that they have more understanding of the life of disability. But we have great friends who pitch in and brought us food when we needed it during postdoc periods or offered help in other ways. You know we have a lot of friends."

All respondents brought up significant changes in their experiences with communication and social relationships during the pandemic. Video calls and social media networks were most mentioned by the participants. Ellen highlighted new habit, a weekly Zoom, instituted in her family during the pandemic. In addition, Denise relates that the digital media has enabled her son to solidify relationships with his extended family since they live far away, and Erick cannot travel because of accessibility barriers. Several participants echoed these sentiments, talking at length about changes in technology use and Zoom fatigue. Marta reports that reliance on virtual rather than in-person communication during the pandemic was difficult because she was going through a period of mourning following her mother's death. During lockdown, she did not have the option of asking her friends to visit her when she was mourning: "I couldn't call one of my friends and be like hey come over and sit with me while I'm sad for a while because I don't know how to process this right now. And you can't comfortably sit in silence with someone over the phone or over zoom or whatever."

Adaptation and Access

Struggles adapting to changing circumstances and advocating for access were discussed by participants in both sets of interviews. This included general adaptation to their changing bodies, making their houses accessible, advocating for medical procedures, dealing their aftermath etc. Such experiences may have created a form of disability-specific expertise that made adjusting to pandemic realities a little easier. In his pre-pandemic interviews Sylvester discussed adapting his routine when his leg was amputated and how his disability expertise enabled him to adapt faster to a variety of conditions throughout his life:

> I figured it out. I figured whatever, you know. One of the good things about it is that you learn to adjust faster, you know. Like I said, they amputated my leg three years ago and I was bopping around pretty fast, because I already knew how to learn, I would teach myself how to walk and stuff, so. I was pretty good at adjusting to whatever.

Unique disability experiences enabled our participants to adapt to the new public health protocols of the pandemic. We can identify the inequalities implicated in the process of adapting to the measures, since the condition and complexity of disability singularities may require extra effort to invent new embodied techniques. In addition, the risk group status of people with complex medical conditions was motivation for the participants to strictly follow all recommendations. Ellen says, "definitely just being mindful and following public health guidelines." Denise expressed living with constant fear and anxiety of her disabled son becoming infected: "We were extremely worried about Erick, in particular, catching it, so we took a lot of extreme measures to stay safe with him. We rarely went anywhere, I think, for months at one point."

Marta's discussed her experience as wheelchair user, always below the field of vision of others, so people approached her without maintaining a safe distance. This happened before the pandemic, but when distancing became a safety practice, such experiences were highlighted and extremely frustrating "The only time I would scream and holler and throw a fit is if you weren't wearing a mask and almost walked into me." All the participants discussed how masking became essential to fighting COVID-19. Sylvester – a Polio survivor – pointed out that "I'm having problems breathing. I gotta figure out a way to do this and then they said well, you could wear a face shield, and that's what I did."

A similar situation occurred regarding Willa's daughter's adaptation to wearing the mask: "she won't wear a mask. So, I don't take her in the grocery store anymore right now, until the mask mandate is lifted, obviously. And when we go to the doctors, when we get on top of the things, the doctor has to tell them that she won't wear a mask." In contrast, Erick's experience with wearing masks was described by his mother as positive, "Erick was OK wearing masks. It wasn't a big deal, and...I sewed some, and then when cloth masks became more available to buy, I bought him stuff once with Darth Vader."

Participants described social isolation as the security measure that most impacted them, as explained by Sylvester:

> Staying at home and staying away from people, I didn't really like it. I wanted to go places and do things with people. You know, I don't, I don't know if we're better off staying away from each other than having this stupid virus sometimes. We're people that need to be next to each other all the time, you know. And then there's people like, I say, have mental health issues, and you're keeping them away from other people, is that a good idea? I mean, from what I understand, suicide has gone way up, you know.

When the disabled person needed personal assistance to ensure their survival, pandemic distancing measures needed to be adapted to allow for a team of health providers to frequent the home. Denise relates her experience of adapting to frequent staff presence in her home. The use of masks in her home was constant, as was the substitution of paper towels in place of cloth towels and the use of sanitizers.

The Barriers and Possibilities of Accessibility

Even before the pandemic, the participants reported difficulties in accessing technologies that would enable learning and social participation. Denise describes the struggle to get appropriate assistive technology for her son's communication. Everything was very expensive and the school did not support and encourage the boy to develop his language: "things cost so much money, so you don't have one computer at home and one at school and the list of complications goes on and on. So, we finally made some progress with this when the eye camera maker got involved, and Medicaid paid for the devices." The barriers caused by the lack of equipment compatible with people's needs become apparent through these interviews, and we also note that accessibility and well-being are interconnected throughout the life trajectories of the disabled participants interviewed.

In a pre-pandemic interview, when asked about what would improve her life, Emily states:

> I think the point is better access. That's why I do what I do. I wouldn't change myself. I wouldn't change my life. You know obviously, we are really social model around here, but I think probably the best way to illustrate it is I just recently won an award for my work, so we were at the event celebrating that...then two days later, I was on a date with a guy at the scene when we were supposed to meet on a street at the city, and instead, we met on the subway platform...because the elevator was broken, and I was stuck down there. So I ended up being carried upstairs by the FDNY. I'd appreciate better access.

Emily's activist approach focuses on a more accessible environment and acceptance of one's own body. Ellen also mentioned access in their pre-pandemic interview, reporting that she has moved house 4 times and had to make several modifications in every area of the house to reduce barriers for herself and her daughter. With the advent of the pandemic, access at home became a central aspect reported by participants. Some of them found that their homes were too small to move around in a wheelchair or to have nurses around all the time. Some participants, Like Ellen, had the means to modify their homes to meet their physical needs and enable strict adherence to the pandemic safety measures, others made do with what they had.

Thus, in the discussion about accessibility, the participants highlighted the complexity of the factors that influence accessibility, for example, Willa reports a severe drop in the number of available services and supports and subtle changes in attitude as disabled children transition into adulthood:

> I think that people with disability if they are kids, it's easy to garner, not sympathy, that is not the word, I think empathy and appreciation. People want to help. People want to be more open to the things that they are going through. But as they get older and transition into adulthood, it's not quite as publicly appealing and the thing is that if you are not careful, everyone, the medical industry, push them to the side a little bit. So, we had to protect against that. The school system starts to, even as they get into high school, the school system pulls away. You know they just don't receive the level of attention and care that they did when they were children.

And virtual supports were no substitute for in person, leaving Willa with the responsibility for her child's engagement and well-being during the pandemic.

Remote work has always been a disability activist agenda item. During their pandemic interviews Emily, Marta and Sylvester noted how workplaces finally acknowledged that working remotely is an efficient and viable possibility for the inclusion of disabled people in the labor market. Marta reports this reality in her interview:

> That's ridiculous, but a small good thing that sticks, that we've learned out of this is that there are more accessibility options. If everyone can do their job over zoom and do college over zoom, then there are no reasons for us to be excluded from spaces anymore because these options are here now. I know a lot of people who have tried to get jobs and their jobs have been like we can't accommodate you that way, we can't let you work from home, we don't have the resources for that. Now we know that's a lie, because everyone did it, you figured it out. So, I hope that remains once all this is over that we can do more and we've proven to do more, so let's just do it.

Respondents discussed how the disability experience is intrinsically connected with the COVID-19 pandemic, Marta addresses this:

> Because of what I do for a living and disability work is my job, it became pretty clear to me quickly that this was going to become a disability issue. There were going to be people who couldn't get their vaccines because of their disabilities, there were going to be people who died because doctors didn't think they were worth saving, there were going to be disability specific long-term consequences to something like this. And I think there are going to be people who become a part of the disabled community because of this and sort of have to be walked through that because they weren't that yesterday, they were able bodied people when they went to sleep

> and they're not anymore. And they have all those preconceptions that able bodied people have about what disabled lives are like and what our lives are worth and what it means to be this way but they don't have the history and the context to comfortably to sit in that. So, I think there's going to be a lot of long-term work in how do we unpack this in a healthy way, that doesn't harm the community more than it has to.

Experiences With Health Care Before and During the Pandemic

All respondents described important experiences with the health system throughout their lives such as surgeries, frequent appointments, and hospitalizations. Marta reports that when she was young, she stayed at the hospital periodically for short and long stays during her childhood:

> ...it didn't occur to me that this wasn't how everyone spent their summer. What I remember about it is like the boredom. I'm like, I want to do things that I wasn't allowed to do...this is summer and I have stuff I want to do...But what do you mean? I can't go do all the stuff I want to do because you just broke my legs or whatever. Like, it doesn't occur to you that surgery is a big deal and you're a little bit older and then suddenly you're like, oh, wait a minute, what?

Ellen discussed one of Emily's childhood surgeries in which, due to her own disability, Ellen needed family support while taking care of Emily in the hospital.

> She was in a halo for 3.5 months after that procedure. For me, with disability, it was definitely a struggle. I needed a lot of family assistance while we were living at the hospital. My niece, who was living in the NYC at the time, came in to help me shower at the hospital while my husband was sleeping, because we were taking shifts. We have never left her alone in the hospital at any time when she was inpatient because there'd just been too many issues.

All participants expressed fears of being separated from family if someone needed hospitalization. These concerns were motivated by fears of not having their needs met without family support, the risk of exposing themselves to COVID-19, and not receiving adequate care. The interviews show that the participants were preoccupied with health care rationing due to the pandemic, that essential items might be rerouted to supply hospitals, and concerns about how fair and accessible their treatment would be if they/their loved one became sick and needed any other kind of care, even if not related to COVID-19. Emily shares, "I was concerned especially regarding the fact that we're both disabled. I was worried about early conversations about health care rationing and generally concerned about how we would fare if we became sick or needed any other kind of care."

Moreover, because of the concern about contagion, most participants reported that they limited medical procedures, appointments and therapies during the COVID-19 pandemic. Denise decided to reduce her son's team of caregivers and health professionals: "I mean, the risk window, you know, we just we got to minimize this."

Telemedicine allowed for some continuity of the treatment routine, though two participants noted it was less effective. Participants expressed discontent with pandemic health policy leaders. As Emily stated: "they left people with disabilities to figure it out for ourselves and help each other when the government wasn't helping us." Similarly, Sylvester expressed his opinion about lack of preparedness for the pandemic, and also his personal experience when he contracted COVID-19:

> I think a lot of the people got sick and died because they didn't have the right care and the money, and we just weren't prepared for it .... When I started getting sick, I went to the hospital right and this was nearby. This was kind of like in the middle of March when I, so I was hearing about it, and I was thinking was just like other flus that they say come over here and that's it. But obviously it wasn't.

Expectations for the Post-Pandemic World

At the time of the pandemic interviews, many of the participants were already vaccinated or scheduled to be vaccinated. When asked about their expectations for a "post-pandemic" world, or a world in which security restrictions are relaxed, they reported anxiety about being in crowds and social situations. Regarding accessibility, the participants hope that decision-makers now realize how easy it is to make things accessible, to let people work from home, to let people Zoom into events, and to make everyone feel included with the new digital tools. As Marta points out, "What I hope we're going to see is that people realize how easy it is to make things accessible. People realized how easy it is to let people work from home, to let people zoom into events, to make everyone more included. Because we've had to do it, so now we know it's possible."

Our participants hope it will be possible to keep doing accessible events, work routines, and schooling and that leaders will be more prepared for future health crises. Emily states:

> I really just want people to be more conscious about what they think about disability and how they understand disability and the rest of the world. Especially because Covid is leading to more disabilities, you never know what could happen and cause you to become disabled if you're not. We need to focus on creating a world where, if something like this happens again, we are not so confused and uncertain by what it means to grapple with disability and with health issues that we end up causing more harm.

DISCUSSION

The data showcased here illuminates the complexity of the relationship between disability experiences and the pandemic context. The disabled people and mothers interviewed felt at higher risk due to ableism in health policies and getting their health needs met. Understanding ableism as structural, our research results demonstrate the impact of the pandemic on the lives of the disabled people with complex medical conditions, whether in their schooling, work, care, physical and mental health, and social relationships.

Historically, social participation has been denied to disabled people, and one of the elements that hinder social participation is ableism (Mello, 2016). Even before the pandemic social isolation was a routine for many disabled people, including several of our participants, given the numerous barriers they had to accessing public environments. However, participation is a human need, and one of the aspects that most affected the mental health of our participants was isolation from community, friends, and family. Other researchers had similar findings; Wickenden et al. (2021) pointed out that their participants experienced lockdowns as exacerbating mental and emotional stress, limiting relational coping strategies, as people lost access to their social networks.

Many of our participants practiced measures to decrease the risk of contagion in the pandemic period, but many of the pandemic safety measures was more difficult for them. For example, social distancing was impossible for those who relied on personal assistance and skilled nursing, and the use of the masks was difficult for those with breathing issues. Pandemic safety measures must take bodily differences into account, requiring inclusive and collective solutions. The pandemic experiences reported by our participants reveals the cruelty of an individualistic, as opposed to a collective, formulations of health, where our attitudes, about masking for example, impact everyone's life (Kochhar, 2020). The COVID-19 pandemic-imposed restrictions, so carefully followed by our participants have been rejected by large portions of the US population, revealing society's ableism, making the barriers to access more visible. Participants repeatedly emphasized that remote access to events, courses, and lectures were routinely denied to them pre-pandemic, and they hope that access does not disappear when the pandemic ends. Aydos et al. (2021) emphasize how strategies applied by employers during the pandemic increased access.

The complexity of access should not be described with simplistic inclusion/exclusion dichotomies. Rather, accessibility is a process that is always relational, situational, and the consequence of improvisational and ever-changing arrangements (Kafer, 2013; Mello & Gaverio, 2019; Piepzna-Samarasinha, 2018). Unfortunately, our participants' narratives indicate that the responsibility for ensuring access to workplaces, schools, and social activities remain with individuals. They report that the process of guaranteeing access, which should be generally available on a societal level, remains an individual concern, not a collective and interdependent responsibility. This is consistent with Mello and Gavério's (2019), discussion of how the social production of disability is also "naturalized" by the dominant knowledge. Meanings that are attributed to disability remain organized in a system of apparently binary oppositional notions of disability and ability, despite the assertions by disability justice activists and Crip theorist that the realities of disabled life are far more complex and interdependent.

Five of the six participants are women, and from an intersectional feminist perspective this category permeates the experiences and realities of the disabled people interviewed. For example, Marta recounts that "I didn't have a doctor ask me if I was having sex until I was twenty-five and married." This account reflects a simplistic conception of a disabled woman as an "eternal child" who needs care, even as an adult (Dantas et al., 2014). In addition, all three caregivers interviewed were mothers. Mello and Nuernberg (2012) report that, in our society, care work is exploited and invisibilized, usually the responsibility of women.

The phenomenon of health care rationing and discrimination against disabled bodies was brought up by participants Emily, Ellen, Denise, and Sylvester in the interviews. When analyzed from the feminist perspective of disability and the ethics of care, the situations of disabled people with complex medical conditions come into sharper focus: according to ableist perspectives, these subjects have unproductive bodies and lives less worthy of being saved (Ferreira & Lopes, 2021). This provokes reflection about which lives supposedly deserve immediate health treatment and eventually will have the privilege of being mourned, as became evident when policies in response to the pandemic are implemented "for all" without regard for groups in need of accommodation. According to Guidry-Grimes et al. (2020) while catastrophic health emergencies require an immediate response, it is important to reflect on how ableism can distort priorities for care in emergencies.

Dire economic impacts of the pandemic were not highlighted by these participants. The six participants who agreed to be interviewed during the pandemic were generally highly educated, and several were employed in professional positions. Those who had the time and willingness to talk to us were likely in a more secure financial position than other people during this time, including our larger pool of participants who interviewed with us before the pandemic. Emily and her mother Ellen acknowledged how privileged they felt having economic stability. This has not been the experience of many, especially in the global south. For example, Das et al. (2021) reported that disabled people in Bangladesh experienced persistent poverty and an inability to secure a stable livelihood in this time.

CONCLUSION

People at the intersections of many identities are at the highest risk during COVID-19 and other pandemics, a reality that has a major impact on the disability community. The long-term implications of the pandemic are still unknown, just as it was not possible to understand the long-term effects of the polio pandemic on individual and social bodies until decades after that pandemic ended. However, we know that countless people are experiencing the onset of new disability, either directly due to COVID-19 virus or as a secondary result of trauma and loss. Thus, it is important to consider the long-term impacts of the pandemic, new disabled bodies with needs that we cannot predict in the long term, the long-haulers.

Our participants pointed out the importance of policymakers and service providers in health services industries incorporating strategies to reduce ableism in health care provision, rationing, and other forms of decision-making. They highlighted the necessity of including leaders with disability in building public policy for disabled people, ensuring that their needs for access and safety are met. They emphasize the importance of thinking about long-term supports for newly disabled people who will continue to experience the effects of the COVID-19 pandemic. New services and interventions will need to be designed keeping in mind the priorities and challenges of disabled people, and their need for support. In addition, adequate education and employment opportunities for disabled people must be ensured, while continuing to expand access options that were available throughout the lockdown. Future safety plans must include everyone, especially our most vulnerable communities: those with food and housing insecurity, without adequate health insurance or employment, racialized communities, women, transgender people, indigenous communities, immigrant communities, and disabled people.

In conclusion, this study allowed us to understand the experience of six participants with disabilities, before and during the pandemic. The results and discussions presented relate to this sample and are not generalizable, though they are consistent with other research collected during this time. We recommend that further studies be carried out in this area, especially in consideration of the "post-pandemic" context and the long-term consequences of COVID-19.

ACKNOWLEDGMENTS

We would like to acknowledge research assistants who helped with interviews: Julie Maury and Alexandra Wagner and transcribed the recordings: Rebecca DePasquale, Daryn Osman, and Shaela Khan. We thank Nancy Speller and Joan Headley for invaluable assistance framing the research project and recruiting participants for "Aging Out of Children's Hospitals." We enact this project to honor the memory of Nick Dupree.

NOTES

1. Mothers were interviewed when communication barriers and intellectual disability prevented their children from doing so.
2. Emily and Ellen, mother and daughter, chose to be interviewed together both before and during the pandemic, but they answered each question separately.
3. Author Block moved from Stony Brook University to Western University and the research ethics permissions were transferred during the course of this research.
4. Regarding the use of pseudonyms: the Letter of Information and Consent states that, unless the participant chooses otherwise, they will be given a pseudonym and their personal information will be kept private. Participants chose whether to use a pseudonym or use their own name. Some who were public figures opted for using their own name. In some cases, we confirmed the choice in subsequent communication.

REFERENCES

Aydos, V., Navarini, D., & Oliveira, B. (2021). The paradox of "remote working" in COVID-19 pandemic times: Disability, inclusion, and accessibility in Brazil. *Disability Studies Quarterly*, *41*(3). https://doi.org/10.18061/dsq.v41i3.8359

Bardin, L. (2010). *Análise de conteúdo* [Content analysis]. Ed 70.

Berger, Z. D., Evans, N. G., Phelan, A. L., & Silverman, R. D. (2020). COVID-19: Control measures must be equitable and inclusive. *The BMJ*, *368*(September 2001), 19–20. https://doi.org/10.1136/bmj.m1141

Block, P., & Diallo, S. (2020). Activism, anthropology and disability studies in times of austerity. *Current Anthropology 61*(21), S68–S75. https://doi.org/10.1086/705762

Block, P., Pereira, E. L., Mello, A. G., & Sakellariou, D. (2021). Introduction to the special issue: Disability and Covid-19. *Disability Studies Quarterly*, *41*(3). https://doi.org/10.18061/dsq.v41i3.8440

Ciciurkaite, G., Marquez-Velarde, G., & Brown, R. L. (2021). Stressors associated with the COVID-19 pandemic, disability, and mental health: Considerations from the Intermountain West. *Stress and Health: Journal of the International Society for the Investigation of Stress*, *23*, 231–241. https://doi.org/10.1002/smi.3091

Dantas, T. C., Silva, J. S. S., & Carvalho, M. E. P. (2014). Entrelace entre gênero, sexualidade e deficiência: Uma história feminina de rupturas e empoderamento. *Revista Brasileira de Educação Especial*, *20*(4), 555–568. https://doi.org/10.1590/S1413-65382014000400007

Das, A. S., Bonny, F. A., Mohosin, A. B., Rashid, S. F., & Hasan, M. T. (2021). Co-exploring the effects of Covid-19 pandemic on the livelihood of persons with disabilities in Bangladesh. *Disability Studies Quarterly*, *41*(3). https://doi.org/10.18061/dsq.v41i3.8377

Diniz, D., Barbosa, L., & Santos, W. R. (2009). Deficiência, direitos humanos e justiça. *Sur. Revista Internacional de Direitos Humanos*, *6*(11). https://doi.org/10.1590/S1806-64452009000200004

Ferreira, C., & Lopes, P. (2021). Deficiências e adoecimento crônico: Permanências e atualizações trazidas pelo coronavírus. *ANPOCS Boletim Cientistas Sociais*, *35*, 651–655.

Fietz, H. (2019). The work of care. *Somatosphere*. http://somatosphere.net/2019/the-work-of-care.html/

Fine, M., & Glendinning, C. (2005). Dependence, independence or inter-dependence? Revisiting the concepts of 'care' and 'dependency'. *Ageing & Society*, *25*, 601–621

Gesser, M., Block, P., & Nuernberg, A. H. (2019). Participation, agency, and disability in Brasil: Transforming psychological practices into public policy from a human rights perspective. *Disability and the Global South*, *6*(2), 1772–1791.

Guidry-Grimes, L., Savin, K., Stramondo, J. A., Reynolds, J. M., Tsaplina, M., Burke, T. B., & Fins, J. J. (2020). Disability rights as a necessary framework for crisis standards of care and the future of health care. *Hastings Center Report*, *50*(3), 28–32. https://doi.org/10.1002/hast.1128

Kafer, A. (2013). *Feminist, queer, crip*. Indiana University Press.

Kochhar, R. (2020). Disability and dismantling: Four reflections in a time of Covid-19. *Anthropology Now*, *12*(1), 73–75. https://doi.org/10.1080/19428200.2020.1761213

Ladau, E. (2021). *DEmystifying disability: What do know, what to say, and how to be an ally*. Penguin Random House.

Mello, A. G. (2016). Deficiência, incapacidade e vulnerabilidade: Do capacitismo ou a preeminência capacitista e biomédica do Comitê de Ética em Pesquisa da UFSC. *Ciênc. Saúde Coletiva*, *21*(10), 3265–3276.

Mello, A. G., & Gaverio, M. A. (2019). Facts of cripness to the Brazilian: Dialogues with avatar, the film. *Anuário antropológico*, *44*(1), 43–65.

Mello, A. G., & Nuernberg, A. H. (2012). Gênero e deficiência: Interseções e perspectivas. *Revista Estudos Feministas*, *20*(3), 635–655. https://doi.org/10.1590/S0104-026X2012000300003

Minayo, M. C. S. (2010). *O desafio do conhecimento: Pesquisa Qualitativa em Saúde* (12th ed.). Hucitec-Abrasco.

Mingus, M. (2022). You are not entitled to our deaths: Covid, abled supremacy & interdependence. https://leavingevidence.wordpress.com/2022/01/16/you-are-not-entitled-to-our-deaths-Covid-abled-supremacy-interdependence/

Pettinicchio, D., Maroto, M., Chai, L., & Lukk, M. (2021). Findings from an online survey on the mental health effects of Covid-19 on Canadians with disabilities and chronic health conditions. *Disability and Health Journal*, *14*(3), 101085. https://doi.org/10.1016/j.dhjo.2021.101085

Piepzna-Samarasinha, L. L. (2018). *Care work: Dreaming disability justice*. Arsenal Pulp Press.

Rohwerder, B., Njungi, J., Wickenden, M., Thompson, S., & Shaw, J. (2021). "This time of Corona has been hard": People with disabilities' experiences of the Covid-19 pandemic in Kenya. https://doi.org/10.19088/IF.2021.005

Seidman, I. (2006). *Interviewing as qualitative research: A guide for researchers in education and the social sciences* (3rd ed.). Teachers College Press.

Tomasini, F. (2019). *Vulnerable bodies: New directions in disability studies*. Palgrave Pivot. https://doi.org/10.1057/978-1-137-31899-2

Wickenden, M., Shaw, J., Thompson, S., & Rohwerder, B. (2021). Lives turned upside down in Covid-19 times: Exploring disabled people's experiences in 5 low-and-middle income countries using narrative interviews. *Disability Studies Quarterly*, *41*(3). https://doi.org/10.18061/dsq.v41i3.8375

World Health Organization. (2020). Mental health and Covid-19. https://www.euro.who.int/en/health-topics/health-emergencies/coronavirus-Covid-19/technical-guidance/mental-health-and-Covid-19

PART II

IMPLICATIONS OF THE PANDEMIC FOR PEOPLE WITH DISABILITIES IN EDUCATIONAL AND WORKPLACE SETTINGS

Chapter 7

INEQUALITY IN THE SCHOOLING EXPERIENCES OF DISABLED CHILDREN AND THEIR FAMILIES DURING COVID-19

Rachel Elizabeth Fish, David Enrique Rangel, Nelly De Arcos and Olivia Friend

ABSTRACT

Purpose: *In this chapter, we examine how the schooling experiences of disabled children have changed during COVID-19, how families' engagement, advocacy and support of their children have shifted during the pandemic, and how race, class, and other axes of inequality shape these processes.*

Methods/Approach: *We used a semi-structured interview protocol with families of disabled children, asking them about their experiences with their children's schools before and during the pandemic. We analyzed the interview data using "flexible coding" and the constant comparative method.*

Findings: *COVID-19 has had wide-reaching effects on disabled children's schooling experiences, yet these effects varied, particularly at the intersections of disability with race, class, linguistic status, and gender. Remote learning and other pandemic-related changes to schools exacerbated extant inequalities in children's educational experiences, as well as in families' ability to effectively advocate for their children in school.*

Implications/Value: *This research provides important information about how the pandemic has exacerbated inequality at the intersection of disability, race, and other axes of inequality. Moreover, it provides a lens to examine ableism and other systems of oppression in schools. The findings have crucial policy implications, pointing to the necessity of equitably allocated, high quality,*

Disability in the Time of Pandemic
Research in Social Science and Disability, Volume 13, 135–153

ISSN: 1479-3547/doi:10.1108/S1479-354720230000013008

inclusive educational services for disabled students, as well as to the need for special education policy that does not rely on individual family advocacy to allocate appropriate services.

Keywords: Disability; race; education; special education; inequality; advocacy

The COVID-19 pandemic has impacted the educational experiences of children around the world through multiple pathways, including school closures, remote learning, and the trauma of illness and death of loved ones. Yet the pandemic has not had uniform effects, as research demonstrates broad inequalities in the pandemic by race, class, and disability (Abedi et al., 2021; Maroto et al., 2021). This is particularly true in education. Disabled,[1] low-income, and racially marginalized children have had less access to in-person instruction – and when in remote schooling, less access to regular, live instruction – than their White, higher-income, and nondisabled peers, due to district offerings, staffing constraints, variation in health and safety concerns, and access to high-speed internet (Belsha et al., 2020; Landivar et al., 2021; Patrick et al., 2021; Szabo, 2021; Zimmer & Zimmerman, 2020, p. 1). These and other pandemic-driven disparities have accumulated and exacerbated extant inequalities by race, socioeconomic status, and disability, such that researchers expect achievement gaps to grow (Bailey et al., 2021; Easop, 2021; Kuhfeld et al., 2020).

Practitioners, researchers, and policymakers consider parent engagement with schools to be crucial for children's academic achievement, particularly for marginalized families, despite evidence that schools perceive and respond differently to such engagement by race and class (Carreón et al., 2005; Lareau & Horvat, 1999; Miller et al., 2016). For disabled students, family engagement, advocacy, and support are of particular importance. Federal law requires parent/guardian involvement in educational decision-making for these students – yet parent resources and strategies for this involvement, as well as schools' responses to families, occurs inequitably by race/ethnicity and class (Blum, 2015; Voulgarides, 2021; Wilson, 2015). During COVID-19, disabled children and their families have experienced isolation from educational and medical professionals, and expanded expectations for involvement and support in their children's schooling (Greer & Pierce, 2021). Examining these families' experiences during COVID-19, with attention to the intersection (as conceptualized by Black Feminist scholars (Crenshaw, 1991)) of disability with race, class, gender, and language is critical to understanding how the pandemic has shaped patterns of inequality. In this chapter, we examine (1) how COVID-19 has shaped the schooling experiences of disabled children through the lenses of their families, (2) how families' engagement, advocacy, and support of their children shifted during the pandemic, and (3) how race/ethnicity, gender, language, and class shape these processes.

INEQUALITY IN THE SCHOOLING EXPERIENCES OF DISABLED STUDENTS

Prior to COVID-19, the role of special education in the production and maintenance of existing inequalities was becoming more apparent. Disability is a key axis of inequality, and disabilities qualifying for special education services are both inequitably deployed and have inequitable effects. Administrative data show racial, socioeconomic, and linguistic disparities in special education receipt (US Department of Education, 2020).

Robust analyses suggest complex relations between disability and other social categories, whereby socially advantaged children have greater access to disability diagnosis and special education services than their peers, particularly for higher-status, more advantageous categories of disability (Fish, 2019). Special education services provide important support, legal protection, and educational benefits for many students, but these services can also stigmatize and exclude students from their peers, reduce access to higher-level content, and even depress academic outcomes (Owens & Jackson, 2016; Schwartz et al., 2021; Shifrer et al., 2013). Disabled children of color are more likely to be labeled with more exclusionary disability categories, with lower access to grade-level content and inclusive social experiences, and higher levels of stigma (Fish, 2019; Saatcioglu & Skrtic, 2019). Methodologically, few studies have been able to identify effects of special education. However, recent research has shown that for children diagnosed with learning disabilities, the most common disability in schools, special education has positive effects on achievement for all students except for Black students (Schwartz et al., 2021). Racially marginalized families report that their children with disabilities have many unmet needs (Iland et al., 2012). English learner students with disabilities have been left out of appropriate, inclusive schooling environments due to an "intersectional gap" in policies and practices for bilingual students and disabled students (Cioè-Peña, 2017). Research examining intersecting inequalities by disability, race, class, gender, language, and other axes of inequality is necessary to understand the schooling experiences of disabled children and special education's stratifying processes.

FAMILY ENGAGEMENT, ADVOCACY, AND SUPPORT OF DISABLED CHILDREN

Family engagement, advocacy, and support are particularly important for students with disabilities. Special education policy and practice are designed to respond to families' advocacy for their child's right to a free, appropriate, public education (Blum, 2015; Carey et al., 2020; Voulgarides, 2021). Families of children with disabilities often navigate complex medical and educational systems to support their children's education and well-being and manage stigma, creating a "burden of care" rooted in scarce resources and structural constraints (Green, 2007; Green et al., 2016). Because management of services and supports for disabled children is treated as the "personal responsibility" of families, who must advocate for their children as individualist consumers, these families are "propelled . . . to become vigilantes" to acquire expertise and resources (Blum, 2015, p. 32). Yet the same legal, medical, and educational structures that have positioned families in this role have also facilitated tensions between families' interests and those of disabled self-advocates, with conflict arising over perceptions of disability and special education services, family engagement and advocacy, and desirable educational outcomes (Carey et al., 2020).

Inequality in Family-School Interactions for Disabled Children

Mirroring broader evidence of inequality in families' school engagement, as well as schools' responses to parent involvement (Carreón et al., 2005; Lareau & Horvat, 1999; Miller et al., 2016), family engagement, advocacy, and support of children with disabilities is also shaped by – and shapes – inequality by race, class, and language (Blum, 2015; Voulgarides, 2021; Wilson, 2015). While the most privileged families can negotiate for special education outcomes that they believe address the needs of their children, socially marginalized families experience various barriers to advocacy and support of their disabled children (Lareau, 2003; Ong-Dean, 2009; Voulgarides, 2021). Families of color and low-income families are less likely than White and middle- or high-income families to have the types of cultural and social capital that educators respond to in Individualized Education Plan (IEP) meetings (Wilson, 2015). They also may feel uncomfortable voicing opinions in these meetings (Lian & Fontánez-Phelan, 2001), preventing them from acquiring desired outcomes for their children.

Family involvement can be constrained by jobs without flexible, autonomous, or predictable work hours, by language barriers, and by family-teacher power dynamics and deficit-based perceptions of families of color (Cooper, 2009; Valenzuela, 1999). For example, Latinx parents' involvement tends to focus more on interactions with their children that support achievement at home, which is largely invisible to teachers (Reese et al., 1995), who thus perceive Latinx families as having low academic expectations (Quiocho & Daoud, 2006).[2]

At the same time, this focus on involvement places greater emphasis on the role of parents and says little about the responsibility of schools to engage families. Prior research has found that schools in under-resourced communities do a poor job engaging parents and that outreach efforts, when not conducted in a culturally sensitive manner, exacerbate constraints on involvement (Rangel & Valdez, 2017; Valenzuela, 1999). In addition, research has shown that schools rebuff racial and ethnic minoritized parents' intervention efforts (Angell & Solomon, 2017), and when these parents demonstrate high levels of involvement, their children do not receive the same educational benefits as their non-minoritized peers (McNeal Jr, 1999).

Policies meant to equalize the receipt of special education services have deepened existing racial and ethnic inequalities (Voulgarides et al., 2021). Specifically, school officials tend to focus on procedural aspects to ensure compliance with the Individual with Disabilities Education Act that, in practice, makes it more difficult for racial and ethnic minoritized parents and children to receive services. Thus, racial and ethnic minoritized and low-income parents must overcome not only constraints on their involvement, but also systems and schools that may deny their autonomy (Evans, 2007).

EXAMINING THE PANDEMIC SCHOOLING EXPERIENCES OF DISABLED STUDENTS AND THEIR FAMILIES' RESPONSES

During COVID-19, children's schooling experiences have been broadly disrupted by remote learning, safety precautions in schools, disruptions to staffing, and the trauma of the pandemic more broadly, with marginalized children experiencing the worst of these effects (Bailey et al., 2021; Easop, 2021). Children with disabilities, in particular, have had less access to in-person or live instruction than their peers, and have been disproportionately affected by staffing shortages, as well as denied the services dictated in their IEPs (Zimmer & Zimmerman, 2020). Disability diagnosis evaluations have been delayed during the pandemic, restricting access to special education services (Bamberger et al., 2020). Families of children with disabilities have experienced heightened anxiety relative to families of nondisabled children, largely due to the loss of routines and support networks, as well as taking on an expanded role in their child's education and therapy while isolated at home (Asbury et al., 2021; Greer & Pierce, 2021). While some of these pandemic effects are becoming more apparent, we know much less about how families' experiences of disabled children's schooling varied by race, class, linguistic status, and other intersecting inequalities, nor do we know how the pandemic has affected families' interactions and advocacy with schools or support at home. Yet it is clear that the pandemic has had the potential to exacerbate extant inequalities and create opportunities for change. Therefore, we examine (1) how COVID-19 has shaped the schooling experiences of disabled children through the lenses of their families, (2) how families' engagement, advocacy, and support of their children shifted during the pandemic, and (3) how race, class, and other axes of inequality shape these processes.

METHODS

This study uses in-depth interviews with families of disabled children to explore their schooling experiences, as well as family advocacy and support, before and during COVID-19. Our convenience sample includes 26 participants from two ongoing research studies on the schooling experiences of children with disabilities in Wisconsin and New York City.[3] There are 21 different schools represented in the sample. Except for seven families, all of whom attend the same school, the rest of the students all attended different schools. Nine of the children attended segregated special education programs; these students were all Black or Latinx. Schools varied by governance (charter, private, public) and setting (rural, urban, suburban). All of the White students attended schools that were majority White

(n = 10), while of the 16 children of color, five attended predominantly White schools, and 11 attended predominantly non-White schools.

Recruitment materials were sent to families through public school teachers, through a listserv for parents of disabled children, and through organizations that support families of disabled children. Parents interested in participating in the study completed an initial interest and consent form and responded to questions about their demographic and family information. The full sample description can be found in Table 1.

The first, third, and fourth authors interviewed families using a semi-structured interview protocol (typically 45–60 minutes), including descriptions of the educational support their child received, if they felt the school met their child's needs, interactions with school staff, support of their child at home, and how they made decisions about their child's schooling during the pandemic – asking about these aspects of their lives prior to the pandemic, during the initial school closures in March of 2020, during the 2020–2021 school year, and during the 2021–2022 school year. The fourth author conducted all interviews with families that preferred Spanish. English interviews were transcribed by the first,

Table 1. Sample Description, as Reported by Families.

Child	*N* 26	Family	*N* 26	Household	*N* 26
Race/Ethnicity		Race/Ethnicity		Socioeconomic status (defined by Pew Household Income Calculator and eligibility for public assistance)	
Asian	1	Asian	1	Upper income	1
Black	7	Black	6	Middle income	13
Indigenous	2	Indigenous	2	Lower income	12
Latinx	6	Latinx	6	Location	
Multi-racial	1	Multi-racial	0	NYC	3
White	9	White	11	Wisconsin, large city	3
Gender		Relationship to child		Wisconsin, mid-sized city	2
Girls	5	Mother	22	Wisconsin, small city	3
Boys	21	Father	2	Wisconsin, suburb	11
One girl and one boy were identified as transgender by their parents. They are included in the gender counts above.		Grandmother	2	Wisconsin, town	1
Primary disability		Language		Wisconsin, rural	2
ADHD	3	English	23	Wisconsin, location not reported	1
Autism	13	Spanish	3		
Emotional-behavioral disorder	1				
Hearing impairment	1				
Orthopedic impairment	2				
Speech/language impairment	1				
Specific learning disability	5				

third, and fourth authors; Spanish interviews were transcribed and translated by a professional transcription and translation service.

To analyze how families made sense of their experiences with schooling before and during the pandemic, we used "flexible coding" (Deterding & Waters, 2018) in Dedoose software: first, we collaboratively indexed coded each transcript and wrote analytic memos summarizing the interview and exploring emergent topics and themes. Index coding involved chunking large amounts of data, which correspond to each section and question of the interview guide. For example, we had codes around the timeline and setting "pre-COVID-19," "spring 2020," and "2021–2022." We also created index codes to capture parents' feelings and experiences with educational concerns, life at home, and schooling experiences. To ensure consistency in coding across the authors, the second, third, and fourth author met weekly for four weeks, each coding the same interview transcript separately and then coming together to discuss our process. Through this process we worked out disagreements until the final week when the coverage of each index coded was similar across each of the authors. The first author reviewed all procedures through Dedoose and provided feedback throughout the initial coding process. Second, we developed an analytic code list, based on emergent themes from the index coding process. Third, we applied analytic codes (the first author monitored all transcripts for interrater reliability); finally, we explored coding validity, examined trends in the data, and refined theory in the memos. Analysis was ongoing during data collection, following the constant comparative method, so that insights could be incorporated and tested with new cases.

FINDINGS AND DISCUSSION

Disabled Children's Pre-COVID-19 Schooling

Pre-COVID-19 schooling experiences were decidedly mixed, with about half of the participants reporting that they were generally happy with their children's experiences, services, and progress in school, and the other half reporting that their children's needs were not being met by their school. Moreover, racial-ethnic differences in the data highlight the disparities in special education by race in the extant literature: while six out of the eight White families perceived their children's pre-COVID schooling and special education services positively, only three of the six Black families, and only one of the six Latinx families, described their children's schooling experiences similarly; the two Indigenous families did not perceive their children's schooling experiences positively overall.

Representative of families who were pleased with how their school supported their child was Savanna,[4] the Black mother of Eve, a fourth-grade girl with autism. She said:

> I feel like their support was not out of obligation, but because they really wanted to help her. Teachers are dealing with 27 kids or more in the classroom all day, but they still found a way to give her the right support and the right amount of attention.

Similarly, Heather, the White mother of Addyson, a fourth-grade girl with a learning disability, called her daughter's special education teacher "amazing … She's got lots of experience." Heather explained that her daughter was thriving in school, in part due to the many accommodations and individualized supports her daughter received since she was diagnosed with a disability. Heather's comment typified those of the families that were pleased with their children's schools and special education services.

Yet many other families felt that schools did not provide appropriate access and support for their children to succeed in school. Some families described basic accessibility issues, such as broken elevators that resulted in Leandro, a Latino 7th grader who uses a wheelchair due to his orthopedic impairment, not attending class for days on end. Many families described IEPs that were not set up to adequately support their children, such as Araceli, the Latina grandmother of Ernesto, an autistic third-grader. Expressing frustration about the mere 15-minute occupational therapy sessions, Araceli said, "what can they do in fifteen minutes?"

Beyond logistical and resource-constrained accessibility difficulties, many families said that schools "didn't have the toolbox" to provide appropriate instruction and support for their children, as Rebecca, the White mother of Micah, a Black first-grade boy with autism said. Rebecca recalled that the teachers "were just a deer in the headlights when he started school. They did not know how to meet his complex needs." Instead, he "just became the behavior problem." Tammy, the Black mother of Parker, an autistic eighth-grade boy, recalled that despite attending a segregated school for disabled students with more specialized and intensive educational supports, he was not working on appropriately modified academic content: "He didn't know what was going on … This [homework] is not modified because he can't do nothing." Tammy expressed her frustration that "a person-centered IEP should be tailored to the person … but everybody has the same IEP." Like Tammy, many families of children whose impairments affected their day-to-day living skills were frustrated by schools focusing on higher-level academic skills. Katie, the White mother of Avery, a third-grade girl with an orthopedic impairment, for example, asked,

> Why are we pushing her to do these things when she should be learning how to be with people in a social setting … Avery doesn't need to know that two plus two equals four. I mean, like that isn't going to be a skill that she's going to need as an adult, but she's going to need to say, "I'm cold, can I have a sweater?"

Special education practitioners and disabled self-advocates may disagree with these family perspectives on academic content. Nevertheless, families were frustrated with schools because they did not teach their children the skills they deemed essential.

Several disabled children and their families had particularly detrimental schooling experiences shaped by multiply marginalized social positions. For example, Patricia, the Indigenous grandmother of Casey, a transgender ninth-grade boy with a learning disability and a chronic health condition, described a long history of transphobia and racism from school board members and school administration, as well as bullying and physical aggression by peers, with no response by school staff to support her grandson. Linguistically marginalized families detailed unique difficulties at the "intersectional gap" (Cioè-Peña, 2017) of bilingualism and special education: Beatriz, the Spanish-speaking Latina mother of Alejandro, a kindergarten boy with autism, explained that she communicates with her son in Spanish and using some signs, but his teachers only used English to communicate with Alejandro, and maintained that he was fully non-speaking. The school's inability to use Spanish harmed Alejandro's experiences and learning in school, and also affected Beatriz's self-efficacy as a parent: "I can't speak English, and I can't take Spanish away from him because that's my language, and that's the way I communicate with him. I can't teach him a language that I don't know." Likely in part due to having no form of communication at school, Alejandro was often stressed and overstimulated at school, causing him to rely on behaviors for self-regulation. Teachers complained to Beatriz about Alejandro's self-regulation but provided little support to help him. Violeta, another Spanish-speaking Latina mother, also recalled her autistic son's teachers complaining about his behavior, yet they did not propose solutions or seem to "know how to support me or how to support my son."

"Remote Schooling is Not for Our Children."

For all but seven participants, COVID-19-era schooling was markedly worse for their children, primarily because, as Tammy said, "remote schooling is not for *our* children." Overall, disabled children and their families experienced new or exacerbated difficulties accessing appropriate instruction. Like pre-COVID schooling experiences, some of these issues were rooted in inaccessible technology, logistical difficulties, or inaccessible physical space. Jeffrey, the White father of Irene, a hard-of-hearing third-grade girl, described remote learning as essentially inaccessible for his daughter, despite trying different types of headphones and other assistive technology. The school relied on auto-captioning during live instruction, and Jeffrey attributed its inaccuracy to the "thick accents" in Wisconsin, teachers speaking too quickly and unclearly, as well as having multiple students with their microphones on. Leandro, the Latino boy with orthopedic impairment described above, needed adequate space to complete his physical therapy tasks during lock-downs, but even the hallway outside of their small apartment was inadequate.

Remote schooling was structured differently for children across the sample, from a full day of live remote instruction to predominantly asynchronous instruction. Both live and asynchronous instruction created new difficulties for children's access to instruction, and additional challenges for their families to navigate. Hours of live instruction required sustained attention to a computer screen with little opportunity for movement, which was particularly challenging for children with ADHD. The majority of the children in the study needed an adult sitting with them all day for live instruction, supporting them in using keyboards and touch screens, understanding directions, and maintaining attention. Meanwhile, when schools used primarily asynchronous instruction, most families described their role as "becoming the teacher." As Carleen, the Black mother of Harrison, an autistic fifth grader, said, "I'm not qualified for this shit. If I wanted to be a teacher, I would have went to school." Carleen, like many families, described feelings of inadequacy and concern for her son's progress because she was "winging it" without training in teaching special education.

About half of the families had perceived inadequate accommodations and modifications for their children prior to the pandemic, while nearly all of the participants described "nonexistent" differentiation (i.e., varying instructional methods and content to support students with different levels of skills, interests, and learning preferences) and accommodations during remote schooling. The overwhelming majority of families felt that teachers were "trying within the best of their ability," but said the schools "weren't focusing on children with special needs." Instruction was typically delivered to the whole class without the supports that would be available in-person. As a result, many families described their children being unable to keep up with the class work or experiencing distress, which resulted in resistance to virtual schooling.

While many children struggled to keep up without differentiated instruction or accommodations, other families described virtual instruction as "a joke," and that "they didn't do the curriculum." Therefore, families often described their children regressing academically and in other domains on their IEPs, due to inaccessible content, content and pedagogy that were too difficult, as well as content that was too easy. Remote schooling was particularly difficult for several linguistically marginalized families. Beatriz, introduced above, struggled with the "intersectional gap" of language and disability for Alejandro, and described difficulty supporting her son's remote instruction:

> I said, "How am I going to teach the child if I don't know anything? How am I going to work with him?" And as I told you, I live in a place where no one speaks Spanish, and all the documents were in English. So, I had to translate the documents [using online translators] and think about how I was going to do the programs with the child.

Unexpected Advantages of Remote Learning

A subset of participants described remote schooling as providing some positive changes for their children. For example, Stephani, the Black mother of Dontrell, an autistic eleventh-grade boy, said that remote-learning prevented Dontrell from becoming overstimulated, and that under her supervision, he could take more breaks during the day than he could in school. Dontrell felt the work was easier, leaving Stephani pleased with Dontrell's academic performance during remote instruction. Several children that attended segregated special education programs prior to the pandemic – or who were provided with small-group services for students with IEPs during the pandemic – received what families perceived as high-quality instruction. These programs are, by definition, exclusionary, and risk higher levels of stigma and lower academic expectations, yet particularly in the context of the pandemic, families often described these services as providing much-needed remediation and targeted instruction for their children.

For several families and their children, remote instruction offered a highly desirable escape, or simply a buffer, from schooling that they believed was harming their children. Melanie, a White mother of an autistic sixth-grade boy, Steven, described her child's teachers as bullies, and believed his special education services were inappropriate for him; when Steven attended remote schooling, she was able to monitor teachers' interactions with him, and buffer him from some of these effects. More dramatically, recall Rebecca, the White mother of Micah, an autistic Black boy, who believed that the school was not supporting her child at all. She called COVID-19 "the best thing that happened in kindergarten because it ended the year for him. He was euphorically happy that it was over. And so was I. I knew then and there, he would never return in person to that school." For some multiply-marginalized children, such as Ellie, a transgender girl with a learning disability, remote instruction offered some relief from micro-level racism or transphobia; her mother described Ellie's relief: "she's like, 'Oh, this is kinda nice. I don't have to be out around people and worry about if somebody knows I'm trans'."

Inequality in Resources to Buffer Pandemic Effects

While the majority of families described negative effects of pandemic schooling, families varied in their resources to buffer their children and themselves from these effects. Nearly all families talked about role expansion during remote instruction (Greer & Pierce, 2021) as they took over the work of teachers and therapists, yet this had varying meaning for families. Above, we describe linguistically marginalized families struggling to understand teachers' instructions. Several families were financially unable to have a parent or other caregiver at home: one mother said her child barely attended school, as his older sister was unable to enforce remote schooling attendance; another parent left her autistic middle-schooler at home with cameras around the house so that she could watch him from work. Meanwhile, families with more resources were often able to work from home and also hire additional help to support their children.

Effects Beyond Remote Schooling

While most families' descriptions of negative pandemic effects focused on remote schooling, broader difficulties with teacher shortages, stress, and trauma associated with the pandemic have also exacerbated the marginalization of disabled children in school. For example, Ernesto, a Latino autistic boy, has been in-person for the 2021–2022 school year, yet as of the December 2021 interview with his mother, he has been without a teacher. His IEP mandates that he attend school in a classroom with two teachers, but his school has only been able to staff the room with two paraprofessionals. Other families noted heightened behavioral difficulties among their children's peers as schools reopened. Michelle, a Black mother of Lamonte, a tenth-grade boy with emotional-behavior disorder, expressed concern about "all this violence going on in school right now," and was worried this increased violence would lead to Lamonte being bullied. She attributed the violence to the school being unprepared to support children's mental health during the pandemic.

In summary, COVID has had wide-reaching – but variable – effects on disabled children's schooling experiences. Across race, class, and other social categories, many children experienced inappropriate instruction and other difficulties due to pandemic-driven changes in schools. When children were multiply marginalized at the intersections of disability with language, race, gender, and class, these effects were largely more negative. Moreover, families varied in their ability to buffer their children from these effects with various forms of capital, including knowledge of educational content and language, as well as financial resources to allow a parent to stay home with a child or to hire help. Next, we will further examine how COVID shaped families' strategies for buffering negative aspects of their child's schooling, as well as their advocacy to improve their child's schooling experiences.

Pre-COVID-19 Family Support, Engagement, and Advocacy for Disabled Children

Echoing Linda Blum's (2015) finding that families of disabled children have found it necessary to become fierce advocates to navigate educational and medical systems for their children, many participants described intensive engagement and advocacy in their children's schooling. Yet variation by social status and other factors was clear. For some families, especially White, middle-class families whose children had relatively straightforward educational needs, like Andrea, little advocacy had historically been necessary pre-COVID. She said that teachers proactively asked her, "what can we do to help Ellie?". Most families did not have this experience, however, and responded with various forms of advocacy, engagement, and support. Middle-class and White families largely described effective advocacy, as schools work to appease these families (Voulgarides, 2021). Natalie, a White mother of a boy with ADHD, said she had to "essentially come up with the whole plan" for her son, resulting in effective supports for her son. Similarly, Tammy, a low-income Black mother of Parker, relied on the social capital of her support group for parents of autistic children; they suggested she bring a binder with his photo on it to IEP meetings, to humanize her son as she advocated for his needs; she also contacted teachers frequently to check in. Stephani, also a low-income Black mother, made her presence known among Dontrell's teachers. She communicated frequently with teachers and often observed the classroom to better advocate for her son, saying, "they [the school] *know* me."

Many other families relied on exit strategies to support their children, to varying degrees of effectiveness, depending on their social position and resources. For example, Joshua, the White, middle-class father of Theodore, a tenth-grade boy with ADHD, described applying for scholarships to send Joshua to a boarding school because the public school was not adequately supporting him. In contrast, Carleen, a Black, low-income mother, had transferred Harrison several times between schools in the mid-sized city where they lived and a nearby suburb, in the hopes of finding a placement that would support him well, but she had yet to find a school that met his needs.

A subset of families – who were predominantly Latinx and Black – had not found success in advocating for their children. Despite adopting strategies to get the school to care about her son, Tammy found it difficult to secure the supports her son Parker needed. She stated,

> I just felt like they were not helping me. I felt like I really speak up for Parker. I don't have a problem with communicating every detail in the emails. I'm not only complaining to the teacher. I'm CC'ing everybody. I'm CC'ing [special education administration]. Like somebody's got to help me get him out of the school.

Echoing research on Latinx families, and especially Spanish-dominant families, the Spanish-dominant Latinx families in this study often relayed discomfort in directly advocating for their children in school (Lian & Fontánez-Phelan, 2001), instead highlighting the ways they supported their children's learning at home.

COVID-19 as a Window to Disabled Children's School Experiences

For many families, remote schooling gave them new insights into their children's education. Beatriz "was able to work better with Alejandro, and understand, and learn more about my son." Many families described this window as helping them see how schools were not meeting their children's educational needs, albeit under the suboptimal remote schooling context. One of several families perceiving negative student-teacher interactions, Violeta said she

> ...started to see how the face-to-face classes were with the teacher. She was yelling at a child, and the child was yelling. It was very ugly to be hearing that. I said thank God I left Santiago here [in remote schooling].

Other families saw more clearly that their children's instruction was not supporting them the way they hoped. For example, Beatriz, who had navigated complex systems to bring private Applied Behavior Analysis (ABA) therapists into the school, said, "I saw what the ABA therapists were like in person, and so I said, 'now I understand why public schools don't want ABA people, because they don't help'."

"COVID-19 Lit a Fire"

This window into their children's schooling shaped many families' engagement, advocacy, and support for many families. For example, Araceli noted the purely academic focus in remote schooling. She decided to teach Ernesto "to read the clock, to count money, because that's what he's going to use in life." Other families became more vigorous advocates because of what they saw in remote schooling. Recall Tammy, who was unhappy with her Parker's schooling prior to COVID. With remote schooling, she got "to see everybody on the Zoom," where she was shocked to see that even in a specialized class of six children, the teachers were not modifying and differentiating for her son.

> I had a conversation with the teacher. I said "you have six kids in a class and only two kids are participating because the other kids don't know the work. But how was this effective if you keep calling the same two kids? What about the other four? Parker is one of the four that don't know anything, just sitting there looking at y'all?" So she said "you know what, you're not the only parent that said that." Yet, but nobody is doing nothing about the other four kids. I was so disappointed in the school system that they will allow my son to sit in school and just not know nothing.

For Tammy, seeing the extent to which her son was struggling pushed her to advocate even more, and to have her son transferred to a class where he would work on "essential life skills." Many families that observed negative educational experiences for their children under remote schooling responded by exiting their current schools. For example, Rebecca, who above described remote schooling as a positive change for her son, decided to homeschool him indefinitely. Others, like Angela, the Latina mother of Leo, an autistic second-grade boy, said "COVID-19 kind of lit a fire. This kid is not going to thrive here. I had to be more vigilant" to advocate for services.

While COVID-19 seems to have served as an inflection point for many families of disabled children to consider the effectiveness of their schooling and revise their interactions with the school, the same inequalities that shaped their pre-COVID-19 schooling experiences continued into the pandemic. Katie, a White, middle-class mother of a third-grader with orthopedic impairment, said "we had Avery's IEP this fall, and I'm like, you guys are not listening to what we want as parents." Katie prepared to fight the school with legal advocacy, saying "this is like a service industry. It really is. You should do what the families feel is best for the kids." Others, like Rebecca, were able to take time away from paid work to homeschool their children, or could move their children to private schools. Several socially advantaged families were able to advocate for accommodations during remote learning, such as several White, middle-class families that told teachers their children could not attend as many remote instruction hours as their peers. Sandra, the Asian middle-class mother of Andrew, also successfully advocated for educational service changes: the school agreed to amend her son's IEP to require the school to provide in-person instruction in the case of a future shift back to remote-schooling. Meanwhile, parents and other caregivers like Beatriz were running out of ways to advocate for their children:

> In a monolingual school, it would be nice if they offered the help of an interpreter. So, when you try to ask for it, the school won't give it to you... They're denying you everything... They're going to deny him aid.

Beatriz had requested a communication tablet for Alejandro, who was non-speaking, but the school insisted he did not need it. She had requested a Functional Behavioral Assessment to support his behaviors, but was told "No. The school can't give him that." She requested the school undergo "autism training, so that the teachers that are around my son know what autism is like, because they have no idea how autism works." Again, the school told her "no." Therefore, while many of the families described the pandemic schooling context as a period that provided them with new information to help them advocate for their disabled children, intersecting inequalities continued to shape schools' responses to family advocacy.

CONCLUSION

Our data illuminate how schools are generally not structured to provide adequate access, support, and instruction for disabled students, even before the pandemic, particularly for multiply marginalized disabled children. Pervasive ableism – and intersections of ableism with racism and other systems of oppression – structures power and access to resources across social domains, and schools are no exception. Schools' ability to support disabled students was shaped by power, privilege, and inequality. In some communities, services for disabled students met the need, and in others, typically those from underresourced and racially and ethnically minoritized populations, services were woefully inadequate. The crisis of COVID-19 has exacerbated these inequalities. Parents described their children being afterthoughts, if considered at all, by schools' pandemic plans for instruction. However, these effects were uneven, not only because of inequalities in schools, but also because of the resources parents were able to provide to supplement their children's schooling. Even for the minority of families who characterized the pandemic and remote schooling as providing unexpected benefits, this largely reflected the ways that their children's schools were not meeting their needs prior to the pandemic.

For many families, the pandemic provided a window into aspects of their children's schooling that were not beneficial. Thus, the pandemic was an inflection point for families to advocate for changes for their children. Yet because racism, ableism, and other systems of inequality structures school organization and resources, as well as family resources, families' agency was bounded (Evans, 2007). Schools attended to White, middle- and upper-class disabled children by providing better supports to them in the first place, and by responding to their families' advocacy. Meanwhile, schools lacked the resources to support socially marginalized disabled children, and were less responsive to family advocacy, even when these families were well-versed in their children's legal right to a free, appropriate, public education. In the context of the pandemic, only the more advantaged families had access to information, financial resources, and better-resourced schools, allowing them to pivot during the crisis, and to acquire more advantageous schooling supports for their children, while marginalized families experienced more constraints.

Mirroring many families' perception of the pandemic as a time to reflect on how schools were serving their children, researchers, policy-makers, and practitioners should examine how schools serve disabled children more broadly. Prior to the pandemic, many disabled children were not receiving appropriate instruction or services at school. Some children attended nominally inclusive classrooms, where educators did not have adequate resources to support disabled students, such as additional staff to support differentiated instruction. Other children attended segregated special education programs, where instruction was targeted, but often mismatched from student needs, in addition to the risks of stigma, lowered expectations, and social exclusions from segregated programs. As schools abruptly shifted to remote schooling, it is not surprising that many teachers struggled to provide appropriate instruction to disabled children, given the extant marginalization of disabled children in schools. The fact that many of the families whose children attended segregated programs spoke highly of them during remote schooling should not be used as evidence to promote segregated programs – rather, it speaks to the need for low student-teacher ratios and organizational supports for differentiation in all classrooms serving disabled children. This requires policy changes to support higher quality, inclusive, equitable special education services, funding for additional teachers and paraprofessionals, professional development for inclusive teaching practices, and administrative support to create and maintain these structures within schools. Yet attending only to disability will not adequately address these inequalities, given the experiences of multiply marginalized disabled students. Rather, improvements to access and inclusion should be prioritized for schools serving racially, linguistically, and socioeconomically marginalized disabled students. In addition to these increased supports, policy-makers should create regulatory structures that hold schools accountable for appropriate educational services for all disabled students, rather than relying on individual parents to advocate for their children.

ACKNOWLEDGMENTS

We thank the reviewers for their helpful advice and feedback. This research was supported by the National Academy of Education and the Spencer Foundation, through the National Academy of Education/Spencer Postdoctoral Fellowship to the first author. The article's contents are solely the responsibility of the authors and do not represent the official views of any supporting agency.

NOTES

1. Language conventions vary in using person-first language (i.e., "people with disabilities") or disability-first language (i.e., "disabled people), with variation across communities with different kinds of disabilities (e.g., disability-first language is more common among Autistic self-advocates, while person-first language is more common among people with intellectual disability), as well as between disabled self-advocates as compared to parents of children with disabilities (Carey et al., 2020). In this chapter, we will largely use disability-first language, with some variation, particularly when capturing the perspectives of families.

2. While people of Latin American descent vary in labels for self-identification, here we use "Latinx" to include people outside of the gender binary (Salinas & Lozano, 2019).

3. This research was reviewed and approved by the Institutional Review Board at New York University.

4. All names are pseudonyms.

REFERENCES

Abedi, V., Olulana, O., Avula, V., Chaudhary, D., Khan, A., Shahjouei, S., Li, J., & Zand, R. (2021). Racial, economic, and health inequality and COVID-19 infection in the United States. *Journal of Racial and Ethnic Health Disparities*, *8*(3), 732–742. https://doi.org/10.1007/s40615-020-00833-4

Angell, A. M., & Solomon, O. (2017). 'If I was a different ethnicity, would she treat me the same?': Latino parents' experiences obtaining autism services. *Disability & Society*, *32*(8), 1142–1164. https://doi.org/10.1080/09687599.2017.1339589

Asbury, K., Fox, L., Deniz, E., Code, A., & Toseeb, U. (2021). How is COVID-19 affecting the mental health of children with special educational needs and disabilities and their families? *Journal of Autism and Developmental Disorders*, *51*(5), 1772–1780. https://doi.org/10.1007/s10803-020-04577-2

Bailey, D. H., Duncan, G. J., Murnane, R. J., & Au Yeung, N. (2021). Achievement gaps in the wake of COVID-19. *Educational Researcher*, *50*(5), 266–275. https://doi.org/10.3102/0013189X211011237

Bamberger, C., Butrymowicz, S., Mader, J., & Preston, C. (2020). *Thousands of families in special education limbo* (p. 2). The Hechinger Report.

Belsha, K., Rubinkam, M., LeMee, G. L., & Fenn, L. (2020). A nationwide divide: Hispanic and Black students more likely than white students to start the year online. Chalkbeat, 11.

Blum, L. (2015). *Raising generation Rx: Mothering kids with invisible disabilities in an age of inequality*. NYU Press. https://www.amazon.com/Raising-Generation-Mothering-Disabilities-Inequality/dp/1479871540

Carey, A. C., Block, P., & Scotch, R. K. (2020). *Allies and obstacles: Disability activism and parents of children with disabilities*. Temple University Press.

Carreón, G. P., Drake, C., & Barton, A. C. (2005). The importance of presence: Immigrant parents' school engagement experiences. *American Educational Research Journal*, *42*(3), 465–498. https://doi.org/10.3102/00028312042003465

Cioè-Peña, M. (2017). The intersectional gap: How bilingual students in the United States are excluded from inclusion. *International Journal of Inclusive Education*, *21*(9), 906–919. https://doi.org/10.1080/13603116.2017.1296032

Cooper, C. W. (2009). Parent involvement, African American Mothers, and the politics of educational care. *Equity & Excellence in Education*, *42*(4), 379–394. https://doi.org/10.1080/10665680903228389

Crenshaw, K. (1991). Mapping the margins: Intersectionality, identity politics, and violence against women of color. *Stanford Law Review*, 1241–1299.

Deterding, N. M., & Waters, M. C. (2018). Flexible coding of in-depth interviews: A twenty-first-century approach. *Sociological Methods & Research*. https://doi.org/10.1177/0049124118799377

Easop, B. (2021). Education equity during COVID-19: Analyzing in-person priority policies for students with disabilities. *SSRN Electronic Journal*. https://doi.org/10.2139/ssrn.3869935

Evans, K. (2007). Concepts of bounded agency in education, work, and the personal lives of young adults. *International Journal of Psychology*, *42*(2), 85–93. https://doi.org/10.1080/00207590600991237

Fish, R. E. (2019). Standing out and sorting in: Exploring the role of racial composition in racial disparities in special education. *American Educational Research Journal*, *56*(6), 2573–2608.

Green, S. E. (2007). "We're tired, not sad": Benefits and burdens of mothering a child with a disability. *Social Science & Medicine*, *64*(1), 150–163. https://doi.org/10.1016/j.socscimed.2006.08.025

Green, S. E., Darling, R. B., & Wilbers, L. (2016). Struggles and joys: A Review of research on the social experience of parenting disabled children. In S. E. Green & S. N. Barnartt (Eds.), *Research in social science and disability* (*Vol. 9*, pp. 261–285). Emerald Group Publishing Limited. https://doi.org/10.1108/S1479-354720160000009013

Greer, M., & Pierce, C. (2021). Examining the impact of the COVID-19 pandemic on caregivers of children with complex and chronic conditions. *Research, Advocacy, and Practice for Complex and Chronic Conditions*, *40*(1), 42–50. https://doi.org/10.14434/rapcc.v40i1.33294

Iland, E. D., Weiner, I., & Murawski, W. W. (2012). Obstacles faced by Latina mothers of children with autism. *Californian Journal of Health Promotion*, *10*(SI-Latino), 25–36. https://doi.org/10.32398/cjhp.v10iSI-Latino.1480

Kuhfeld, M., Soland, J., Tarasawa, B., Johnson, A., Ruzek, E., & Liu, J. (2020). Projecting the potential impact of COVID-19 school closures on academic achievement. *Educational Researcher*, *49*(8), 549–565. https://doi.org/10.3102/0013189X20965918

Landivar, L. C., Ruppanner, L., Rouse, L., Scarborough, W. J., & Collins, C. (2021). Research note: School reopenings during the COVID-19 pandemic and implications for gender and racial equity. 12.

Lareau, A. (2003). *Unequal childhoods*. Univ of California Press. http://books.google.com/books?id=3rmmj3lKATAC&printsec=frontcover&dq=inauthor:lareau+(2003+intitle:unequal+childhoods)&hl=&cd=1&source=gbs_api

Lareau, A., & Horvat, E. M. N. (1999). Moments of social inclusion and exclusion race, class, and cultural capital in family-school relationships. *Sociology of Education*, 37–53

Lian, M.-G. J., & Fontánez-Phelan, S. M. (2001). Perceptions of Latino parents regarding cultural and linguistic issues and advocacy for children with disabilities. *Journal of the Association for Persons with Severe Handicaps*, *26*(3), 189–194. https://doi.org/10.2511/rpsd.26.3.189

Maroto, M. L., Pettinicchio, D., & Lukk, M. (2021). Working differently or not at all: COVID-19's effects on employment among people with disabilities and chronic health conditions. *Sociological Perspectives*, *64*(5), 876–897. https://doi.org/10.1177/07311214211012018

McNeal, R., Jr. (1999). Parental involvement as social capital: Differential effectiveness on science achievement, truancy, and dropping out. *Social Forces*, 117–144.

Miller, H., Valentine, J. L., Fish, R. E., & Robinson, M. (2016). Is the feeling mutual? Examining parent- teacher relationships in low-income, predominantly Latino schools. *American Journal of Education*, *123*, 37–67.

Ong-Dean, C. (2009). *Distinguishing disability*. University of Chicago Press. http://books.google.com/books?id=EHvmW85vg3sC&printsec=frontcover&dq=inauthor:ong+dean+distinguishing+disability&hl=&cd=1&source=gbs_api

Owens, J., & Jackson, H. (2016). Attention-deficit/hyperactivity disorder severity, diagnosis, & later academic achievement in a national sample. *Social Science Research*, 1–15. https://doi.org/10.1016/j.ssresearch.2016.06.018

Patrick, S. K., Grissom, J. A., Woods, S. C., & Newsome, U. W. (2021). Broadband Access, district policy, and student opportunities for remote learning during COVID-19 school closures. *AERA Open*, *7*. https://doi.org/10.1177/23328584211064298

Quiocho, A. M., & Daoud, A. M. (2006). Dispelling myths about Latino parent participation in schools. *The Educational Forum*, *70*(3), 255–267.

Rangel, D. E., & Valdez, C. R. (2017). A culturally sensitive approach to large-scale prevention studies: A case study of a randomized controlled trial with low-income Latino communities. *The Journal of Primary Prevention*, *38*(6), 627–645. https://doi.org/10.1007/s10935-017-0487-2

Reese, L., Balzano, S., Gallimore, R., & Goldenberg, C. (1995). The concept of educación: Latino family values and American schooling. *International Journal of Educational Research*. http://ezproxy.library.wisc.edu/login?url=http://www.library.wisc.edu/

Saatcioglu, A., & Skrtic, T. M. (2019). Categorization by organizations: Manipulation of disability categories in a racially desegregated school district. *American Journal of Sociology*, *125*(1), 184–260.

Salinas, C., & Lozano, A. (2019). Mapping and recontextualizing the evolution of the term *Latinx*: An environmental scanning in higher education. *Journal of Latinos and Education*, *18*(4), 302–315. https://doi.org/10.1080/15348431.2017.1390464

Schwartz, A. E., Hopkins, B. G., & Stiefel, L. (2021). The effects of special education on the academic performance of students with learning disabilities. *Journal of Policy Analysis and Management*, *40*(2), 480–520. https://doi.org/10.1002/pam.22282

Shifrer, D., Callahan, R. M., & Muller, C. (2013). Equity or marginalization? *American Educational Research Journal*, *50*, 656–682.

Szabo, J. (2021). Online or in-person instruction? Factors influencing COVID-19 schooling decisions among Latinx families in houston, Texas. *AERA Open*, *7*. https://doi.org/10.1177/23328584211053323

US Department of Education. (2020). *41st annual report to congress on the implementation of the individuals with disabilities education act 2019*.

Valenzuela, A. (1999). *Subtractive schooling: US-Mexican youth and the politics of caring.* State University of New York Press. http://scholar.google.com/scholar?q=related:86Rm2c0WhicJ:scholar.google.com/&hl=en&num=30&as_sdt=0,5

Voulgarides, C. (2021). Equity, parental/caregiver 'Power,' and disability policy in the US Context. *International Journal of Inclusive Education, 19.* https://doi.org/10.1080/13603116.2021.1937345

Voulgarides, C., Aylward, A., Tefera, A., Artiles, A. J., Alvarado, S. L., & Noguera, P. (2021). Unpacking the logic of compliance in special education: Contextual influences on discipline racial disparities in suburban schools. *Sociology of Education, 94*(3), 208–226. https://doi.org/10.1177/00380407211013322

Wilson, N. M. (2015). *Question-asking and advocacy by African American parents at individualized education program meetings: A social and cultural capital perspective* (p. 15).

Zimmer, A., & Zimmerman, A. (2020). *NYC's staffing crunch takes a big toll on students with disabilities, report finds.* Chalkbeat (p. 1).

Chapter 8

"EVERYBODY THROWN INTO THE DEEP END AT THE SAME TIME": REFLECTIONS ON FAMILY-SCHOOL PARTNERSHIP IN A TIME OF COVID-19

Julia Jansen-van Vuuren, Danielle Roberts, Grace L. Francis, Colleen M. Davison, Sharon Gabison and Heather M. Aldersey

ABSTRACT

Purpose: *COVID-19 has affected families across the globe with far-reaching consequences, particularly in regard to children's education. The pandemic has exacerbated existing inequalities for families of students with disabilities in particular. This chapter explores families' perspectives on how COVID-19 affected partnerships between families of students with disabilities and their schools in Ontario, Canada.*

Approach: *We interviewed 18 parents of students with disabilities in K-12 Ontario schools. Using a reflexive thematic analysis approach, we analyzed interviews to develop themes inductively.*

Findings: *Participants shared varied experiences of partnerships with their schools both before and during the pandemic. However, all participants described additional challenges as a result of COVID-19. Frequent, open, and personalized communication was emphasized as essential for effective*

Disability in the Time of Pandemic
Research in Social Science and Disability, Volume 13, 155–174

Published under exclusive licence by Emerald Publishing Limited
ISSN: 1479-3547/doi:10.1108/S1479-354720230000013009

partnerships; however, this was often lacking. Participants shared various ways they were involved in schools, including advocating for their child, and needing to balance multiple roles during COVID-19. Overwhelmingly, participants expressed an inadequacy of support during the pandemic related to online learning and a lack of human resources (e.g., Educational Assistants, therapists), negatively affecting partnerships. However, they also described positive experiences of family-school partnerships, as well as hope for effective future partnerships.

Implication/Value: *This research gives voice to families of students with disabilities to deepen our understanding of barriers and facilitators to positive family-school partnerships. Findings help to direct appropriate policies and practices that can improve partnerships during COVID-19 and beyond, and ultimately enhance education and quality of life for students with disabilities and their families.*

Keywords: Family-school partnership; disability; family; education; COVID-19; Ontario; Canada

Internationally, COVID-19 disrupted education, affecting students' academic progress, mental and physical health, and overall wellbeing, as well as the routines and wellbeing of families more broadly (Calarco et al., 2020, 2021; Gallagher-Mackay et al., 2021; Kinsey et al., 2020). Students in Ontario, Canada, experienced school closures, with some regions extending over 12 months, resulting in physical isolation from loved ones, teachers, and community networks (Engzell et al., 2021). Such experiences resulted in loneliness and increased mental health needs due to loss of daily routines and face-to-face social interactions, as well as cancellations of important events (Cost et al., 2021; Loades et al., 2020). Furthermore, COVID-19 affected special education delivery, increasing the risk of further educational disparities for children with disabilities, as many relied on school-based services such as structured learning environments, specialized educators, and assistive technologies (Fredman, 2021; Masonbrink & Hurley, 2020).

Respectful, trusting, and reciprocal family-school partnerships support students' emotional, social, and academic needs (Daniel, 2015; Haines et al., 2015; Hands, 2013). Positive family-school partnerships are linked to improved student behavior, reduced absenteeism, higher student achievement, and decreased maternal stress (Burke & Hodapp, 2016). Conversely, negative attitudes from school staff toward family involvement, poor communication, intimidating school environments, and inadequate support for children can create barriers to family-school partnerships (Baker et al., 2016; Burke & Hodapp, 2016). However, Lareau and colleagues argue that not all parent involvement in schools is positive and can, instead, create challenges for both families and schools (Lareau, 1994; Lareau & Muñoz, 2012). Parents and school staff may have different perspectives on how or when they should be involved, even when family-school relationships are considered important (Harry & Ocasio-Stoutenburg, 2018; Posey-Maddox & Haley-Lock, 2020).

Research also demonstrates that sociocultural factors influence family-school partnerships. For example, families from higher socioeconomic backgrounds tend to engage more with schools and schools often privilege and cater to more affluent families (Calarco, 2020; Lareau & Calarco, 2012; Lareau & Ferguson, 2018). In contrast, lower socioeconomic or racial minoritized families are often less involved because they may not have the time, resources, or knowledge of how to advocate for their children. Although they may genuinely care about their children's education, schools can perceive them as disinterested or "bad" parents. Lareau (1987) described this as "cultural capital" where some families have more resources (e.g., knowledge, skills, competence) to invest in school partnerships and therefore, usually experience more positive outcomes. Harry and Ocasio-Stoutenburg (2018) have discussed the importance of true collaboration (e.g., shared knowledge, goals, resources, power, and trust) with *all* families, and the key role of school leadership at all educational levels, for effective family-school partnerships to flourish. In addition, the onset of COVID-19 has affected how families interact with the school system. For instance, Ocasio-Stoutenburg and Harry (2021) described diverse families' experiences of advocating for their children in special education, including navigating the challenges of COVID-19. They also highlighted how systemic bias in the educational system related to race and socioeconomic status influenced parents' participation and advocacy efforts for their children both before and during the pandemic.

FAMILY-SCHOOL PARTNERSHIPS IN ONTARIO

"The Participant Engagement Policy for Ontario Schools" envisions the enhancement of student education through welcoming and respecting parents as valuable partners in the school community (Ontario Ministry of Education, 2010). The Ontario government provided strategies and an action plan – including school, board, and ministry-specific actions – to reach the policy's goals. However, the implementation of government policies to support parent engagement is insufficient or ineffective and additional initiatives are needed (Hands, 2013). In a survey of families of students with intellectual disabilities in Ontario schools, some parents reported that schools discouraged attendance at Identification, Placement and Review Committee (IPRC) or Individual Education Plan (IEP) meetings and that they were not informed about their rights (Reid, 2018). Furthermore, Reid (2018) identified multiple challenges that students with disabilities in Ontario experience including, staffing shortages, transportation schedules, and missing behavioral support plans. Inadequate resources and support also negatively affect Canadian teachers' time and energy to engage in training around inclusion (Lord, 2020). Unwelcoming, intimidating school environments can negatively affect family involvement (Baker at al., 2016), resulting in parents serving as staunch advocates for their children (Bennett et al.,

2020; Burke & Hodapp, 2016; Reid, 2018; Ryan & Quinlan, 2018). Unsurprisingly, the onset of COVID-19 has created additional challenges for family-school partnerships.

COVID-19, EDUCATION, AND FAMILY-SCHOOL PARTNERSHIPS IN ONTARIO

To limit the spread of COVID-19, the Canadian government implemented public health measures such as school and business closures, travel restrictions, and stay-at-home orders in early 2020 (Wu et al., 2020). During the 2020–2021 school year, educational delivery varied, including fully remote, fully in-person, and blended in-person and online learning, causing disruption to student learning (Gallagher-Mackay et al., 2021). Some families had no access to resources or digital literacy skills needed for remote learning (Di Pietro et al., 2020; Gallagher-Mackay et al., 2021). This upheaval to the education system resulted in additional strains placed on families as they took on many roles (e.g., parent, teacher, employee). However, positive family-school partnerships can potentially alleviate some of these stresses and challenges. The purpose of this study was to explore the impact of COVID-19 on family-school partnerships from the perspective of families of students with disabilities in public schools in Ontario, Canada. The study answered the following questions: (1) what are the family-school partnership experiences of families of students with disabilities enrolled in (K-12) public schools in Ontario and (2) how has COVID-19 affected partnerships between families and their schools?

METHODS

Study Design

This study was part of a larger research project using an online survey and interviews to understand family-school partnerships during COVID-19 in Ontario public schools. We obtained university ethical clearance prior to data collection and number identifiers were used for participants to maintain confidentiality.

Research Team

Our research team included (1) two family members of students with disabilities who attend/ed school in the Ontario public system, (2) a family member of persons with disabilities outside of Ontario, and (3) two former Ontario public school educators. All team members were also students or faculty members in the fields of Rehabilitation, Public Health, Global Development, and Special Education. Further, one team member was a representative of the study partner, the Family Alliance Ontario, which provides resources and support to individuals with disabilities and their families.

Participants

Interview participants were recruited from survey respondents who volunteered to be contacted for an interview (see Francis et al., 2021 for survey information). The researchers used maximum variation sampling (Farrugia, 2019) based on participant demographics (e.g., income, age, gender, child's age). Forty-five participants were contacted by email with an information letter and invitation to participate, and 18 participated in interviews (representing a total of 22 children with disabilities). The children had various specific diagnoses (the majority having autism spectrum disorder [ASD]), but all of them had some form of developmental disability, sometimes in combination with other diagnoses. Table 1 provides participant demographic information. All participants received a CAD30 Amazon gift card in appreciation of their time.

Data Collection

Three members of the research team collaborated to create a semi-structured protocol based on the survey and family-school partnership literature (e.g., Haines et al., 2017). A pilot interview was conducted with a member of the

Table 1. Demographic Characteristics of Study Participants.

	n (%)		*n (%)*
Age of participant (years)		Relationship to children with disability	
26–30	1 (5.6)		
31–35	1 (5.6)	Mother	17 (94.4)
36–40	3 (16.6)	Father	1 (5.6)
41–45	3 (16.6)	Age of children with disability (years)	
46–50	5 (27.7)		
51–55	4 (22.2)	5–10	11 (50.0)
Not stated	1 (5.6)	11–15	6 (27.3)
Sex of participant		16–20	5 (22.7)
Female	17 (94.4)	Sex of children with disability	
Male	1 (5.6)	Female	4 (18.2)
Approximate annual family income (CAD)		Male	18 (81.8)
<20,000	3 (16.6)		
21,000–40,000	3 (16.6)		
41,000–60,000	1 (5.6)		
61,000–80,000	2 (11.1)		
81,000–100,000	3 (16.6)		
101,000–120,000	2 (11.1)		
121,000–140,000	2 (11.1)		
>141,000	2 (11.1)		

Family Alliance Ontario to ensure social validity and clarity of interview questions. Four of the authors used teleconferencing software to conduct interviews between September and December 2020. Interviews lasted between 45–90 minutes, were audio-recorded and transcribed verbatim.

Data Analysis

Following data collection, transcripts were analyzed using reflexive thematic analysis techniques (Braun & Clarke, 2006). The researchers familiarized themselves with the transcripts before commencing inductive coding with NVivo qualitative software. Two authors independently coded two transcripts before meeting to discuss the codes and clarify discrepancies. After initial coding, three authors further discussed and refined the codes into themes and subthemes.

FINDINGS

The researchers inductively developed four major themes related to experiences of family-school partnerships and effects of COVID-19: (1) communication facilitating or impeding partnerships, (2) inadequate support for student learning, (3) participant involvement in family-school partnerships, and (4) ideal family-school partnerships. Child age/school level and family income did not appear to shape family-school partnerships. Participants described other factors, such as: (1) the attitude and level of support and flexibility from principals, teachers, and support staff; (2) participant teaching experience, and (3) support from family and community, which resulted in greater empathy for school staff and positively influenced family-school partnerships

Communication Facilitating or Impeding Family-School Partnerships

This theme includes two subthemes: open lines of communication and unhelpful/ lack of communication. Some participants discussed how open, regular contact with the school resulted in good relationships, while others felt that the school was not open to communicating or unavailable/inaccessible, leading to strained partnerships.

Open Lines of Communication

Prior to COVID-19, some participants spoke of open lines of communication with school staff. This communication included daily communication books, emails, phone calls, apps, and in-person conversations. The amount of communication varied among participants, with some speaking to school staff daily to less frequently, but all still felt communication was available when needed. Participants appreciated school staff who informed them of concerns and collaborated to address their child's educational needs (e.g., "If I had an issue she would meet with me, I would just go in early before school and she would meet with me a couple times just to kinda run through things, or if she thought something was up." P4).

Some communication was eliminated during COVID-19 (e.g., daily communication books, face-to-face interactions) and instead, communication occurred through emails, phone calls, text messages, video calls, and online learning platforms. Some participants found school staff accessible, available as needed, or proactive in checking-in: "I got a little email or text … 'Hey, just checking in how's [Child]? No pressure…We just wanted to let you know we're thinking of you.' So they were awesome with keeping in touch" (P7).

Unhelpful/Lack of Communication

Participants shared negative experiences communicating with school staff prior to and during COVID-19, which inhibited effective collaboration to support children's needs. Such experiences included school staff resistance to talking with participants outside of designated times such as report card meetings: "[teachers] don't really want to have a conversation with you, unless it's parent interviews" (P14). Before COVID-19, one participant described a strained relationship, believing the school was unwilling to build a positive partnership after conflicting in views. Another participant described how the school's negative assumptions about them (e.g., they must be "bad" parents for allowing their son to live in a group home) created resistance in communication. Both before and during the pandemic, participants described feeling dismissed by school staff when they tried to communicate their child's needs, including staff ignoring requests: "When I asked if we could do an IEP or adapt some of the things that weren't really being very successful with him there was a kind of like, oh don't worry, he's fine" (P6). Participants also felt distressed when schools focused on or only contacted them to discuss negative information: "The problem is we only hear when there's problems. We don't hear the good" (P10). Further, a low-income, single mother of a primary-level child, lacked confidence communicating with higher level school staff because of their deficit focus and a lack of trust; however, she acknowledged that her own mental health challenges contributed to sub-optimal communication.

Participants found it unhelpful when emails/newsletters were sent to the whole school board, school, or class; instead desiring individual check-ins during the pandemic: "Now with COVID, you call … everything just goes to voicemail … you never reach anybody, so it's hard" (P4). One participant reported how she received no communication from the teacher after her child returned to in-person learning, leaving her wondering how her son was progressing.

Inadequate Support for Student Learning

Participants discussed navigating technology and online learning, as well as the inadequacy of human resources. They described how lack of supports, both before and during COVID-19, sometimes led to regression and/or impeded their child's potential. During COVID-19, minimal school support resulted in many participants feeling abandoned and left to educate their child alone. This was particularly challenging when students had severe impairments or difficult behaviors, regardless of specific disability diagnosis.

Navigating Technology and Inadequacy of Online Learning

Every family experienced online learning at some point, specifically at the start of the pandemic when schools closed to in-person learning. Participants described difficulties accessing technology, navigating online learning, and the overall inadequacy of online learning during COVID-19. Participants felt that their children's education was not supported and online options were inappropriate or insufficient:

> I think [teachers] were not at all prepared … how do you teach children outside of the mainstream when you're not in a school setting and doing hands on learning with them, how do you make that work without them falling behind, getting lost, losing more time than they already have and putting them even further developmentally behind? (P9).

One participant expressed frustration in securing a device they needed for online learning, as education staff believed they were not responsible for providing the device: "If you guys are going to get wrapped up in your politics and your bureaucracy, I'm going to find somebody else" (P1). This negatively affected the child's ability to participate in online learning with peers. Another participant waited for a Chromebook prior to COVID-19 and were never updated on when they would receive it; they believed that if their child could work on the device in class, transferring to online learning would be easier if schools closed again. Similarly, another participant spoke of poor Internet access as a barrier to online learning. Additionally, participants reported that learning platforms were too difficult to navigate: "There was like 10,000 virtual platforms for doing everything which was completely mind boggling for me and I couldn't make heads or tails of it" (P6). None of the participants reported receiving any technology training from their schools.

Some participants felt that their children were being left behind and were not prioritized because online learning was not modified. Further, this lack of modification left participants to teach their children alone. For example, one participant was provided a 65-page document from which they were expected to pick instructional activities to implement: "I think that's the biggest learning curve for COVID, is as a parent, I had to learn how can I just do this all myself" (P1).

In addition, participants engaged in different forms of online learning (i.e., synchronous and asynchronous). Some participants used both approaches, whereas others were only given one option (which did not support their child's needs). Participants expressed confusion regarding what was expected of their child. Other participants felt that the available online options were below their child's learning abilities (e.g., coloring sheets, dance, yoga videos), so they saw little point in participating: "It almost was many times too easy or way too difficult for him" (P2).

Inadequate Human Resources

Participants spoke of limited access to human resources for collaboratively supporting their children before and during COVID-19. They described how schools were short-staffed due to a lack of funding, affecting their child's access to essential support. Participants shared how lack of Educational Assistant (EA) support led schools to prioritize students with behavioral issues, while others fell through the cracks: "I think there's 200 kids at the school that need one-on-one. This is in a school of 1,000 kids and there's one person that comes a couple hours every week... a lot of kids are really unsupported in their needs" (P16).

During COVID-19, participants described being unable to access EA support or only receiving wellness checks and/or reading to their child, feeling that this undermined their child's abilities. One participant whose husband was an EA acknowledged that their role had changed to providing health and safety support rather than educational support, therefore "EAs had their hands tied on what they could do to support" (P2). Some participants chose not to ask teachers for more support, acknowledging that teachers had heavy workloads and minimal resources. Several participants described challenges transitioning back to in-person school due to limited collaboration with teachers and support staff. Some children were not even able to return because schools could not guarantee their safety: "The transition back to school was probably the worst part of all of the COVID issues" (P12). Further, secondary students in work experience programs were unable to continue their placements due to health and safety policies.

Prior to COVID-19, participants accessed various paraprofessionals such as specialized education teams, physiotherapists, occupational therapists, and speech language pathologists. During COVID-19, these professionals were not allowed into the school and were unavailable online. Participants viewed these professionals as important to their child's education and overall development, and, as a part of the IEP, their absence reinforced the notion that students with disabilities were disregarded. Their absence also affected schools' ability to understand children's current needs and create education plans. Some participants desired home-based support services, but acknowledged this was not possible due to COVID-19 policies. One participant noticed that without these support services, the school expected less from their child, ultimately impeding his potential: "Now they're just happy if he does coloring and I'm like, oh God, he can do so much more than that" (P6).

Parent Involvement in Family-School Partnerships

Participants discussed how they had to advocate for their children both before and during COVID-19. They also described the increased expectations placed upon them during COVID-19, as they were forced to take on multiple roles.

The Need for Parental Advocacy

Prior to COVID-19, participants had opportunities to attend their children's assemblies, holiday concerts, volunteer in the classroom, or participate in school councils and committees. Additionally, participants discussed advocating both before and during COVID-19: "I am the biggest advocate for my kid and that's the way it is now and that's the way it will always be. And if I don't do it, nobody else will" (P9). Participants engaged in different levels of advocacy: some discussed their child's needs with school staff, while others approached higher authorities (e.g., school board directors, union representatives).

Before COVID-19, participants advocated for their children in various ways, including: (1) obtaining assistive devices, (2) ensuring schools followed recommendations from their child's psychological assessment, (3) remaining at the same school for consistency despite moving out of the catchment area, (4) accessing EA support, (5) securing bus transportation, and (6) obtaining curriculum modifications. In some cases, participants' advocacy was unsuccessful, and their children suffered as a result. One mother recounted her frustration when the school did not follow her son's IEP despite advocating for a doctor to come and explain her son's needs to school staff:

> You know this [IEP] is a legal binding document ... They know it. We've talked about it ... they presented like they understood, and they didn't do half of what was even talked about. So [my son] had to suffer and he was let down time after time after time ... I said, what is wrong with you people? It was devastating and yet he still managed to come out ok grade wise, but not without a lot of mental health challenges (P3).

After the initial school closures at the onset of COVID-19, schools opened up options for students to return to in-person learning. Participants had to decide whether to follow the online learning option provided to them or return to in-person learning, otherwise some were told their child would be taken off the school roster. Several participants attempted to advocate for an alternate solution, recognizing that their children struggled to engage in online learning, but could not be guaranteed a safe return to in-person learning; however, participants were unsuccessful due to inflexible school board policies. Further, many secondary students in work experience programs lost their right to their placements. In several cases, participants acknowledged that systemic barriers (e.g., government health policies) lead to schools' inflexibility: "I think that [schools] were doing the best they could...the ministry was giving them very little to go on. I would have liked the ministry to step up and do more planning for the special ed students" (P5).

Balancing Roles During COVID-19

Participants spoke of the challenges they faced with changing roles during COVID-19, and they became responsible for facilitating their children's learning: "Basically I had to take over the complete teacher role, it's hard to put a teacher hat on and a mom hat" (P17). Due to COVID-19, many participants described the devastating absence of critical support such as in-home services (e.g., respite workers, care providers, friends, and family). Furthermore, while schools were closed many extra-curricular activities were also canceled. This was often upsetting or confusing for children.

Participants described difficulties having their children at home 24/7, trying to facilitate their learning (and often the learning of siblings), and balancing other roles such as parenting and their employment: "I feel insanely guilty. Because I just, I don't feel that I can do enough for [my daughter] right now . . . [tears up] without having to do my other stuff and take care of myself . . . and my family . . . we're going to muddle through, we'll get through it" (P8). Some participants had to quit their jobs, reduce hours, or find alternative, more flexible employment: "I left everything for [my son], my job, my work and everything" (P13). Some participants felt fortunate that their educational background supported their child's learning, while others felt unable to facilitate their child's learning: "I was having to work . . . I just had to let him go into that little world where he's happy and comfortable doing his Roblox video game . . . he basically spent six months lying on the couch doing his video games" (P6). Balancing these roles with minimal support negatively impacted participants' wellbeing: "I don't have it in me to keep having that battle. I just . . . it was mentally and physically exhausting . . . watching her regress, watching her get dropped by a system that I thought supported her" (P18).

Ideal Family-School Partnerships

One participant described consistently positive family-school partnerships throughout their child's 10 years of schooling. Other participants spoke about specific times in their child's education when they experienced positive relationships with school staff who stood out. In addition, participants shared hopes for family-school partnerships, including positive, consistent, and open communication.

Positive Experiences of Family-School Partnerships

Participants reported positive experiences of family-school partnerships before and during COVID-19 when school staff had an inclusive mindset, accepted their child with a disability, and were open to accommodating their needs: "[The teacher] seems very open to having, you know, somebody who's different in the classroom" (P1). One parent of a child in a congregate school described consistently positive interactions with the school: "Every single year we've had a teacher who has simply gone above and beyond what I expected" (P14). Participants valued teachers who worked with them to identify how to best support their child's education. However, they described facing frequent resistance or unwillingness from school staff to collaborate on accommodating students' needs, specifically regarding IEPs. Participants spoke of particularly positive experiences when school staff initiated and responded to students' needs by developing and tracking goals within students' IEPs: "She's the only teacher I've ever known who's actually like, followed an IEP, checked in with the IEP to see where we were on track with goals . . . she was really, really a brilliant teacher and quite unusual from a lot of other teachers" (P6).

During COVID-19, participants described positive partnership experiences when schools worked collaboratively to create reentry plans that supported individual children's needs and promoted a smooth transition back to in-person learning; this included school visits prior to starting in-person leaning, communicating with participants on how to safely transition, modifying academic demands, and supporting a gradual transition back to school. Participants appreciated school staff who got to know their child on a one-on-one basis and were therefore able to recognize both their strengths and limitations. By doing this, school staff were able to make appropriate accommodations to support student learning, such as sensory breaks, seating arrangements, modified curriculum delivery, and adaptive equipment. Participants valued educators providing educational opportunities that matched their child's abilities: "She really understood him, and she was sure to make sure that he was doing the work that all the other kids were doing ... saying that he was able to take sensory breaks if he needed it" (P4).

Hope for Family-School Partnerships

Participants expressed their hopes for the future during COVID-19 and beyond, believing it was important for school staff to have open and accepting mindsets to support children's unique needs by collaboratively addressing barriers in the curriculum and classroom environment. As one participant noted:

> I think one of the pieces I kind of find missing in the education system is that the parent knows their child best and if a parent is telling you that's not going to work for them, it's probably true, and if they're saying they need something else that's also probably true. If they don't know what that something else might be, then that's where you step in and say, well, hey, maybe as a school we need to try this with him, or maybe as a teacher I need to work on that with him, or maybe as a board we need to research this a bit more. (P9)

Furthermore, participants emphasized how a universal lens would benefit all students, as everyone is unique and learns differently: "I think personality is a big thing, assigning somebody who is open to changing the way they teach or adapting the way they teach or just looking at teaching with a different lens, of a more like a universal design lens versus a label lens" (P1). Participants wished all teachers understood different disabilities, how to modify curriculum and environments, and how to write special education forms: "[I wish] that all the teachers would be trained in special education. That they would all have knowledge of, and tailor the education to each student. I know the IEPs are supposed to do that, but it doesn't happen right" (P11). Participants acknowledged that this required involvement from the government and school boards and indicated that schools need more funding for resources and staff training (e.g., how to write IEPs or special equipment claims, using accessible learning apps). Furthermore, participants emphasized the need for school staff to collaboratively support and share the workload of teachers. They also reported that teachers were unable to access important documents, such as Ontario Student Records, creating a barrier to supporting students.

Although participants indicated a willingness to be flexible and acknowledged that teachers are busy, they wished for consistent communication throughout the school year, not just during assigned times (e.g., after report cards). They desired school staff who could help them navigate school systems and available resources; recognizing that this cannot fall on teachers' shoulders, as they are already overworked. In addition, participants hoped for more one-on-one support for their children and called for greater flexibility from schools to support each family's unique needs: "All I'm asking is if you see I'm struggling and I'm asking for a life preserver, please don't just close me out" (P7).

DISCUSSION

Participants shared diverse experiences of their partnerships (or lack of) with schools before and during COVID-19. Many participants indicated partnerships were on shaky ground prior to COVID-19. It was unanimous, however, that the pandemic exacerbated challenges to partnerships. Participants emphasized frequent, open, and personalized communication as essential for effective partnerships with schools; however, this was often lacking in their experiences. Participants shared various ways that they were involved in schools, including advocating for their child, as well as needing to balance multiple roles during COVID-19 (e.g., parent, educator, therapist, employee). Overwhelmingly, participants expressed an inadequacy of support during COVID-19 related to online learning and a lack of human resources (e.g., EAs, therapists), negatively affecting partnerships. However, they also described positive experiences of family-school partnerships, as well as hope for effective future partnerships.

COVID-19 and Family-School Partnerships

Although our research focused specifically on Ontario schools, our findings aligned with other research in similar high-income contexts (Hong et al., 2021). COVID-19 created significant disruptions and challenges for families of children with disabilities (Fredman, 2021; Middleton, 2020; Smith, 2021). Our participants felt inadequately supported during the pandemic, as schools closed and services were reduced/suspended, leaving participants to assume additional roles to support their children (Greenway & Eaton-Thomas, 2020; Skipp, 2021; Smith, 2021). Many participants were also frustrated trying to access and navigate online learning, finding no differentiation/modification for their children, and unclear guidelines (Embregts et al., 2021; Greenway & Eaton-Thomas, 2020).

Additionally, participants described challenges during transitions (e.g., return to in-person learning; Smith, 2021). Research also reflects participant fears for their children's safety and psychological wellbeing, resulting in participants weighing the risks and benefits of keeping their children at home or sending them back to school (Embregts et al., 2021; Greenway & Eaton-Thomas, 2020). Similar to our findings, international researchers have reported that families experienced inadequate support and resources, resulting in children with complex needs being unable to return to school while home education support simultaneously reduced (Brandenburg et al., 2020; Smith, 2021). Conversely, our participants shared how regular communication, earlier school visits, and modifications to learning, facilitated smooth transitions.

Promoting Positive Family-School Partnerships During COVID-19 and Beyond

Effective family-school partnerships are crucial for positive learning and development outcomes for students with disabilities as well as for their families and schools during COVID-19 and beyond (Jones & Forster, 2021). Haines et al.'s (2017) "Sunshine Model" for family-professional partnerships provides a useful framework for practically promoting family-school partnerships. The principles outlined in this model (i.e., communication, respect, professional competence, commitment, equality, advocacy, and trust) allow for effective collaboration across five main partnership activities (i.e., determining and meeting needs; obtaining services and support; monitoring services and support; connecting home, school, and community; and advocating for systems improvement). In the following paragraphs, we discuss key principles based on our findings that are important in each of these partnership activities and which correspond to the principles of partnership.

Our findings align with global literature highlighting the pivotal role of effective, open, frequent, culturally sensitive, and creative communication for developing and maintaining positive family-school partnerships (Francis, Blue-Banning, Haines et al., 2016; Francis, Blue-Banning, Turnbull et al., 2016; McKenzie et al., 2021; Tremmel et al., 2020). Consistent with this study, Greenway and Eaton-Thomas (2020) found that COVID-19 affected the frequency and approach of communication, and many families were dissatisfied with the amount of contact from schools. Our participants confirmed this, describing frustration when feeling sidelined or when schools only focused on negative aspects of their child. Instead, school staff should initiate communication and reach out to families personally, emphasizing the strengths of children and families as well as collaboratively identifying needs and addressing challenges. This study reinforces literature that calls for schools to discuss their preferred mode of communication and maintain a friendly and approachable demeanor by engaging families in reciprocal information sharing (Francis, Blue-Banning, Haines et al., 2016; Francis, Blue-Banning, Turnbull et al., 2016; Haines et al., 2017).

Closely connected with positive communication, creating a welcoming and inclusive environment for families of children with disabilities is paramount for fostering family-school partnerships, where families feel accepted as valuable team members in their child's education (Francis, Blue-Banning, Haines et al., 2016; Francis, Blue-Banning, Turnbull et al., 2016; Reid, 2018). Our participants shared positive experiences when school staff were accepting and accommodating and took initiative to know children personally and adhere to IEPs. Several authors note that school leadership plays a crucial role in facilitating a welcoming environment, where administrators are approachable, accessible, knowledgeable about disability, committed to attending IEP meetings, show a personal interest in the child, actively listen to parents and authentically care (Francis, Blue-Banning, Haines et al., 2016; Francis, Blue-Banning, Turnbull et al., 2016; Reid, 2018; Shelden et al., 2010). School leadership should develop a culture of partnership before crisis events that can support all stakeholders during crisis. This could involve proactively bringing together relevant stakeholders who support children with disabilities (e.g., families, school staff, paraprofessionals) to collaboratively discuss and develop individual crisis-support plans.

Our findings showed that families expressed a desire for more engagement with their schools. However, families need to be encouraged and empowered to take an active role in partnering with schools, as some participants expressed fear of speaking out, consistent with studies where schools emphasize compliance rather than collaboration and parents are expected to acquiesce or are labeled as troublemakers (Bennett et al., 2020; Harry, 2008; Xu, 2020). As COVID-19 restrictions begin to lift, schools can provide opportunities for families to partner in their child's education (e.g., volunteer in classrooms with appropriate health precautions) as well as to develop leadership skills and influence policy development/change (e.g., participate in committees) (Francis, Blue-Banning, Haines et al., 2016; Francis, Blue-Banning, Turnbull et al., 2016; Rossetti et al., 2020). Families should be considered key stakeholders and actively engaged in developing and reassessing IEPs. For example, Mueller and Vick (2019) discussed how facilitated IEP meetings can promote meaningful collaboration for IEP development and implementation, including conflict prevention and resolution.

In light of the pandemic's ongoing effects, several researchers emphasize the need for schools to holistically support students with disabilities and their families, focusing on social-emotional wellbeing before academics (Mann et al., 2021; Minkos & Gelbar, 2021). As study participants highlighted, COVID-19 affected whole families, sometimes leading to breakdowns between families and schools or service providers, underscoring the need to consider family-centric supports (Skipp, 2021). While our participants did not highlight the role of siblings, Hagiwara et al. (2019) have described the importance of considering siblings and their essential role in enhancing family-school partnerships. In terms of holistic support, study participants lamented school rigidity and unwillingness to creatively and compassionately partner with them to address barriers to their child's ability to thrive. This forced some participants to advocate more assertively and approach higher levels of authority, leaving them exhausted. Therefore, school boards, schools, and educators, must consider ways to holistically and respectfully listen and collaborate with families to identify solutions and promote students' wellbeing (Bennett et al., 2020; Minkos & Gelbar, 2021). The pandemic has shown that schools can adapt and creatively address barriers. However, these attributes need to continue beyond COVID-19 and promote deeper partnerships between families, schools, and the broader community (Mann et al., 2021).

Participants recognized that teachers and schools were unprepared for COVID-19 (Middleton, 2020) and educators were not solely to blame for poor partnerships, acknowledging the effect of broader constraints and limited resources. Cavendish et al. (2020) have discussed how, even prior to the pandemic, special education teachers were often frustrated by limited support and resources for them to effectively support students, highlighting the importance of collaboration and partnerships between schools, families, and the community. Participants in this study also expressed empathy for school staff despite their frustrations. When considering the future, participants hoped for increased funding and resources to support students with disabilities. Therefore, policy changes are needed to increase support staff to provide more one-on-one support and for "reforming educational structures, systems, resources, and incentives to support whole child learning, health, recovery, and success" (Mann et al., 2021, p. 449). In the aftermath of the pandemic, educational policies will need to consider the unique needs of children who will require a range of different, targeted supports (Mann et al., 2021; Minkos & Gelbar, 2021). Families also acknowledged that existing staff need more support and understanding around disability, including training and professional development for *all* school staff that emphasizes inclusion and practical skills in supporting students with disabilities and their families (Hands, 2013; Lord, 2020).

Limitations

This study is not without limitations. Firstly, virtual interviews have the potential for lost rapport compared to in-person interviews. Additionally, despite purposefully seeking diversity in experiences, the sample consisted primarily of white mothers of children with developmental disabilities. A more diverse sample could reveal different or deeper insights around family-school partnerships, particularly in relation to the influence of socio-economic status and race. Most participants were already staunch advocates for their children, perhaps reflecting a recruitment bias whereby more educated, vocal parents are more likely to volunteer for interviews, and this may not reflect the experience of all families. Although school boards across Ontario have different policies, the researchers did not analyze the interviews according to their school boards. Finally, hearing from students with disabilities themselves would add an important dimension to understanding experiences of family-school partnerships.

CONCLUSION

Like families globally, many Ontarian families of children with disabilities experienced significant family-school partnership challenges prior to COVID-19, and the pandemic exacerbated these challenges. Participants demonstrated empathy toward teachers, principals, and school boards, while desiring improvements in family-school partnerships for the ultimate benefit of their children. Study findings demonstrate the need for the Ontario provincial government to foster an environment whereby schools are required and supported to make families trusted and meaningful partners in charting the pathway toward a positive post-COVID-19 future.

REFERENCES

Baker, T., Wise, J., Kelley, G., & Skiba, R. (2016). Identifying barriers: Creating solutions to improve family engagement. *School Community Journal*, *26*(2), 161–184. http://www.schoolcommunitynetwork.org/SCJ.aspx

Bennett, S., Specht, J., Somma, M., & White, R. (2020). Navigating school interactions: Participants of students with intellectual disabilities speak out. *Current Developmental Disorders Reports, 7*(3), 149–154. https://doi.org/10.1007/s40474-020-00203-z

Brandenburg, J. E., Holman, L. K., Apkon, S. D., Houtrowd, A. J., Robert, R., & Scholas, M. G. (2020). School reopening during COVID-19 pandemic: Considering students with disabilities. *Journal of Pediatric Rehabilitation Medicine*, 1–7. https://doi.org/10.3233/PRM-200746

Braun, V., & Clarke, V. (2006). Using thematic analysis in psychology. *Qualitative Research in Psychology, 3*(2), 77–101. https://doi.org/10.1191/1478088706qp063oa

Burke, M. M., & Hodapp, R. M. (2016). The nature, correlates, and conditions of parental advocacy in special education. *Exceptionality, 24*(3), 137–150. https://doi.org/10.1080/09362835.2015.1064412

Calarco, J. M. (2020). Avoiding us versus them: How schools' dependence on privileged "Helicopter" parents influences enforcement of rules. *American Sociological Review, 85*(2), 223–246. https://doi.org/10.1177/0003122420905793

Calarco, J. M., Anderson, E., Meanwell, E., & Knopf, A. (2020). "Let's not pretend it's fun": How COVID-19-related school and childcare closures are damaging mothers' well-being. SocArXiv papers. https://doi.org/10.31235/osf.io/jyvk4

Calarco, J. M., Meanwell, E., Anderson, E. M., & Knopf, A. S. (2021). By default: How mothers in different-sex dual-earner couples account for inequalities in pandemic parenting. *Socius, 7*, 1–15. https://doi.org/10.1177/23780231211038783

Cavendish, W., Morris, C. T., Chapman, L. A., Ocasio-Stoutenburg, L., & Kibler, K. (2020). Teacher perceptions of implementation practices to support secondary students in special education. *Preventing School Failure: Alternative Education for Children and Youth, 64*(1), 19–27. https://doi.org/10.1080/1045988X.2019.1628000

Cost, K. T., Crosbie, J., Anagnostou, E., Birken, C. S., Charach, A., Monga, S., Kelley, E., Nicolson, R., Maguire, J. L., Burton, C. L., Schachar, R. J., Arnold, P. D., & Korczak, D. J. (2021). Mostly worse, occasionally better: Impact of COVID-19 pandemic on the mental health of Canadian children and adolescents. *European Child & Adolescent Psychiatry*. https://doi.org/10.1007/s00787-021-01744-3

Daniel, G. (2015). Patterns of participant involvement: A longitudinal analysis of family-school partnerships in the early years of school in Australia. *Australasian Journal of Early Childhood, 40*(1), 119–128. https://doi.org/10.1177/183693911504000115

Di Pietro, G., Biagi, F., Costa, P., Karpinski, Z., & Mazza, J. (2020). *The likely impact of COVID-19 on education: Reflections based on the existing literature and recent international datasets.* Publications Office of the European Union. https://doi.org/10.2760/126686

Embregts, P., Heerkens, L., Frielink, N., Giesbers, S., Vromans, L., & Jahoda, A. (2021). Experiences of mothers caring for a child with an intellectual disability during the COVID-19 pandemic in the Netherlands. *Journal of Intellectual Disability Research, 65*(8), 760–771. https://doi.org/10.1111/jir.12859

Engzell, P., Frey, A., & Verhagen, M. D. (2021). Learning loss due to school closures during the COVID-19 pandemic. *Proceedings of the National Academy of Sciences, 118*(17), 1–7. https://doi.org/10.1073/pnas.2022376118

Farrugia, B. (2019). WASP (Write a Scientific Paper): Sampling in qualitative research. *Early Human Development, 133*, 69–71. https://doi.org/10.1016/j.earlhumdev.2019.03.016

Francis, G. L., Blue-Banning, M., Haines, S. J., Turnbull, A. P., & Gross, J. M. S. (2016). Building "Our School": Parental perspectives for building trusting family-professional partnerships. *Preventing School Failure: Alternative Education for Children and Youth, 60*(4), 329–336. https://doi.org/10.1080/1045988X.2016.1164115

Francis, G. L., Blue-Banning, M., Turnbull, A. P., Hill, C., Haines, S. J., & Gross, J. M. S. (2016). Culture in inclusive schools: Parental perspectives on trusting family-professional partnerships. *Education and Training in Autism and Developmental Disabilities, 51*(3), 281–293. http://www.jstor.org/stable/24827524

Francis, G. L., Jansen-van Vuuren, J., Guarav, N., Aldersey, H. M., Gabison, S., & Davison, C. M. (2021). Family-school collaboration for students with disabilities in Ontario, Canada. *Network for International Policies and Cooperation in Education and Training NORRAG, 6*, 48–52.

Fredman, S. (2021). A human rights approach: The right to education in the time of COVID-19. *Child Development, 92*(5), 900–903. https://doi.org/10.1111/cdev.13654

Gallagher-Mackay, K., Srivastava, P., Underwood, K., Maltsev, A., Perkhun, A., Steiner, R., Barrett, K., & Sander, B. (2021). COVID-19 and education disruption in Ontario: Emerging evidence on impacts. *Science Briefs of the Ontario COVID-19 Science Advisory Table*, *2*(34). https://doi.org/10.47326/ocsat.2021.02.34.1.0

Greenway, C. W., & Eaton-Thomas, K. (2020). Parent experiences of home-schooling children with special educational needs or disabilities during the coronavirus pandemic. *British Journal of Special Education*, *47*(4), 510–535. https://doi.org/10.1111/1467-8578.12341

Hagiwara, M., Palmer, S. B., Hancock, C. L., & Shogren, K. A. (2019). Sibling roles in family-school partnerships for students with disabilities during transition planning. *Career Development and Transition for Exceptional Individuals*, *42*(3), 194–200. https://doi.org/10.1177/2165143418792045

Haines, S. J., Francis, G. L., Mueller, T. G., Chiu, C.-Y., Burke, M. M., Kyzar, K., Shepherd, K. G., Holdren, N., Aldersey, H. M., & Turnbull, A. P. (2017). Reconceptualizing family-professional partnership for inclusive schools: A call to action. *Inclusion*, *5*(4), 234–247. https://doi.org/10.1352/2326-6988-5.4.234

Haines, S. J., Gross, J. M. S., Blue-Banning, M., Francis, G. L., & Turnbull, A. P. (2015). Fostering family-school and community-school partnerships in inclusive schools: Using practice as a guide. *Research and Practice for Persons with Severe Disabilities*, *40*(3), 227–239. https://doi.org/10.1177/1540796915594141

Hands, C. (2013). Including all families in education: School district-level efforts to promote participant engagement in Ontario, Canada. *Teaching Education*, *24*(2), 134–149. https://doi.org/10.1080/10476210.2013.786893

Harry, B. (2008). Collaboration with culturally and linguistically diverse families: Ideal versus reality. *Exceptional Children*, *74*(3), 372–388. https://doi.org/10.1177/001440290807400306

Harry, B., & Ocasio-Stoutenburg, L. (2018). Leadership and collaboration in home-school partnerships. In J. B. Crockett, B. Billingsley, & M. L. Boscardin (Eds.), *Handbook of leadership and administration for special education* (2nd ed., pp. 243–264). Routledge.

Hong, J. Y., Choi, S., Francis, G. L., & Park, H. (2021). Stress among Korean immigrant parents of children with diagnosed needs amid the COVID-19 pandemic. *School Community Journal*, *31*(2), 31–51. https://www.adi.org/journal/2021fw/HongEtAlFW21.pdf

Jones, C., & Forster, C. (2021). Family-school partnerships in the age of Covid-19: Reasons for optimism amidst a global pandemic. *Practice*, 1–11. https://doi.org/10.1080/25783858.2021.1927159

Kinsey, E. W., Hecht, A. A., Dunn, C. D., Levi, R., Read, M. A., Smith, C., Niesen, P., Seligman, H. K., & Hager, E. R. (2020). School closures during COVID-19: Opportunities for innovation in meal service. *American Journal of Public Health*, *110*(11), 1635–1643. https://doi.10.2105/AJPH.2020.305875

Lareau, A. (1987). Social class differences in family-school relationships: The importance of cultural capital. *Sociology of Education*, *60*(2), 73–85. https://doi.org/10.2307/2112583

Lareau, A. (1994). Parent involvement in schooling: A dissenting view. In C. L Fagnano & B. Z. Werber (Eds.), *School, family, and community interaction: A view from the firing lines* (pp. 61–73). Routledge. https://doi.org/10.4324/9780429305375-6

Lareau, A., & Calarco, J. M. (2012). Class, cultural capital, and institutions: The case of families and schools. In S. T. Fiske & H. R. Markus (Eds.), *Facing social class: How societal rank influences interaction* (pp. 61–86). Russell Sage Foundation.

Lareau, A., & Ferguson, S. (2018). Sociology of education. In J. M. Ryan (Ed.), *Core concepts in sociology* (pp. 86–89). Wiley/Blackwell.

Lareau, A., & Muñoz, V. L. (2012). "You're not going to call the shots": Structural conflicts between the principal and the PTO at a suburban public elementary school. *Sociology of Education*, *85*(3), 201–218. https://doi.org/10.1177/0038040711435855

Loades, M. E., Chatburn, E., Higson-Sweeney, N., Reynolds, S., Shafran, R., Brigden, A., Linney, C., McManus, M. N., Borwick, C., & Crawley, E. (2020). Rapid systematic review: The impact of social isolation and loneliness on the mental health of children and adolescents in the context of COVID-19. *Journal of the American Academy of Child & Adolescent Psychiatry*, *59*(11), 1218–1239. https://doi.org/10.1016/j.jaac.2020.05.009

Lord, P. (2020). Access to inclusive education for students with autism: An analysis of Canada's compliance with the United Nations Convention on the Rights of Persons with Disabilities. *Canadian Journal of Disability Studies*, *9*(5), 328–346. https://doi.org/10.15353/cjds.v9i5.700

Mann, M. J., Smith, M. L., Kristjansson, A. L., Daily, S., McDowell, S., & Traywick, P. (2021). Our children are not "behind" due to the COVID-19 pandemic, but our institutional response might be. *Journal of School Health*, *91*(6), 447–450. https://doi.org/10.1111/josh.13016

Masonbrink, A. R., & Hurley, E. (2020). Advocating for children during the COVID-19 school closures. *Pediatrics*, *146*(3). https://doi.org/10.1542/peds.2020-1440

McKenzie, J., Shanda, N., & Aldersey, H. M. (2021). Family–teacher partnerships: Families' and teachers' experiences of working together to support learners with disabilities in South Africa. *British Journal of Special Education*, *48*(1), 26–49. https://doi.org/10.1111/1467-8578.12337

Middleton, K. V. (2020). The longer-term impact of COVID-19 on K–12 student learning and assessment. *Educational Measurement, Issues and Practice*, *39*(3), 41–44. https://doi.org/10.1111/emip.12368

Minkos, M. L., & Gelbar, N. W. (2021). Considerations for educators in supporting student learning in the midst of COVID-19. *Psychology in the Schools*, *58*(2), 416–426. https://doi.org/10.1002/pits.22454

Mueller, T. G., & Vick, A. M. (2019). Rebuilding the family–professional partnership through facilitated Individualized Education Program meetings: A conflict prevention and resolution practice. *Journal of Educational and Psychological Consultation*, *29*(2), 99–127. https://doi.org/1080/10474412.2018.1470934

Ocasio-Stoutenburg, L., & Harry, B. (2021). *Case studies in building equity through family advocacy in special education: A companion volume to "meeting families where they are"*. Teachers College Press.

Ontario Ministry of Education. (2010). Participants in partnership: A participant engagement policy for Ontario schools. http://www.edu.gov.on.ca/eng/participants/involvement/FS_PE_PolicyEn.pdf

Posey-Maddox, L., & Haley-Lock, A. (2020). One size does not fit all: Understanding parent engagement in the contexts of work, family, and public schooling. *Urban Education*, *55*(5), 671–698. https://doi.org/10.1177/0042085916660348

Reid, L. (2018). Inclusion means everyone, why not me? https://www.inclusiveeducationresearch.ca/docs/why-not-me.pdf

Rossetti, Z., Burke, M. M., Rios, K., Rivera, J. I., Schraml-Block, K., Hughes, O., Lee, J. D., & Aleman-Tovar, J. (2020). Participant leadership and civic engagement: Suggestions for the next individuals with disabilities education act reauthorization. *Journal of Disability Policy Studies*, *31*(2), 99–111. https://doi.org/10.1177/1044207319901260

Ryan, C., & Quinlan, E. (2018). Whoever shouts the loudest: Listening to participants of children with disabilities. *Journal of Applied Research in Intellectual Disabilities*, *31*(S2), 203–214. https://doi.org/10.1111/jar.12354

Shelden, D. L., Angell, M. E., Stoner, J. B., & Roseland, B. D. (2010). School principals' influence on trust: Perspectives of mothers of children with disabilities. *Journal of Educational Research*, *103*(3), 159–170. https://doi.org/10.1080/00220670903382921

Skipp, A. (2021). Learning from the COVID crisis for educating children and young people with SEN/disabilities; Section 2: Special education during lockdown: Provider and participant experiences. *Journal of Research in Special Educational Needs*, *21*(2), 168–184. https://doi.org/10.1111/1471-3802.12513

Smith, S. (2021). Learning from the COVID crisis for educating children and young people with SEN/disabilities; Section 3: Participants' perspectives: What we can learn from COVID crisis education for students labelled with SEND. *Journal of Research in Special Educational Needs*, *21*(2), 168–184. https://doi.org/10.1111/1471-3802.12513

Tremmel, P., Myers, R., Brunow, D. A., & Hott, B. L. (2020). Educating students with disabilities during the COVID-19 pandemic: Lessons learned from commerce independent school district. *Rural Special Education Quarterly*, *39*(4), 201–210. https://doi.org/10.1177/8756870520958114

Wu, J., Tang, B., Bragazzi, N. L., Nah, K., & McCarthy, Z. (2020). Quantifying the role of social distancing, personal protection and case detection in mitigating COVID-19 outbreak in

Ontario, Canada. *Journal of Mathematics in Industry*, *10*(1), 15–15. https://doi.org/10.1186/s13362-020-00083
Xu, Y. (2020). Engaging families of young children with disabilities through family-school-community partnerships. *Early Child Development and Care*, *190*(12), 1959–1968. https://doi.org/10.1080/03004430.2018.1552950

Chapter 9

SOL EXPRESS IN THE TIME OF COVID-19: REFLECTIONS FROM A CREATIVE ARTS PARTICIPATORY RESEARCH PROJECT

Madeline Burghardt, with Natalie Breton, Maya Findlay, Irene Pollock, Matt Rawlins, Kathleen Woo and Cheryl Zinyk

ABSTRACT

Purpose: *Stay-at-home and lock-down orders issued by the Ontario government at the beginning of the COVID-19 pandemic led to the closure of many community-based programs for people labelled/with intellectual disabilities. L'Arche Toronto Sol Express, an interdisciplinary arts program located in Toronto, is one example of a program that rapidly changed its program delivery to an online format so that participants could remain engaged and collaborative projects could continue. Similarly, participants had to adapt to new programs with virtual formats, and to accessing programs from their own homes as opposed to gathering with others in the community.*

Methods/Approach: *To reflect on these changes, Sol Express members and creative facilitators together conducted a participatory research project which considered the impact of the online format on individual participants and the group as a whole. Following the principles of emancipatory and participatory research, a research team was established and focus groups were held to explore people's experiences.*

Disability in the Time of Pandemic
Research in Social Science and Disability, Volume 13, 175–192

Published under exclusive licence by Emerald Publishing Limited
ISSN: 1479-3547/doi:10.1108/S1479-354720230000013010

Findings: *Our findings suggest that while there were many difficult aspects to the pandemic, people also experienced situations of learning and growth. However, our project also points to issues of inequity in the pandemic's effects, such as the inability for technology to incorporate diverse communication methods, and concerns regarding members of the extended community who remain disengaged or 'lost' due to a lack of technological and personal support.*

Implications/Value: *Although our research focused on an arts group for people labelled/with intellectual disabilities, our findings can be applied to the broader community, especially regarding the benefits of in-person gathering and what is lost when programs are held exclusively online.*

Keywords: Disability arts programs; COVID-19 restrictions; online programs; participatory research; pandemic effects; L'Arche Toronto Sol Express

INTRODUCTION

L'Arche Toronto Sol Express is an interdisciplinary arts program for people with intellectual disabilities located in Toronto, Ontario.[1,2] Established in 2007, Sol Express uses an interdependent approach that incorporates the leadership, ideas and gifts of all members to create original artistic and stage productions. The group's unique creative and collaborative process facilitates personal growth and confidence in its members and has led to meaningful connections between participants and the broader community. Before the onset of the COVID-19 pandemic in early 2020, Sol Express participants met frequently, sometimes several times a week, to work on large projects with established completion dates, including theatre performances such as *Birds Make Me think about Freedom* and art gallery installations.[3,4]

In March 2020, Sol Express's regular meetings were brought to an abrupt halt when national and local governments issued restrictions on gatherings in attempts to curb the spread of the COVID-19 virus. Community-based programs normally delivered in person hastily altered their formats or ceased altogether due to concerns regarding the virus being spread in groups of people in close proximity, obliging participants, their families and supporters to quickly adapt to online or discontinued programming (Alphonso, 2021; Community Living Toronto, 2020; Hole & Stainton, 2020; Yoshida et al., 2021). Sol Express's creative facilitators altered how their programs were offered so that participants could remain engaged and so that collaborative projects could continue. Participants, as well as their families and supporters, had to adapt to new programs with virtual formats and to accessing programs from their own homes as opposed to gathering with others in the community. New online programs were created, as well as an off-line, phone-based program for those without internet access.[5]

In answer to the call to submit work to this peer reviewed volume, Sol Express facilitators and participants decided to explore the impact of these changes. We set up a research project to learn how Sol Express participants experienced the shift to an online format during the COVID-19 pandemic. Our aim was to create a safe virtual space where people could share both negative and positive aspects of their online Sol Express experience. In addition, we committed to using a participatory and equity-based approach. Drawing from the inspiration of Mike Oliver (1992) who called for emancipatory methods in all research involving disabled people – designed, led by and accountable to people with disabilities – we decided to use a collaborative model, with the aim of creating knowledge as equitably as possible. It was for these reasons that we established a seven-person research team including Sol Express's creative facilitators as well as two of its regular participants, in order to contribute to collaborative decision-making and knowledge production.

The aim of this chapter is twofold. The first is to discuss what we learned in our project, following the two general questions 'What was hard about Sol Express being online?' and 'What was good about Sol Express being online?' The second aim is to share the methods that we used in order to add to the growing literature concerning research conducted by people of varying gifts and abilities working together. We begin, however, with a brief description of the history and development of arts programs for people labelled/with intellectual disabilities in order to position Sol Express within the bigger field of disability arts and to provide a backdrop for the learnings from our project and how they might contribute to other arts-based initiatives. We then move to a discussion of our methods and their theoretical framing, which in turn sets the stage for our discussion of what we learned in the project.

Context: Disability and the Arts

The disability art and theatre movement emerged from the Disability Rights Movement in the UK, Europe and North America in the mid-late twentieth century (Gorman, 2007; Stöckl, 2014). While the movement initially foregrounded artistic engagement as an avenue toward individual and communal self-expression, it also signalled the use of art as a medium to express disability pride, culture, identity and empowerment (Fox, 2015; French & Jones, 2019; Newsinger & Green, 2016). Since its emergence, members of the disability arts community have challenged mainstream assumptions of art by disabled artists, including the notion that artistic work with and by disabled people is inherently therapeutic in nature, thus minimizing the creation of art for art's sake, an assumption generally not directed at non-disabled artists (Gold, 2021; Maconi, 2020; Nyqvist & Stjerna, 2017). Others have challenged the apparent need within the non-disabled community to identify when art has been created by someone with a disability (Fox, 2015), as well as the failure by the non-disabled community to recognize the valuable contributions that art by disabled people makes to society in general (French & Jones, 2019; Gold, 2021).

Prior to the founding of Sol Express, Cheryl Zinyk, one of its founders (and a member of the research team), spent time with disability art and theatre groups in Canada, the UK, Germany and Ukraine, and used her experiences to inform Sol

Express's goals and methods. Sol Express prioritizes interdependent collaboration both between members and with outside professionals, grounded in the idea that group members who have an intellectual disability offer an essential perspective to art- and theatre-making. The group works collaboratively to create original work that reflects the current concerns and artistic ideas of the group members. In its respect of individual needs as well as each person's strengths, Sol Express thus encapsulates what Swain and French (2000) describe as the 'affirmative model' of disability, which asserts that disability is neither problematic, needing to be 'rehabilitated' through medical or professional intervention, nor is it adequately defined as a social construction. Rather, Sol Express moves beyond this fundamental tension in disability studies and recognizes instead the importance of valuing individual and collective creativity within the supportive milieu of a caring and respectful community.

In light of these both tangible and intangible elements, our reflection on how Sol Express managed during the pandemic may be useful to other arts groups. The forced closure of Sol Express's regular meeting place revealed an essential question, one relevant not only to disability arts groups: to what extent is a physical space needed in order for the benefits of the program – both artistic and interpersonal – to be realized? In other words, which essential, positive elements remained in spite of the online format, and what was lost? Reflecting together on these questions led us to a deeper understanding of the effects of online programming, such as the limits of virtual formats in facilitating access and inclusion. In addition, our thinking together revealed the extent to which interpersonal benefits were harmed by the online format, this lack thus affirming the existence of less visible, underlying benefits of arts programs that involve social interactions in physical space, beyond the creative work they engender. Reflection on what happens, and what does not happen, when physical gathering is not possible and when spaces are transformed into virtual ones thus reveals some of the less quantifiable benefits of being physically together, a lesson that can be applied to other work and social situations.

'I'm Ready That I Can Do It': Aiming for Equity-Informed Research

Following Sol Express's tradition of creating original works with input from all members, we felt it was important to incorporate those methods in our reflection on people's experiences of Sol Express during the pandemic, and to include ways that participants could take active leadership and decision-making roles.

In articulating this desire, we follow the lead of disability studies researchers who have prioritized participatory and emancipatory research. Mike Oliver's 1992 statement on the need for emancipatory research called for a radical shift in the 'social relations of research production' in order to break down and invert the traditional barriers between 'expert' researchers and disabled research subjects. Oliver noted that not only do traditional research methods contribute to the ongoing oppression encountered by disabled people (102), but they also *produce* disability (101) by articulating it as a particular entity or condition that requires classification, categorization and study.

Oliver's call for disabled people to reclaim the research process has been taken up by others in the field (see, e.g., Aubrecht et al., 2021; Buettgen et al., 2012; Iriarte et al., 2014). All of these projects prioritize the inversion of traditional power relationships as a principal research goal, including the equitable sharing of leadership tasks and assisting in the data collection and analysis, resulting in participants having a greater sense of ownership and control over the process. As Fudge Schormans et al. (2018) point out, participatory and collaborative research is thus a political act owing its attempt to stop the traditional exclusion and silencing of people with disabilities. Participants' involvement in the articulation of the research question means that it is more likely to be of concern in their lives and to be an 'accurate and authentic reflection' (Buettgen et al., 2012, p. 609) of their social reality. In addition, Aubrecht et al. (2021) point out that the co-researchers in their project, which described the situations of young disabled people living in long-term care, provided 'ethical checks' (7) and 'critical insights' (Aubrecht et al., 2021) regarding participants' contributions, reflections that might otherwise have been missed had the research been conducted solely by a non-disabled research team. Perhaps most importantly, all of these projects describe the enhanced individual and communal empowerment that can result from the establishment of a diverse research team with varying abilities, experiences and insights.

However, researchers have also pointed out the difficulties that persist in spite of these emancipatory goals. Rios et al. (2016) note that despite an increase in the inclusion of underrepresented groups in research, such as women, people from racial and ethnic minorities and children, disabled people remain excluded from most research processes. Coons and Watson (2013) note that although the intention to utilize emancipatory and participatory research methods is well-documented, evidence of research meeting these transformative objectives remains scarce, particularly with people labelled/with intellectual disabilities. They observe that research that claims to be participatory in nature but neglects to include disabled participants in forming the research questions and analysing the data ultimately perpetuates the oppression the research is attempting to address (19). Fudge Schormans et al. (2018) share this perspective, and note that while participatory methods are meant to challenge traditional power imbalances, an imposed and un-nuanced approach even within a participatory frame can paradoxically reinforce traditional oppressions and unbalanced power relations between disabled and non-disabled people. In another project which examined people's perspective on their individual and collective rights, Iriarte et al. (2014) found that while the study generated insights regarding people's living conditions and understandings of their rights, and while personal changes such as increases in self-confidence occurred due to the use of participatory and egalitarian methods, the translation of these gains to broader social and political change has been limited. Finally, scholars note the difficulty of conducting participatory research with input from all members of a team within the confines of output-driven, neoliberal institutions owing the increased time that is often needed to ensure true collaboration and agreement (Fudge Schormans et al., 2018).

Upon reflection, we feel that our project achieved many of the participatory and emancipatory goals described above. We shared group leadership and project design between disabled and non-disabled participants, and together we determined how we would enact this research. This included assigning the various tasks for each week's large-group online session on a rotating basis with each member of the team, such as leading an icebreaker or warm-up activity, leading the main activity and doing the conclusion or summing up what we accomplished that day. This sorting through of roles and responsibilities and the empowerment that resulted was demonstrated through an email exchange within the team prior to one of the large-group meetings. Two members of the team were scheduled to lead the main activity that week. When one person indicated that she could not attend, the other team member remained committed to the task, stating that she was willing to lead the activity on her own, writing 'Just a thought, I could try and lead the activity myself. I'm ready that I can do it'. Similarly, on a different occasion, another team member indicated that she would like to have support while leading an activity. We welcomed this as a reminder that all types of leadership are needed: while taking on solo leadership was important for one person, being able to ask for someone to share that responsibility was important to another.

In addition, the sharing of responsibilities meant a recalibration of how academic research is typically done with regard to communication styles and timelines. We slowed down the research process, scheduling research team meetings in between each of the larger group sessions (described below) so that each step of the process could be discussed and decided upon. Decisions were made by consensus only – including when meetings would take place – to ensure that decisions were never imposed, and that people felt that they were part of the decision-making process. Care was taken to write all communication in plain language. At the beginning of each meeting, we incorporated focusing exercises and ice-breakers to bring everyone together, and we were faithful to the timelines we had established, ending our meetings at the agreed-upon time, even when our work was not completely finished. Each of these steps took time, and our embrace of that time countered standard expectations of punctuality and productivity.

Interestingly, the fact that our group remained under pandemic restrictions at the time of the project resulted in a small but nevertheless meaningful reduction in typical power imbalances. Due to ongoing social distancing measures, the research was conducted online and thus everyone participated from their own home. This resulted in a lessening of the inequity that can occur when researchers choose the location for research projects, locations in which the participants may feel less comfortable and may feel that they cannot, or should not, express their opinions or exert personal agency.

Similar to other researchers in the field (French & Jones, 2019), we also encountered obstacles in our journey toward emancipatory and participatory research, and did not necessarily meet all of the criteria as described above. Specifically, the research question was primarily decided upon by three members of the research team. Reasons for this include the fairly specific parameters outlined within the call for papers, as well as the relatively tight time frame within which to complete the project. However, although the research question was predominantly predefined – to investigate the effects of Sol Express's online format on participants – we were committed to allowing as wide an expression of experiences as possible, encouraging participants to use the modality with which they felt most comfortable (e.g., drawing, painting, voice, actions, etc.). In alignment with some of the literature outlined above, our group also experienced the way in which time constraints can make participatory work more challenging, due to the tension between ensuring that everyone's voices were heard adequately and that all participants had input into various drafts of the paper while simultaneously respecting the need for completion. Despite these difficulties, however, our group felt that important insights were made due to the group's diverse membership. This was especially evident when we were discussing how best to describe ourselves, which is discussed below.

METHODS, ETHICS AND LIMITATIONS

In all, there were 12 participants in the project: seven team members and five additional participants from Sol Express.[6] Three people initiated the project: two were creative facilitators with Sol Express, and one is an academic who is a friend and former contributor to the group. Research team members and the remaining participants were recruited using a general invitation that was sent to all Sol Express members. Participants were also verbally invited at one of Sol Express's regular online sessions.

All of the participants had been part of online programs prior to the research and thus were familiar with Zoom technology as well as the email communication that was used to relay meeting details. The group that was recruited, therefore, was engaged and knowledgeable and had the skills and support needed to connect consistently for the duration of the project. This indicates another of the project's limitations: due to the degree of technical competence needed and the ability to participate in a group that required some degree of focus, group skills and sharing of experiences, whether verbally or through other media, this project reached those who already possess a certain degree of technical competence, or who had enough support people around them to assist with technological challenges. It also reached those who were already connected to programs, and thus potentially did not reach those who have been more removed from regular connection due to pandemic restrictions. This includes people who are not well-supported or for whom Zoom technology does not suit their communication methods. Thus, we are aware that although Sol Express and its members experienced significant challenges due to the pandemic, there are many people who have been completely disconnected from social programming for its duration, many of whom might still be unable to participate, two years on. In addition, little is known about this disconnected group: in situations without adequate support or follow-up, people have become 'lost' to program organizers and have become invisible in the broader community, a point that is discussed in more detail below.

The team had two planning meetings at the beginning of the project. These were followed by four large-group meetings, the 'heart' of the project, at which the research team and all participants were in attendance and during which participants shared their experiences of Sol Express moving to an online format. At the first large-group meeting, a consent form written in plain language with accompanying explanatory illustrations (see Kidney & McDonald, 2014) was displayed and explained to the group, and the various methods that participants could use to complete and return it were also explained.[7,8] In the week following, group leaders communicated individually with each participant to determine whether or not they wished to continue; in the end, all of the original participants either signed the consent form or gave oral consent to continue with the project.

Each of the four large sessions was devoted to a different question, beginning with more general questions (i.e., What was hard about the pandemic? and What was something good that came from the pandemic, or something that you learned?) to more specific questions (What was hard about Sol Express moving online? and What was good, or what did you learn from Sol Express moving online?). Participants were encouraged to use whatever medium they wished to share their responses and experiences. Participants used a range of techniques, including spoken reflections, drawings, paintings, song, the sharing of objects, sculptures and poems.

All of the meetings took place online, using Zoom technology. Notes for each meeting were taken by two members of the research team which were then cross-checked and collated. Meeting notes were emailed to all members of the research team within 24 hours of the meetings' completion. Team members were asked to give feedback to the written notes and to make note of any errors or misunderstandings.

The four large groups were followed by two additional meetings at which the findings, the writing process and drafts of the paper were discussed. At the first meeting, the research team reflected on participants' contributions in breakout rooms and then identified major themes as well as any unique or thought-provoking findings. At the second meeting, the entire group gathered to review a draft of the paper and to provide feedback and input. During the revisions stage the group met three more times to discuss changes to the original paper.

Throughout this final stage of the writing process, the group had to make decisions regarding how and by whom the final paper would be written. As a group that was trying to adhere to principles of equity, we needed to determine how best to communicate the learnings from our project to an academic audience while remaining faithful to the principles of emancipatory and participatory research. In the end, the group decided that one person (Madeline) would take leadership with the formal writing due to her writing experience. However, the group agreed early on that drafts should be distributed to all participants, and that these should be discussed in follow-up meetings to ensure that the writing accurately reflected participants' contributions and that the writing remained accessible. We know we are not alone in our attempts to fulfil all of Oliver's requisites for emancipatory research (see, e.g., Buettgen et al., 2012), and our project points to the need for ongoing discussion of the tension between preparing work for broader dissemination while maintaining true, as opposed to token, inclusion.

Finally, part of our discussion during the writing process concerned the question of how best to describe ourselves. This resulted in a lively exchange that ultimately touched on bigger questions of individual and communal identity. As a group, we acknowledged that there are many ways that are used to describe people of varying abilities, but we all agreed that it is important to respect each person's position in their own journey of self-identity. For example, for some people, stating 'I have Down Syndrome' is a statement of identity and pride; others might choose another way to refer to themselves. In addition, we question whether it is even necessary to use words like 'disability' and 'impairment', as these are terms that non-disabled people use to describe presumed levels of dis/ability; we prefer, rather, to describe ourselves by the roles that we assumed in this project and to the roles that we assume in life more generally, such as actor, artist and playwright. While not a stated goal of our project, our discussion revealed the need to question the (generally) ongoing academic practice of indicating whether or not someone on the research team has a disability.

FINDINGS: WHAT WE LEARNED

Initially, we had expected our findings to fall under the two principal themes with which we had started the project: that we would learn about both the difficult and positive aspects of Sol Express moving online. However, when we carefully reviewed people's contributions, an interesting pattern emerged in which the major themes contradicted but also balanced each other out. That is, what most participants found difficult about doing Sol Express online was met by an equal and opposing effort to compensate for that deficit. In the discussion that follows, we explain some of these contradictory but balanced findings; we then move on to discuss a few stand-alone findings that are not so neatly categorized but deserve attention nonetheless.

Physical Connection: Checking in and Checking out

First, participants described the lack of physical connection as one of the hardest aspects of online programming. Participants spoke of missing being in the presence of others and doing activities together in a shared space. One of the participants compared the online connection to a glass apple: while it is beautiful in some ways and looks like the real thing, it is not real; it does not nourish and leaves one feeling empty. Another participant explained that he found it very difficult that the group 'could not connect through our bodies ... we are a theatre group. We have our hands on each other's bodies and move at the same time ... and are used to being close together. Now, with Covid, it's hard to do that'.

In an insight that goes beyond this notion of the importance of connecting physically with each other, one participant indicated that his usual way of 'checking in' with himself is through the presence of others, and that this had been taken away. He explained that he often determines how he is feeling through interpersonal encounters, and that communal experiences act as a barometer for his emotional self-awareness (and often reminds him that he feels better when in the presence of others). Zoom's focused, intentional and targeted nature prevents the shared, rhizomatic and sometimes-messy interactions that are a normal part of everyday life, and, in this case, was an obstacle to his self-determination of how he was doing. Doing everything online and in separate spaces also prevented the spontaneous banter and side-chatter that typically happens when the group gathers. These observations pose questions for the broader public: What has been lost, both in skill and comfort in our encounters with the 'other', due to this sudden shift in how we share space, or not, with each other? To what extent have all of us lost some of our own self-awareness due to our lack of contact with others?

However, participants also observed that despite its limitations, Zoom technology provided at least some human connection during the long months without in-person contact. Many described it as 'better than nothing', and admitted that the connection it offered, while not physical, still allowed them to see each other and to do things together each week. One participant went so far as to describe the online sessions as 'a lifesaver... like throwing a life raft out to save somebody... even though it's different, we can still dance with each other. Even in the singing sessions, we can share our voices together'. Ultimately, however, participants were unanimous in their hope that the online format will be temporary, a placeholder until in-person programming can begin again.

Adaptation and Problem-Solving

Another example of the ways in which the positive and negative features of online programming offset each other were the ways in which individual and communal feelings of frustration led to sometimes-surprising creative adaptation and problem-solving. This was experienced in many ways, including figuring out ways to enhance people's access, and learning how to create art while alone yet together on Zoom. Both the leaders and participants of Sol Express learned, sometimes surprisingly, how much is still creatively possible even when people are not sharing the same art table or when they are not moving their bodies together in the same space to create dance or movement. Although Sol Express members could not experience the energy of being creative while in the physical presence of others, many spoke of learning how to adapt, to become comfortable drawing and singing and dancing alone/together. Some even described doing more artwork and more singing than they had before the pandemic, as the forced alone time granted them more space in their lives to do so.

Technology: Access, (Dis)Empowerment and Exclusion

A further example of a feature of the online programming that had both positive and negative outcomes concerns technology. For some, Zoom had positive features, including the possibility to participate from multiple locations: inside, outside, at one's home, at a summer home outside of the city, etc. As one participant said, 'you could take it anywhere!' Some described a significant improvement in their technology skills, such as learning how to manage email, PowerPoint, sharing their screen, using the Zoom 'reactions', etc., and described the increased confidence that resulted. However, others pointed out that the need to have access to the required technology and to the systems that support it, such as a strong internet connection, could be a source of frustration and disempowerment. Rather than people's participation being dependent on their own volition and getting to the program site, people were now reliant on services and networks over which they had little, if any, control. Difficulties accessing and navigating the required technology led some participants to turn to support people such as family members or residential staff. This need to rely on helpers meant some participants had less independence than they had enjoyed before the pandemic, and in some cases, may have prevented some people from participating at all.

In addition, a participant who is partially-sighted and uses other senses to get information noted that access to technology, as well as the ways in which information is presented online, tend to be predominantly visual in nature and can thus exclude people whose ways of receiving information and communicating relies on senses other than sight. Zoom does not make it easy to gather information using senses such as hearing, as exhibited by, for example, how difficult it is to discriminate between the origins of different sounds when on Zoom, and the control of the 'mute' function by meeting leaders. Zoom technology's favouring of visual over auditory communication meant that this participant sometimes needed to ask for clarification from other participants, or used a magnifier, both of which required more time and could be frustrating. His participation required extra work in other ways as well: although it did not initially seem relevant to him that he use his camera or adjust his screen so that others could see him, he made the effort to do so after other participants expressed their appreciation at being able to see him during online groups. His reflections highlight that without careful facilitation, virtual formats such as Zoom can present obstacles to equitable access and can paradoxically result in exclusion.

Sol Express Participants: Online Losses, Geographic Expansion

A final example of counterbalanced experiences concerns the broader issue regarding who is being reached by online programming and who is being 'lost' in the absence of in-person contact. Interestingly, Sol Express's online format did not necessarily result in large decreases in the numbers of people participating. The online format was mostly manageable for those who already knew and trusted each other, and the program also recruited new participants whose usual programs were cancelled outright due to the pandemic, some of whom decided to stay. However, some people decided not to remain with the program, including some of the new participants who had not had the opportunity to develop trusting and familiar relationships, as well as those who felt that they did not benefit from the online format. It was not always possible to maintain contact with those who left the program, resulting in a sense that there are people who have become 'lost' due to the pandemic, the online format making it even more difficult to know who is missing (Pettinichio et al., 2021). Sol Express's creative facilitators have always been aware that the program can only reach a small number of people relative to the total number that might benefit in a city the size of Toronto. Thus, this phenomenon of people missing out on programs that are offered in the community is something that pre-existed the pandemic yet has since been brought into sharper focus. As other scholars have noted, including teachers whose classes were conducted online for much of the pandemic's first year, students and participants who stopped attending online classes or sessions often 'disappeared' into a void of communication and the lack of physical contact made it even more difficult to determine exactly who was missing (Gallagher-McKay et al., 2021; Wong, 2021).

In counterbalance to the losses, some participants noted that being forced to conduct programs online meant that Sol Express was able to extend its geographic reach. People were able to participate from as far away as Nova Scotia, British Columbia and the United Kingdom, something that would not have been possible using an in-person format. This expansion is something that Sol Express leadership would like to reflect upon as the program emerges from pandemic restrictions in the coming months, as a possible way to provide access to those who are not able to attend in person.

Life in a Pandemic: A Shared Suffering

On a less positive note, without counterbalance, some of the participants remarked on the loss of being 'out in the world'. In addition to not seeing each other, people missed walking or taking public transit to their programs and activities. The sense of 'belonging in the world' that we all experience when we move outside of our immediate surroundings and immerse ourselves in our communities, among others who might be strangers yet are sharing in the common pursuit of seeking meaning in our day, was taken away. This was of course not unique to Sol Express participants; however, people's remarking on it in our project is a reminder that everyone, disabled and non-disabled alike, has suffered from the loss of connection and immersion in the human family due to the pandemic.

People also described feeling burdened by the almost constant decision-making and risk assessment that have accompanied pandemic life. We have all been living under imposed regulations and have experienced the emotional and cognitive weight of navigating the constantly-shifting rules that have characterized official attempts to minimize the spread of the virus. Individuals have had to deal with the task of constantly weighing the risk of exposing oneself or those in one's circle to the possibility of contagion versus trying to maintain a sense of personal wellness through human connection and contact. The burden of trying to make the best decision in different situations is especially amplified for those who support others, especially those who live with heightened vulnerability.

Finally, several participants shared that it was hard to think of something 'good' that came out of the pandemic. Although we have all learned from this time, including acquiring new skills and learning how to make the best of a difficult situation, we realize that it is because we are all experiencing a terrible phenomenon – a worldwide pandemic that has killed millions of people – that we have had to do this. Although we have adapted, we are aware that the online format was necessary due to a bad situation and that many, many people have suffered. All of us would have preferred that the learning that we have acquired throughout this time had happened as a result of different, less difficult circumstances.

CONCLUSION

In this chapter, we have presented the findings from a participatory research project that reflected on one group's experience of being part of an online creative arts program during the COVID-19 pandemic. With regard to the research process, all of the participants felt that we embraced important tenets of a participatory approach, particularly when it came to sharing and discussing the research findings, yet there were some aspects of the project where power distribution and leadership remained uneven. The most notable example of this was that the research question did not emerge from the group itself, but was pre-established by three non-disabled members of the research team. Further, much of the writing and some of the key organizing was also done by non-disabled members of the research team, often for reasons of time. On these points, our project aligns with some of the previously identified tensions in participatory research and signals the need to continue to explore ways to do research 'from the ground up' such that all members of the project can contribute as equitably as possible. Rather than this being daunting, however, we prefer instead to consider participatory methods a form of research activism, a political act (Fudge Schormans et al., 2018) in which the parameters and relationships typically attached to knowledge production are challenged.

With regard to the effects of online programming, the principal finding from our project concerns the ways in which the pandemic's effects have been simultaneously experienced as something difficult, and as something from which we learned new skills, new ways of being and creating together, and about our own inner capacities and abilities to adapt. We learned that an online format can have positive effects, such as increasing a program's geographic reach and offering a chance for people who live far away to participate, as well as opportunities for people to continue to develop new technological skills and to connect despite being instructed to remain distant from each other. These interesting, sometimes surprising positive outcomes have the potential to be included in future considerations regarding Sol Express programming, as they open up possibilities for skill development that can happen in non-urgent situations and not only as an emergency response.

We also learned, however, that in spite of its 'life-saving' features, an online format cannot replace in-person contact and the benefits it offers, such as casual conversation, checking in with other people, and drawing from the energy of others when engaged in creative pursuits. Additionally, we learned that without careful monitoring, the technology that aims to offer increased access can paradoxically exclude some people due to the degree of competence required, the need for technological and personal support, and the favouring of some communication methods over others. While this does not necessarily mean that online programs should be discouraged, it does suggest that program designers need to hear how people experience them and work toward ameliorating their negative effects. This point is a reminder of the ways in which the pandemic has affected people differentially. There is no one experience of the pandemic, and the diverse range of experiences in our group demonstrates the need for nuanced and sensitive assessments of its short- and long-term effects.

Aside from these observations regarding concurrent positive/negative effects is the fact that there are many people about whose experience we know nothing. Individuals lost due to the disconnect that was inherent to pandemic protocols remain, to a large degree, unaccounted for, and this is the group about which Sol Express's creative facilitators, as well as other on-the-ground program leaders, remain most concerned. As pandemic restrictions loosen and we slowly resume the ability to gather together, Sol Express's resumption of in-person programs will not only involve picking up where we left off, but determining how to seek out and re-establish connection with those who remain hidden due to pandemic restrictions.

Finally, our time together provided an opportunity for us to reflect on the broader phenomenon of the pandemic and its effects around the world. Several participants referred to the idea of 'the human family' and used images or artefacts of the globe as a reminder of our connection to the global community in spite of the many months of isolation and disconnection. As one participant noted, although this has been very hard, there has been a strange comfort in knowing that we have not been alone in our struggle to remain connected.

ACKNOWLEDGMENTS

Research Team

Natalie Breton has been working and volunteering at Sol Express for over 20 years. She is currently in the role of Artistic Assistant at Sol Express Toronto with L'Arche Toronto. She brings extensive experience with her from having worked as an actor/creative facilitator in theatres both nationally and internationally.

Maya Findlay studied Theatre Production at Metropolitan University. She specialized in arts management and costume, with a minor in dance. She joined Sol Express in 2018 for their production of *Birds Make Me Think About Freedom* and is honoured to be part of this team. Maya lives in Toronto with her partner and dog, Toast.

Irene Pollock is a theatre artist based in Toronto. Recent projects include Sol Express productions *Journey to the Greatest Gift, Red Nose: A Play on Words*, and *Birds Make Me Think About Freedom*, as well as the *Importance of ROI* video. She has performed in musicals including *Grease*, and has led creative workshops at the University of Toronto. Irene works at *The Coffee Shed.*

Matt Rawlins has been an artistic facilitator at Sol Express since 2010. As part of its creative performance team, he has staged theatre productions including *Birds Make Me Think About Freedom* and *Red Knows: A Play on Words*, both of which have featured at the Toronto Fringe Festival, and has contributed to several community art exhibits, including the *Disabilities Arts Showcase* at the Art Gallery of Ontario. Matt is involved with various art-based collaborations in Toronto, including audio, visual, film, print, photography and design work.

Kathleen Woo is an artist, musician, photographer, swimmer and athlete who loves spending time with dogs, family and friends. She has won numerous awards including the Debbie Burns Memorial Award (2018–2019) and Athlete of the Year (2013–2014). Kathleen is part of the L'Arche Toronto Sol Express community where she creates art.

Cheryl Zinyk is the co-founder of Sol Express, L'Arche Toronto, a multidisciplinary arts program for artists who have an intellectual disability. Cheryl has consulted with academics engaging in community-based research for social change at McMaster University School of Social work, and at Metropolitan University School of Disability Studies. She is trained in voice, clown, improvisation, and community-based theatre facilitation.

Co-researchers

Rachel Boardman is a theatre artist, dancer, swimmer and dedicated part of the Coffee Shed team. Rachel has a black belt in TaeKwonDo and won two silver medals at the 2018 Canadian Special Olympics. Rachel loves the art of performing, has been part of Sol Express for many years, and has performed numerous times at the Toronto Fringe Festival.

Naomi Cho loves to move and dance. She has competed at national and provincial levels in rhythmic gymnastics and competes in Special Olympics swimming and alpine skiing. She enjoys spending time with her family and friends, cooking, watching movies, going out to eat, Zumba and dancing. She is looking forward to living independently with her friends in the future.

Robert Gray is a Toronto-based actor. He has performed at the Toronto Fringe Festival in *Seasons*, *Birds Make Me Think About Freedom*, and *Red Knows: A Play on Words.* Robert does voice-over work and was consultant for blind and partially-sighted artists in the production *In Between*. Robert co-facilitates workshops for positive change. A skilled cartographer, Robert is interested in history and geography and enjoys listening to basketball, baseball, football and hockey on the radio.

Nicholas Herd is a founding member of L'Arche Toronto Sol Express and has a love for art, performing, hosting and creating. Nicholas was Creative Director for *Free-bird*, an animated short film long-listed for the Academy Awards. He has worked with

Dramaway and Soulpepper Theatre, and has been featured on *Innowave, Employable Me*, and CBC Gem's *You Can't Ask That*. He created and hosts The Disability Channel's *Keeping It Real with Nick*, and currently works with L'Arche Canada in communications.

Andreas Prinz is an actor, playwright and advocate from Toronto. Over the last 19 years, Andreas has trained and performed with George Brown, L'Arche Toronto Sol Express, Rare Theatre Company, and Drama Way. Andreas performed at the Toronto Fringe from 2017–2020. Andreas is currently working on his play *Anthony's Journey*, supported by the Ontario Arts Council.

NOTES

1. L'Arche Toronto Sol Express is the creative arts program of the L'Arche Toronto community. For simplicity, hereafter it will be referred to as Sol Express.

2. A note on language: Different words to denote people with disabilities are used in this paper, depending on the context and the wishes of the speaker. For example, when discussing the emancipatory research methods proposed by Mike Oliver and other disability studies researchers, we use the term 'disabled people' in alignment with the social model principle that people are disabled by social and political obstacles. At other points, we use the term 'people labelled/with intellectual disabilities' to acknowledge that differently-abled people are often 'labelled' for bureaucratic purposes. We are aware and respectful of the varying ways that people choose to describe themselves, and in light of ongoing discussions regarding peoples' preferences, have devoted part of the methodology section of the paper to explaining our process of deciding how best to describe ourselves.

3. *Birds Make Me Think About Freedom* was a Sol Express theatre production (created in collaboration with Victoria Freeman and Jumblies Theatre) that was performed at the 2019 Fringe Theatre Festival in Toronto, Ontario and in other locations. Guided by interviews and story-sharing with survivors of one of Ontario's large institutions for people labelled/with intellectual disabilities, Sol Express members created a play which explored the experiences of institutional survivors and of the family breakages that often result.

4. For example, *A Part of Me; A Part of Us*, 2018, Todmorden Mills, Toronto.

5. Some of the new online programs include *Text & Technique, Song & Story, Movement & Dance, Visual Art Technique*, and *Voice & Singing*.

6. The higher number of leaders can be explained by a few factors: one of the team members is transitioning to a new role from her former leadership within Sol Express. She remained in the project owing her long history with the group and her relationships with many of the participants. Thus, both she and her replacement were involved. In addition, we were committed to having co-researchers in the project; this also raised the number of people on the leadership team.

7. The consent form explained the purpose of the project, what was expected of each participant, the risks and benefits of participating, that the findings from the project might be published at some point in the future, and that participants could withdraw at any time during the project without any repercussions. It also indicated that each participant would receive an honorarium in the form of a gift card.

8. Participants could print off the consent form, sign it, scan it or take a photo of it, and return it by email; or could use an e-signature. For those participants who did not feel comfortable completing, or did not have adequate resources or support to complete the consent form on their own, team leaders followed up with an individual phone or Zoom call in order that the participant could provide their consent orally. Again, this process reiterates the project's limitation in that it reached people who had either a certain level of competence, or had sufficient support, either from the research team or from members of their household, to work through the informed consent process.

REFERENCES

Alphonso, C. (2021, March 7). For parents of kids with complex needs, Covid-19 school disruptions means losing a lifeline of key supports. *The Globe and Mail*. https://www.theglobeandmail.com/canada/article-for-parents-of-kids-with-complex-needs-covid-19-school-disruptions/

Aubrecht, K., Barber, B., Gaunt, M., Larade, J., Levack, V., Earl, M., & Weeks, L. (2021). Empowering younger residents living in long-term care homes as co-researchers. *Disability & Society*, *36*(10), 1712–1718. https://doi.org/10.1080/09687599.2021.1976112

Buettgen, A., Richardson, J., Beckham, K., Richardson, K., Ward, M., & Reimer, M. (2012). We did it together: A participatory action research study on poverty and disability. *Disability & Society*, *27*(5), 603–616. https://doi.org/10.1080/09687599.2012.669106

Community Living Toronto. (2020, March 16). Covid-19 updates. Retrieved from https://cltoronto.ca/coronavirus/

Coons, K., & Watson, S. (2013). Conducting research with individuals who have intellectual disabilities: Ethical and practical implications for qualitative research. *Journal on Developmental Disabilities*, *19*(2), 14–24. https://www.proquest.com/openview/773a6f0741189988d8b4b7ad358e7cd2/1?pq-origsite=gscholar&cbl=28903

Fox, A. (2015). Invigorating disability aesthetics through art and performance: A report from the Bodies of Work festival of disability arts and culture 2013. *Journal of Literary & Cultural Disability Studies*, *9*(3), 349–355.

French, J., & Jones, L. (2019). Positive You: A self-advocate's arts-based approach to building self-esteem. *Disability & Society*, *34*(2), 189–203. https://doi.org/10.1080/09687599.2018.1539649

Fudge Schormans, A., Wilton, R., & Marquis, N. (2018). Building collaboration in the co-production of knowledge with people with intellectual disabilities about their everyday use of city space. *Area*, *51*(3), 415–422. https://doi.org/10.1111/area.12492

Gallagher-McKay, K., Srivastava, P., Underwood, K., Dhuey, E., McCready, L., Born, K. . . . Sander, B. (June 16, 2021). Covid-19 and education disruptions in Ontario: Emerging evidence on impacts. *Science Briefs of the Ontario COVID-19 Science Advisory Table*, *2*(34). https://doi.org/10.47326/ocsat.2021.02.34.1.0

Gold, B. (2021). Neurodiversity and interdependent creation: Breaking into Canadian Disability Arts. *Studies in Social Justice*, *15*(2), 209–229.

Gorman, R. (2007). Whose Disability Culture? Why we need artist-led disability Critical Disability Arts Networks. *Fuse*, *34*(3), 46–51.

Hole, R., & Stainton, T. (2020). Covid-19: The precarity of families and disability. *Child & Youth Services*, *41*(3), 266–268. https://doi.org/10.1080/0145935X.2020.1834997

Iriarte, E. G., O'Brien, P., & Chadwick, D. (2014). Involving people with intellectual disabilities in research teams: Lessons learned from an Irish experience. *Journal of Policy and Practice in Intellectual Disabilities*, *11*(2), 149–157. https://doi.org/10.1111/jppi.12081

Kidney, C., & McDonald, K. (2014). A toolkit for accessible and respectful engagement in research. *Disability & Society*, *29*(7), 1013–1030. http://dx.doi.org/10.1080/09687599.2014.902357

Maconi, M. L. (2020). More than therapy: Conformity and resistance in an organizational narrative of disability and the performing arts. In S. Green & D. Loseke (Eds.), *New narratives of disability: Constructions, clashes and controversies, research in social science and disability* (Vol. 11, pp. 123–136). Emerald.

Newsinger, J., & Green, W. (2016). Arts policy and practice for disabled children and young people: Towards a 'practice spectrum' approach. *Disability & Society*, *31*(3), 357–372.

Nyqvist, H., & Stjerna, M.-L. (2017). Artistry and disability—Doing art for real? Affordances at a day activity centre with an artistic profile. *Disability & Society*, *32*(7), 966–985. https://doi.org/10.1080/09687599.2017.1337563

Oliver, M. (1992). Changing the social relations of research production? *Disability, Handicap & Society*, *7*(2), 101–114. https://doi.org/10.1080/02674649266780141

Pettinichio, D., Maroto, M., Chai, L., & Lukk, M. (2021, February 24). Findings from an online survey on the mental health effects of COVID-19 on Canadians with disabilities and chronic health conditions. *Disability & Health Journal*. https://doi.org/10.1016/j.dhjo.2021.101085

Rios, D., Magasi, S., Novak, C., & Harniss, M. (2016). Conducting accessible research: Including people with disabilities in public health, epidemiological, and outcome studies. *American Journal of Public Health*, *106*(12), 2137–2144. https://doi.org/10.2105/AJPH.2016.303448

Stöckl, A. (2014). Common humanity and shared destinies: Looking at the Disability Arts Movement from an anthropological perspective. *Anthropology in Action*, *21*(1), 36–43.

Swain, J., & French, S. (2000). Towards an affirmation model of disability. *Disability & Society*, *15*(4), 569–582.

Wong, J. (2021, April 7). Teachers warn that some students have 'checked out' of school and that it will be hard to get them back. *CBC News*. https://www.cbc.ca/news/canada/education-pandemic-missing-students-1.5971911

Yoshida, K., Fudge Schormans, A., Niles, C., & Mahipaul, S. (2021, April 21). Covid-19 amplifies the complexity of disability and race. *The Conversation*. https://theconversation.com/covid-19-amplifies-the-complexity-of-disability-and-race-157933

Chapter 10

EVERYDAY LIFE OF STUDENTS WITH DISABILITIES USING ASSISTANCE SERVICES IN POLAND: LESSONS FROM THE PANDEMIC

Ewa Giermanowska, Mariola Racław and Dorota Szawarska

ABSTRACT

Purpose: *We examine the impact of the COVID-19 pandemic on the functioning of university students with disabilities using assistant support services in Poland. The study aims to (1) reveal the role existing university-based assistant services play in students' lives and (2) examine the impact of the pandemic on assistant services by students with disabilities.*

Methods/Approach: *We gathered and analyzed 25 interviews with students with disabilities from across Poland, from public and nonpublic higher education institutions.*

Findings: *The assistant support service at universities introduced in Poland proved to be fragmentary and limited only to the educational process, which resulted in the exclusion of people with complex disabilities and those requiring support in self-care activities. The pandemic has exacerbated previously observed dimensions of segregation and inequalities leading to disproportionate isolation of students with disabilities. It also highlighted the limited understanding of personal assistantship functioning in the academic context and the need for urgent development of universal access to assistance services across Poland. At the same time the forced move to distant,*

Disability in the Time of Pandemic
Research in Social Science and Disability, Volume 13, 193–210

Published under exclusive licence by Emerald Publishing Limited
ISSN: 1479-3547/doi:10.1108/S1479-354720230000013011

internet-based learning, at least for some students, gave them a sense of self-reliance and independence.

Implications: *This research adds to the understanding of the consequences of the COVID-19 pandemic for students with disabilities in the case of Poland. It also calls for a reexamination of what personal assistance should mean in the context of higher education and beyond.*

Keywords: Disability; assistance services; higher education; COVID-19 pandemic; Poland; personal assistants

INTRODUCTION

The COVID-19 pandemic upended entire communities. As basic support institutions, such as healthcare centers, nurseries, schools, social care severely reduced or suspended their operations, everyday life became much more of a challenge. In the context of a lockdown, there was limited contact between family members and friends, home-based work, and education. People with disabilities were even more affected by the pandemic, as not only some of them were more vulnerable to the virus, but their measures of support, such as home help, assistant services, were severely limited. In this chapter, we explore the situation of some of them in the context of two gateways to independent living: personal assistance and support services in higher education. We do so through the analysis of interviews with students with disabilities, as well as persons running support offices at higher education institutions across Poland.

Independent living is the notion that people with disabilities have a right to exercise control over their own lives and make all decisions that affect them. It is also a social movement of people with disabilities to pursue that right (DeJong, 1979). Personal assistance has long been recognized as a key element in achieving independent living by people with disabilities. So much so that it is one of the measures listed in the United Nations Convention on the Rights of Persons with Disabilities (UN CRPD) (art.19) necessary for independent living and social inclusion.

In general, assistance services at universities are not defined as personal assistance (in the sense of Independent Living) – but as educational/didactic, note-taking/transportation, laboratory, organizational/communication assistance. The role of an assistant at a university refers primarily to the academic context, helping students with disabilities to find their way around their studies. This is one of the many forms of support for students with disabilities that are provided at universities by the Support Offices for Persons with Disabilities. The availability of services at universities varies (for students, doctoral students, academic staff). Universities employ from a few to several dozen assistants. These services are most often provided based on a civil law agreement between the Support Office and the assistant in consultation with the person with a disability. These are fixed-term contracts, the number of hours per month, the type of assistant services, hourly rates are determined, and wages are paid based on monthly work cards accepted by the person with a disability. The Support Offices avoid employing family members as assistants and follow the philosophy of preparing people with disabilities for independent living – the person with a disability is to manage the contract (work cards) and the service provided by the assistant(s).

This is an important issue that existed prior to the pandemic because Poland lacks systemic solutions concerning the availability and financing of personal assistance services, as defined in the UN CRPD. They are carried out "randomly" by nongovernmental organizations and some local governments, only based on project activities. As a result, students in need of assistantship support in activities not related to the process of studying do not receive the necessary support. Also at the end of their studies, outside the walls of the university, they generally do not have access to assistantship services, according to the principle "the end of studies, the end of support."

Personal assistance services in the academic environment is a logical step in furthering the independent living of students with disabilities, which also diversifies the student body, and strengthens equal opportunities. Indeed it is argued that "From the perspective of the individual with a severe physical disability, the lack of personal assistance services in higher education may become the deal-breaker for entering and being successful in the post-secondary environment and in future career endeavors" (Stumbo et al., 2009, p. 13). This is because in some cases personal assistance is needed 24 hours a day, 365 days per year (Stumbo et al., 2009, p. 12) to facilitate independent living. But we observed that many of the disability-related supports available to students in their learning environment in Poland, which tend to be present in other countries such as Sweden and the United States (Järkestig et al., 2016), cannot be called personal assistance in the full meaning of the word. Rather, if assistance-like measures are present, they are called academic or educational assistance. This consists narrowly, for example, of note-taking, help in moving around the campus, assistance in laboratories. While they do not necessarily meet all the student's needs, they can contribute to disabled students' access to university education, sense of achievement, social integration, etc.

We focus on higher education because it is often recognized as a way out of poverty, social exclusion, and as means of becoming employed. This also applies to students with a disability, particularly in relation to employment (Riddell et al., 2005). Furthermore, attending an institution of higher education is meaningful for both disabled and able-bodied students. It is a time of growing independence, gaining new friends, skills, a time of developing one's identity as an adult (Goode, 2007). Nonetheless, academic articles dealing with disabled students' experience at University tend to focus on barriers (e.g. Brandt, 2011; Fuller et al., 2004; Hewett et al., 2021; Papasotiriou & Windle, 2012). This literature shows that some of the barriers result from insufficient or inappropriate support systems in higher education.

Measures supporting students with disabilities in higher education are often introduced following the adoption of nationwide laws related to equal opportunities and non-discrimination. That was so in the USA (Americans with

Disabilities Act 1990), Australia (Disability Discrimination Act 1992), the European Union including Poland (EU Charter of Fundamental Rights, art. 21, 26, EU ratified UN CRPD), and Norway (Discrimination and Accessibility Act) among other countries. However, this does not mean that all higher education institutions introduce such solutions in equal measure. Some universities support students better than others.

In Poland, students with disabilities are a diverse group in terms of impairment, and they are not likely to share the same experience of university education (see also Aquino et al., 2017). We suggest the aim of support measures should be to facilitate the academic and social integration of students with disabilities in the university environment. We argue that such measures are more likely to be successful if they are part of an overall effort to address diversity in higher education.

Students with disabilities are not a homogenous group and it is impossible to generalize about the impact of the COVID-19 pandemic on their lives. What can be safely said is that all students with disabilities, just like all able-bodied students, felt the impact of the pandemic on their education and daily living. However, in the case of students with disabilities when considering that impact, one has to factor in the disability. For students who require personal assistance for daily living activities, or those who require assistance when using computers, the impacts of the pandemic can be more specific and profound as assistance often involves closeness, proximity with others and is therefore a risk factor. The COVID-19-related mass transfer of university education to distance learning also reduced the availability of assistance services normally provided on-site to students with disabilities. Our aims were to understand the consequences of COVID-19 related to the lack of or reduced assistantship on education and independent living.

The Institutional Context of Supporting Students With Disabilities at Polish Universities Before and During the Pandemic

After the change of the political system in Poland from communism to democracy in 1989, market mechanisms were introduced to the economy. As a result, changes also took place in Poland in the area of access to higher education. Young people's educational aspirations, which had been hampered in the prior economy by limited access to universities, could finally be satisfied thanks to the dynamic development of both public and private education. Young people with disabilities, who were practically absent from higher education under the previous regime, could now enter. In the initial period, universities were not prepared for the presence of students with disabilities in the academic environment. There were problems with infrastructure, methods of instruction, as well as attitudinal barriers. Legislative and organizational changes concerning the conditions of studying for students with disabilities and financial support for universities gradually led to the adoption of measures supporting students with disabilities (Giermanowska et al., 2015). According to the Polish Central Statistical Office (GUS, 2021) in the academic year 2020–2021, there were 19,600 students with disabilities (certified disabled) (1.6% of the total number of students). 5,200 people with disabilities graduated (1.8% of the total number of graduates, from the academic year 2019–2020). Among doctoral students, 3.3% were people with disabilities (800people).

The Act of 18 March 2011 (Journal of Laws 2011, No. 84, item 455), introduced in Poland a reform of science and higher education including issues of accessibility. The Regulation of 8 August 2011 to the Act (Journal of Laws No. 179, item 1068) defines the procedure for awarding funds to higher education institutions supporting the education of students who are disabled. As a result, universities gained new opportunities to help students with disabilities.

In addition, Poland ratified the UN CRPD in 2012, which also contributed to legislative change in various sectors. But the reforms appear to be uncoordinated. While Universities more or less managed to introduce educational assistant services, at the moment there is no state run personal assistant services available. Currently, the basic tasks of universities include creating conditions for people with disabilities (candidates for studies, students, doctoral students, and employees) to fully participate in the process of admission to the university for education, during their education (at university, in doctoral schools) and in conducting research-related activities. Universities receive subsidies from the state budget for these purposes, and they can also use their own funds. According to the information posted on the official webpage of the Polish Ministry of Education and Science funds can also be spent on other tasks, such as sign language courses for students or university staff, specialized training, including enabling spatial orientation within the university for undergraduate and postgraduate students with disabilities, the purchasing of specialist equipment and devices to support the teaching process, the purchase of specialist and scientific literature for university libraries for the needs of persons with disability, or other adaptations to infrastructure or other forms of support. It is worth emphasizing that expenditures on behalf of persons with disabilities can be allocated to persons with and without a confirmed disability certificate from the State. For this purpose, universities draw up internal regulations, in which they define the qualification criteria and forms of assistance for undergraduate and postgraduate students and employees conducting research. Moreover, students with disabilities may receive financial support in the form of a special scholarship for persons with disability and other forms of material support.

Funds from the subsidies that universities receive can be used to finance or co-finance many different forms of support, including the service of a personal assistant for a person with a disability. But these assistant services at universities in Poland are relatively new, unevenly spread, and not yet available to the extent that they are needed. The presence of assistants for persons with disabilities at universities is one of the instruments supporting the educational process of persons with disabilities, enabling them to participate more fully in the educational process and social life. The model of an educational assistantship at universities performs both supportive and compensatory functions (Chrząszcz, 2016). The introduction of assistance services at universities was due to, among other things, the lack of universal and accessible personal assistance services for all people with disabilities. The Personal Assistance Services Act has still not been implemented today, and one of the barriers is the lack of sufficient funding to meet the needs of all individuals with disabilities in their daily functioning.

Prior Research on Pandemic Effects on Disabled College Students

The adverse impact of the COVID-19 pandemic on students with disabilities is illustrated by other research publications. In a study conducted in the USA, the impact of the pandemic on students with disabilities was found to be significant and disproportionately large compared to students without disabilities (Sutton, 2021).[1] Students with physical, learning, neurodevelopmental and cognitive disabilities were more likely than their peers to experience financial hardship, food, and housing insecurity. A greater proportion of students with disabilities (53–70%) reported major depressive disorders which could be related to the pandemic, compared to 34% of students without a disability. Students with ADHD often indicated that the home environment was too distracting, students with major depressive disorder experienced high levels of isolation and loneliness, students with anxiety disorders faced a much higher level of anxiety due to the ambiguity around the pandemic and uncertainty about the future of their education (Sutton, 2021). In the UK, as in our study, at least part of the problems faced by students with disability stemmed from a lack of appropriate institutional response. Between March and June 2020 out of the 104 higher education institutions surveyed by Newman (2022, p. 9), only 15% issued new advice to academics on the impact of the new learning environment on students with disability. This shows that the integration of students with disabilities is only skin deep.

Prior Research on Student Utilization of Supports in Poland Before and During the Pandemic

Prior research among students with disabilities at Polish universities, conducted in the 2015–2016 academic year, focused on student experiences with these assistants. It showed that young people expect their assistants to both "prosthetize" them in terms of their impairment-related requirements (e.g., help in taking notes, help in moving around, pushing a wheelchair, translating didactic materials for students with sensory disabilities, helping to organize work or translating into sign language), as well as accompanying them in social situations (e.g., when establishing contacts with a peer group or support in conflict situations) (Chrząszcz, 2016).

In March 2020, the situation at universities changed dramatically due to the declaration of a national lockdown, linked to the coronavirus pandemic. As in many countries, including Poland, it was a shocking event for society. It caused a wave of shock among politicians, the media, and the public (Kauffmann et al., 2016). Apart from the clear threat to human life and health associated with the emergence and spread of an unknown virus in Poland, new social risks also emerged, i.e.: an increasing multi-level crisis of trust (in global, national, and local relations), a possible crisis of democracy and return to closed nation-states, economic crisis and long-term economic downturn, social polarization and stratification, increased tendency for individualistic rather than community behavior (Auleytner & Grewiński, 2020, pp. 11–16). The emergence of an immediate threat to physical survival and new risks resulted in a sense of anxiety and chronic stress in many Polish residents.

It also affected the functioning of universities and the welfare of students. A national survey of students conducted by a student organization (the Independent Students' Union) indicated that during the first period of the introduction of national lockdown (March–April 2020), the situation of many young people deteriorated (Białas et al., 2020). A large number of vulnerable students were not informed about the possibilities of financial support during the pandemic, and some lost the opportunity to live in student residences and access to their belongings left there. Maintenance grants for poor students were not paid on time. The universities did not have adequate equipment and facilities to ensure that all students had access to remote education. Approximately a quarter of the students surveyed received free psychological support during this period, which indicates the extent of mental health needs (Białas et al., 2020). The latter finding is confirmed by research conducted among academic youth in other countries. Their results were summarized by Federica Cielo, Randi Ulberg, and Dina Di Giacomo: "The COVID-19 outbreak has globally affected and is still affecting youth mental health. [. . .]The psychological impact was related to the experience of several intensive stressors, such as academic perspectives, massive e-learning adoption, economic obstacles, social restrictions, and daily living side effects related to the COVID-19 outbreak" (Cielo et al., 2021, p. 13).

Public authorities and universities also took countermeasures at the start of the pandemic, although they have been insufficient and problematic. From March 2020, the rules for the functioning of Polish universities were changed. Based on, inter alia, Regulation of the Minister of Science and Higher Education of 23 March 2020 on the temporary limitation of the operation of certain entities of the higher education and science system in connection with preventing, counteracting, and combating COVID-19 (Journal of Laws of 2020, item 511) and the Act of 20 July 2018 – Law on higher education and science (Journal of Laws of 2020, item 85, as amended) universities began to introduce solutions related to work and study aimed at protecting employees and students and limiting the spread of the pandemic. This meant going online. During the height of the pandemic, university employees (both academic staff and nonacademic staff) were not required to work on university premises, except when necessary to ensure the continuity of university operations. Higher education institutions were not closed down, but instead operated remotely. Remote mode of studying and administrative service using electronic communication was introduced for students, doctoral students, employees. Restrictions on accommodation have also been introduced in student dormitories.

A nationwide study on distance learning conducted in Poland after the first few months of the pandemic showed that young people were quite critical, indicating that lecturers were more demanding of students during online learning, and at the same time learning in this mode was less effective than on-site learning

(94% of students surveyed said that on-site learning was more effective) (Muda, 2020). Poor contact with the lecturer and disorganization of social life were identified as the main disadvantages (Muda, 2020).

Hastily introduced legal regulations, without sufficient consultation with the academic community and the existing lack of equipment, software, and skills to work/learn in the form of remote communication among students and employees caused many problems and chaos. Universities gradually improved the competencies of staff by introducing training and purchasing appropriate hardware and software. Successive waves of the pandemic prolonged the restrictions on education and work at universities, which persist into the present (Spring 2022). In September 2021, the Ministry of Education and Science published a document entitled. "Guidelines for the safe operation of universities and other entities of the higher education and science system during an epidemic" (2021). It is a set of recommendations, advice, and suggestions that should be applied taking into account the changing legal situation, the local number of cases, the dynamics of epidemic development, the assessment of key risk factors as well as organizational and technical conditions of a given university.

During the pandemic period and in this wider context of on-site schooling being suspended, universities also withdrew or reduced many additional services offered to students, including assistance services. Our focus is on how, given the prior literature and context of how universities responded to the pandemic, to better understand the consequences for disabled students. The pandemic and responses to it triggered new processes of inequality in education and on the labor market, and affected undergraduate and postgraduate students with disabilities in specific ways. Through interviews, we examine the period before the pandemic and compare this to the changes that occurred during the pandemic.

METHODOLOGY

To better understand disabled students experiences, qualitative interviews with students who use assisted services at universities and interviews with experts from the Offices for Persons with Disabilities (BON) were carried out between June and September 2020.[2] As a research team, we had already planned research on assistance services at universities before the pandemic. But when embarking on this research in 2020, we had to cope with a new situation. The lockdown of universities in Poland took place in March 2020. It led to changes in the conditions for studying and affected the functioning of university support services. Distance learning had become the dominant form of conducting classes and also covered the next academic year 2020–2021. Events unforeseen at the time of planning the research prompted us to take them into account. As a result, we introduced additional questions about the impact of the pandemic on study conditions and the use of support services to the previously prepared interview scenarios with students and experts. We, therefore, focus on these parts of the interviews in this chapter.

Data Collection

Data collection began with 25 individual interviews were conducted among young people with disabilities studying at university, 19 with women and 6 with men. Interviews were conducted with learners at all three levels of academic education (bachelor's, master's and doctoral studies), from all modes of education (full-time, evening and extramural studies) of various universities in Poland (including: in Warsaw, Białystok, Lublin, Gdynia, Rzeszów, Gdańsk, Kraków, Łódź). The interviewees included 14 students (male and female) from public and non-public universities and 11 PhD students. Informants with various types and degrees of disability, including movement, sensory (hearing, vision), and neurological disabilities were recruited for the interviews. In Poland, students in Bachelor's, Master's, and Doctoral programs simply have the status of students and there are no differences between them in terms of the availability of disability support. Hence, we discuss their experiences together.

The interview schedule included approximately 25 questions focused on the following issues: experiences with university or personal assistance services during the studies, perceptions, and opinions about the functioning of the system of (university, personal) assistance services at universities and in the future workplace, the role of personal assistance in the implementation of the demands of independent living, especially in the areas of education and professional work, the impact of the COVID-19 pandemic on the possibility of using (university, personal) assistance services, quality of life and the course of studies.

We also conducted four interviews with people who have experience in managing Disability Support Services at universities in Warsaw, Poznań, Łódź, and Zielona Góra. We started the selection of such experts with a research reconnaissance at our home university – the University of Warsaw. Based on the information obtained regarding the involvement of universities in the development of assistance services at universities, we obtained several competent informants.

All of the interviews were conducted by five interviewers recruited from among young researchers with previous experience in interviewing persons with disabilities. Due to the pandemic, interviews were primarily conducted by telephone or remotely using video conferencing platforms like Zoom. There were also exceptions. One respondent with hearing impairment chose a written form of answering the questions, in another case due to technical reasons only a telephone interview was conducted. We reached students using the snowball method. We gained access to the sample through contacts with Disability Support Offices at universities, the Section of Sociology of Disability of the Polish Sociological Association, academics, and doctoral students dealing with the phenomenon of disability.

Data Analysis

All of the interviews were recorded and we obtained written consent from all our interviewees to record and disseminate the results of the analysis. The interviews were transcribed and analyzed using NVivo 12. We coded the data as a team. An eclectic coding strategy was employed combining descriptive and structural coding. Initial codes were determined by the overall framework of our research project: independent living, assistant services, the working relationship between students with disabilities and their assistants, and the COVID-19 pandemic. Following the initial coding of two interviews (one with a student with a disability, one with an expert), further codes were developed, adding more detail to the general themes.

FINDINGS

Structural Problems Affecting Assistance Services at Universities

The main problem reported by experts about the functioning of assistantship services at universities was their limited scope in covering only tasks related to the study process. Narrowing the service only to the academic context limited the normal functioning of students with disabilities when they were outside the university. Given the context in Poland where personal assistant services are not universally available, this has negative consequences for the realization of students' professional aspirations, access to the labor market, and employment.

> "...given that there is such a lot of systemic gaps, I have this feeling that universities have dealt quite well with the subject of disability, and that overall works quite well. But the thing is, there is nothing after [the studies]. The labor market, PFRON subsidies for employment and salaries, I do not know if it has any motivational dimension [E_Poznań].[3]

In other words, universities were potentially having to make up for a broader lack of access to personal assistance services. This creates inequalities among students and graduates with disabilities because it mainly affects people with complex disabilities and functional limitations that require the support of a personal assistant (Giermanowska et al., 2022, forthcoming).

When asked whether providing personal assistance should be the role of the university, one of the experts replied:

> I am not sure if this is a task for the university, i.e. I think that every person with a disability, regardless of whether they are at university or not, should have such an assistant. I assume that such a student should come to university already with a personal assistant who will help them not only at university but also in other situations, in their personal life, in taking care of their health, etc [E_Poznań].[4]

At the same time, it is worth emphasizing that some universities, noticing gaps in the existing solutions, made their own decisions to extend the scope of university assistance services, e.g. to include hygiene-related activities, which increased the access of students with disabilities to the education process:

> We introduced, I am talking about the University, about the Office for Persons with Disabilities, for example, assistant services consisting in support in toilets, and this caused many people to come to these studies or to stay there, who in the previous model would not have had a chance to function, because we did not manage, for example, to arrange schedules

> so that a person could have one class in the morning, one in the evening, and go home in the middle [E_Warszawa].

Another area that was the area of reflection of students and experts is the possibility of fulfilling professional aspirations by students with disabilities. Before the pandemic, students often emphasized the role of education in the process of them becoming independent, getting a job, and leading an independent life. However, this process had its limitations, as the opening of universities to students with disabilities was not accompanied by the opening of the labor market to disabled people (Giermanowska & Racław, 2014).

While the introduction of assistance services at universities made previously impossible opportunities for further education and professional activity possible, these assistance services outpaced the universal access to personal assistance services in everyday life and on the labor market. The result was the emergence of a category of so-called "eternal students" where people did not want to leave the walls of the university because it meant giving up assistant services and the loss of independence:

> In the end, after defending the thesis and receiving the diploma we can hang it on the wall, and in 90% of cases, not much happens with this diploma, with this knowledge. No, we are not going any further. [W1]

The students interviewed had career plans, but knew that they could be difficult to pursue due to the lack of systemic solutions. "Currently, there is no adapted workplace for me in Poland because the employer would have to hire a personal assistant along with me" [W21].

COVID-19 and Support Services at Universities Once They Went Remote

The change in the mode of operation of universities, due to the pandemic and the nationwide quarantine, affected the organization of the teaching process through the shift to remote teaching. This also affected the social life of universities, which came to be marked by isolation of staff and students and the disappearance of direct or in-person social contact. Consequently, assistance services sometimes seemed unnecessary, so some universities took official decisions to suspend them:

> The university ordered the suspension of assistants of people with disability, but the Rector's Plenipotentiary (...) asked [the assistant - editor's note on] to ask me (...) if I have any problems. (. . ..) I have not used his services at all since mid-March [W18].

Students themselves indeed confirmed the lack of need to use the services of an assistant in the compensatory role in the situation of remote learning. As one of our respondents emphasized: "There is no problem of dependence in the laboratory, there is no problem of the need for help" [W1].

Some of the people managing the university support office also noted that during the initial period of the pandemic and the introduced lockdown, universities lost control over the functioning of the assistantship services. They were going on spontaneously, based on developed relationships between lecturers, students, and their assistants:

> I have little contact. I know that they work, the lecturers tell me that they work with these assistants because they get what they should get from these assistants, and they send the assistant what they should give to the disabled person. So I know they are working. So that's all I can say for today [E_Zielona Góra].

The transition from site-based learning to learning with digital platforms for some students with disabilities was not always difficult. It was preferable for some and they were digitally competent and proficient in the online space. We already know that digital platforms are used mainly by younger people with disabilities (age brackets: 16–24, 25–34) and that they tend to be better educated, professionally or educationally active, and living in cities (Królewski et al., 2014). Prior research also shows that internet users in Poland are over-represented among people with moderate and severe certified disabilities compared to people with mild disabilities (Królewski et al., 2014, p. 344).

A prior study that surveyed students with disabilities showed that for many the Internet "is a tool whose functionality (and also usefulness) could eliminate barriers resulting from disability to a greater degree than it is in overcoming the typical time and space limitations among non-disabled people" (Królewski et al., 2014, p. 344). This suggests a potential positive effect of introducing the national quarantine – namely the popularization of remote work. This mode of work is desirable for some young people with disabilities. Thus, many considered the ongoing normalization and destigmatization of remote work to be a kind of socioeconomic achievement: "So undoubtedly, social quarantine for the entire nation has pros and cons. The undeniable upside, however, is the demystification of remote work as such, which I am very happy about" [W1].

But there were also the negative phenomena associated with the transition to distance learning. Respondents indicated weariness with the lack of social contacts and an increased sense of isolation and fatigue resulting from the need to change routine practices:

> I used to have a set mode that I go to work from Monday to Friday, go to rehabilitation on Wednesday after work, then on Saturday I go shopping with my assistant and go for a walk. And here this Covid just messed everything up (...) At the moment, studies are simply remote, so there is no such contact with people, which I have always cared about (W22).

> It was in March that I really felt that I am a disabled person, even though I have been disabled for twenty-some years. Well, it was impossible to go out, I could not meet anyone (W19).

The state of social isolation, limitation of contact (in Poland called social distance) was interpreted by the respondents as a forced lesson in social education for all Poles, sensitizing them to the experience of disability:

> The undoubted advantage of these restrictions and national quarantine is that all people, regardless of their social status, could at least for a moment try to feel like disabled people, like dependent people [W1].

> Actually at the moment, I don't feel that I have any disability, just as if I were a completely able person [W18].

During the lockdown periods, all were "prisoners in their own home" with limited social contact and limited external relationships. The situation of loneliness, immobility, the necessity to be outside the group in the real world, became a reality for both able-bodied and disabled students. For some, their online contacts meant they felt less alone. "I did not feel it because we worked a lot online" [W19]. Yet all of the students had to limit their freedoms and independence for the sake of the common good. Therefore, some of the respondents indicated that while in the pandemic period the most important role of the assistant was providing emotional support, changing the quality of their relationship with the assistant:

> The bond between me and this assistant grew even stronger (...) being able to hear the assistant's voice gave me a sense of security because everyone during the pandemic was confined to their homes, sometimes feeling stranded by it. [W4]

For some students the transition to distance learning gave them a sense of being just like all the other students: "Actually at the moment, I don't feel that I have any disability, just as if I were a completely able person" [W18]. Moreover, some coped very well with the situation, which gave them a sense of independence:

> You know, everything changed because I had remote classes, we did most things remotely, online,. through email, instant messaging, and I didn't need an assistant for such things on a daily basis I would do these online classes at home without any help because after all, I don't need help at home. [W 17]

The transition to distance learning and the suspension or limitation of assistance services at universities for some categories of students was extremely painful. Deaf or hard of hearing, blind and partially sighted people, those in the autism spectrum, have often been excluded from learning and social relationships. But this had been mitigated by the provision of assistance at the university and now this was lost: "Students were cut off from a source of direct contact... from the only way of entering life and contact with society" [W12]. Educational and social isolation resulted in a variety of coping mechanisms like minimization of needs: "The epidemic is very much affecting the quality of my studies because I find it difficult to participate in remote classes. I have severely limited my use of attendant services because I am afraid to allow strangers who come in contact with people with disabilities, into my home" [W21].

It also lead to a decrease in motivation to learn: "Well, also from the psychological point of view, sitting at home made me bored and lazy. Oh, I'll say that, because there's a lot of material to study, and there's less mobilization when you're at home all the time and you don't have any fixed hours" [W6].

Finally, if students lost their assistant in the pandemic, the support that was previously provided by them was taken over by a family member. Interviewees stated that, *mother is the assistant, since last Friday there are classes, my mother takes notes for me* [W21]. These changes were experienced as a loss of independence, self-determination, autonomy by the student with disabilities, and a return to paternalistic relationships.

DISCUSSION

As our results show, the introduction of assistance services as one of the instruments to support students has contributed to equal opportunities but the loss of them during the pandemic affected disabled students in particular ways. In the above section, we described structural problems, in Poland, where there is no systemic supply of personal assistance, and those who need it, rely on family members, NGOs, and occasional local government projects, limitation of any assistant services, including educational assistance, has an impact on the autonomy of students with disability. Our research confirms the need for seamless integration of personal assistance with educational assistance, where possible. At the same time, the COVID-19 pandemic revealed a lack of procedures and emergency solutions for students with disabilities, which shows that their presence and integration at higher education institutions is often only superficial. What is also clearly needed are health-related procedures in the context of assistant services. We believe that personal assistance is an essential service, and there must be a way in which it may remain operational even during a pandemic, provided precautions are taken.

Secondly, distance learning forced by the COVID-19 pandemic shows that personal assistance is of primary importance in relation to educational assistance, in terms of autonomy and social integration, and that the pandemic affected people with different impairments in different ways. Most of our respondents were able to manage distance learning with no or minimal support from educational assistants. But a major impact of the situation was isolation and dependence related to daily tasks. While educational assistants were unable to help with the latter during the pandemic, they worked to lessen the isolation of students with disabilities.

CONCLUSION

Despite the formal implementation of the UN Convention, people with disabilities in Poland still face significant barriers in accessing health care, education, employment and recreation, and participation in political life. They are more at risk of poverty or social exclusion than non-disabled people, and more than half of them feel discriminated against (Union of Equality. Strategy for the Rights of Persons with Disabilities 2021–2030, 2021, pp. 4–5).

The COVID-19 pandemic and its impact on the functioning of the economy and society have exacerbated pre-existing barriers and inequalities, particularly for people with disabilities in high-risk groups and we would argue those relying on personal assistance (see also Banks et al., 2021). Zoe Meleo-Erwin et al. (2021, p. 3), building on their study of colleges and universities in the NYC metropolitan area, emphasize that: "What COVID-19 has made plain, however, is that the outcomes and impacts of unprecedented infectious, contagious disease are fundamentally connected to and magnified by inequalities during 'precedented' time." In the event of unforeseen disasters, as already demonstrated by the aftermath of Hurricanes Katrina, Irene, and Sandy, people with disabilities were disproportionately affected due to overlapping and mutually reinforcing factors such as impairment, inequalities in the social determinants of health, and the failure of local, state, and federal agencies to adequately consider accessibility needs in disaster planning (Meleo-Erwin et al., 2021, p. 3). As the cited researchers argue, citing the words of activist Adrien Weibgen, disadvantage or discrimination against people with disabilities in times of risk, danger or social uncertainty is not necessarily the result of direct, purposeful hatred and bigotry. It may be the result of "benign neglect", which, however, "involves a choice to value some lives more than others" (Meleo-Erwin et al., 2021, p. 3).

In Poland, as we emphasized earlier, difficulties with the functioning of assistance services at universities are exacerbated by the model of support for people with disabilities that is incompatible with the UN CRPD. At the same time, popularization of remote education and work facilitated, in the case of some students with certain types of disabilities, more participation in the process of education and work. But it did not prevent social isolation, which in the case of people with disabilities is of key importance for the process of social inclusion. These phenomena have been superimposed on the lack of systemic solutions regarding access to personal assistance services beyond the walls of the university. Students studying remotely and deprived of university support services often became dependent on their families and "trapped" in their places of residence.

Yet, there is a growing awareness among disabled students in Poland of their rights, including the right to support in the form of personal assistance services and the right to independent living. The demand for assistance services at universities will grow. It is influenced by an increase in educational aspirations, awareness of one's rights, the need for independence, and an increase in mental disorders (also after COVID-19). However, additional changes in public policies are needed, including systemic solutions in the form of personal assistance services beyond the educational process and the university walls.

NOTES

1. About 30,000 students in 9 large public universities were surveyed, the survey was conducted between May and July 2020.
2. The interviews were conducted as part of an internal grant from the Institute of Applied Social Sciences, University of Warsaw.
3. PFRON – the State Fund for the Rehabilitation of the Disabled, is a fund created from contributions made by employers who do not employ the required number of disabled people (in Poland it is 6%, with some exceptions), the funds of which are used, among others, to support professional activity of people with disabilities.
4. In parentheses, we indicate the designation of interviews with experts from the Offices of Disabled People at universities [E_ city name] and people with disabilities [W interview number].

REFERENCES

Aquino, K. C., Alhaddab, T. A., & Kim, E. (2017). Does disability matter?. Students' satisfaction with college experiences. In E. Kim & K. C. Aquino (Eds.), *Disability as diversity in higher education: Policies and practices to enhance student success* (pp. 47–60). Routledge.

Auleytner, J., & Grewiński, M. (2020). Pandemia koronawirusa i ryzyka społeczne z nią związane a chaos w zarządzaniu państwem–dokąd zmierzamy? Coronavirus pandemic and related social risks and chaos in the management of the state – Where we are going to? In N. G. Pikuła, M. Grewiński, E. Zdebska, & W. Glac (Eds.), *Wyzwania dla polityki społecznej w kontekście pandemii koronawirusa* (pp. 11–25). Scriptum.

Banks, L. M., Davey, C., Shakespeare, T., & Kuper, H. (2021). Disability-inclusive responses to COVID-19: Lessons learnt from research on social protection in low-and middle-income countries. *World Development*, *137*, 105178. https://doi.org/10.1016/j.worlddev.2020.105178

Białas, K., Glaba, P., Hanusko, K., Serafin, P., Waryszak, M., & Zdral, S. (2020). *Sytuacja studentów w czasie epidemii koronawirusa. Raport NZS (National Students' Union Report)*. https://nzs.org.pl/wp-content/uploads/2020/04/NZS_Sytuacja-studentow_w-czasie_epidemii_koronawirusa.pdf. Accessed on September 30, 2020.

Brandt, S. (2011). From policy to practice in higher education: The experiences of disabled students in Norway. *International Journal of Disability, Development and Education*, *58*(2), 107–120. https://doi.org/10.1080/1034912X.2011.570494

Chrząszcz, K. (2016). Asystent edukacyjny–pomoc czy droga w kierunku bezradności studentów z niepełnosprawnością?. *Niepełnosprawność–Zagadnienia, Problemy, Rozwiązania*, *3*(20), 23–35.

Cielo, F., Ulberg, R., & Di Giacomo, D. (2021). Psychological impact of the COVID-19 outbreak on mental health outcomes among youth: A rapid narrative review. *International Journal of Environmental Research and Public Health*, *18*(11), 6067. https://doi.org/10.3390/ijerph18116067

DeJong, Gerben, M. P. A. (1979). Independent living: From social movement to analytic paradigm. *Archives of physical medicine and rehabilitation*, *60*(10), 435–436.

Diagnoza potrzeb osób z niepełnosprawnością w kontekście modyfikacji istniejących i zaproponowania nowych instrumentów włączenia społecznego. (2021). *[(Diagnosis of the needs of people with disability in the context of modifying the existing and proposing new instruments of social inclusion 2021)], Aggregate Report*. Fundacja im. Królowej Polski św. Jadwigi, Puszczykowo 2021. https://www.malopolska.uw.gov.pl/doc/Diagnoza%20potrzeb%20os%C3%B3b%20z%20niepe%C5%82nosprawno%C5%9Bci%C4%85.pdf

EMPL, D. (2021, March). Union of equality: Strategy for the rights of persons with disabilities 2021–2030. EDF: European Disability Forum.

Fuller, M., Healey, M., Bradley, A., & Hall, T. (2004). Barriers to learning: A systematic study of the experience of disabled students in one university. *Studies in Higher Education*, *29*(3), 303–318. https://doi.org/10.1080/03075070410001682592

Giermanowska, E., Kumaniecka-Wiśniewska, A., Racław, M., & Zakrzewska-Manterys, E. (2015). *Niedokończona emancypacja. Wejście niepełnosprawnych absolwentów szkół wyższych na rynek pracy*. Wydawnictwa Uniwersytetu Warszawskiego.

Giermanowska, E., & Racław, M. (2014). Pomiędzy polityką życia, emancypacją i jej pozorowaniem. Pytania o nowy model polityki społecznej wobec zatrudnienia osób niepełnosprawnych. *Studia Socjologiczne*, *2*(214), 107–127.

Giermanowska, E., Racław, M., Szawarska, D. (2022, forthcoming). Personal assistance services in Poland during the period of higher education: Paving the way for independent living. In S. Meyers, M. McCloskey, & G. Petri (Eds.), *Hierarchies of disability human rights. Interdisciplinary disability studies book series*. Routledge Press.

Goode, J. (2007). Managing disability: Early experiences of university students with disabilities. *Disability & Society*, *22*(1), 35–48. https://doi.org/10.1080/09687590601056204

Hewett, R., Douglas, G., & McLinden, M. (2021). "They were questioning whether I would even bother coming back". Exploring evidence of inequality in "access", "success" and "progression" in higher education for students with vision impairment. *Educational Review*, 1–23. https://doi.org/10.1080/00131911.2021.1907315

Järkestig Berggren, U., Rowan, D., Bergbäck, E., & Blomberg, B. (2016). Disabled students' experiences of higher education in Sweden, the Czech Republic, and the United States–A comparative institutional analysis. *Disability & Society*, *31*(3), 339–356. https://doi.org/10.1080/09687599.2016.1174103

Kaufmann, M., Lewandowski, J., Choryński, A., & Wiering, M. (2016). Shock events and flood risk management: A media analysis of the institutional long-term effects of flood events in The Netherlands and Poland. *Ecology and Society*, *21*(4), 51. https://doi.org/10.5751/ES-08764-210451

Królewski, J., Masłyk, T., Migaczewska, E., Stojkow, M., & Żuchowska, D. (2014). Potencjał Internetu i jego (nie) wykorzystanie w kontekście potrzeb osób niepełnosprawnych. In B. Gąciarz & S. Rudnicki (Eds.), *Polscy niepełnosprawni. Od kompleksowej diagnozy do nowego modelu polityki społecznej* (pp. 335–376). Wydawnictwa AGH.

Meleo-Erwin, Z., Kollia, B., Fera, J., Jahren, A., & Basch, C. (2021). Online support information for students with disabilities in colleges and universities during the COVID-19 pandemic. *Disability and Health Journal*, *14*(1), 101013. https://doi.org/10.1016/j.dhjo.2020.101013

Muda, R. (2020). *Jak studenci postrzegają nauczanie zdalne? Ogólnopolskie badanie opinii studentów na temat nauczania zdalnego*. Report prepared by FLOW Centrum Badawcze. https://www.pum.edu.pl/__data/assets/pdf_file/0011/179093/Studenci-a-COVID_FLOW-Centrum-Badawcze.pdf. Accessed on September 30, 2020.

Newman, I. (2022). COVID-lockdown in English higher education March–June 2020. Were disabled students' needs forgotten? *Perspectives: Policy and Practice in Higher Education*, 1–11. https://doi.org/10.1080/13603108.2021.2000516

Papasotiriou, M., & Windle, J. (2012). The social experience of physically disabled Australian university students. *Disability & Society*, *27*(7), 935–947. https://doi.org/10.1080/09687599.2012.692027

Riddell, S., Tinklin, T., & Wilson, A. (2005). *Disabled students in higher education: Perspectives on widening access and changing policy*. Routledge. https://doi.org/10.4324/9780203087121

Stumbo, N. J., Martin, J. K., & Hedrick, B. N. (2009). Personal assistance for students with severe physical disabilities in post-secondary education: Is it the deal breaker? *Journal of Vocational Rehabilitation*, *30*(1), 11–20. https://doi.org/10.3233/JVR-2009-0449

Sutton, H. (2021). COVID-19 disproportionately impacts students with disabilities across all sectors. *Disability Compliance for Higher Education*, *26*(6). 9. https://doi.org/10.1002/dhe.30973

WEBSITES

GUS. (2021, December 02). Osoby niepełnosprawne w 2020 roku. https://stat.gov.pl/obszary-tematyczne/rynek-pracy/pracujacy-bezrobotni-bierni-zawodowo-wg-bael/osoby-niepelnosprawne-w-2020-roku,33,2.html

Ministerstwo Edukacji i Nauki () Wsparcie niepełnosprawnych studentów i doktorantów. https://www.gov.pl/web/edukacja-i-nauka/wsparcie-niepelnosprawnych-studentow-i-doktorantow. Accessed on February 01, 2022.

LEGAL ACTS

Rozporządzenia Ministra Nauki i Szkolnictwa Wyższego z dnia 23 marca 2020 r. w sprawie czasowego ograniczenia funkcjonowania niektórych podmiotów systemu szkolnictwa wyższego i nauki w związku z zapobieganiem, przeciwdziałaniem i zwalczaniem COVID-19 (Dz.U. 2020 poz. 511). [Regulation of the Minister of Science and Higher Education of 23 March 2020 on the temporary limitation of the operation of certain entities of the higher education and science in relation to the prevention, counteraction and combating COVID-19 (Journal of Laws 2020, item 511).

Rozporządzenie Ministra Nauki i Szkolnictwa Wyższego z dnia 8 sierpnia 2011 r. w sprawie trybu udzielania oraz zasad i trybu rozliczania dotacji na dofinansowanie lub finansowanie kosztów realizacji inwestycji uczelni publicznej (Dz. U. Nr 179, poz. 1068) [Regulation of the Minister of Science and Higher Education of 8 August 2011 on the procedure for awarding, and the rules and procedure for accounting for, subsidies to co-finance or finance investment costs of a public higher education institution (Journal of Laws No. 179, item 1068)].

United Nations. (2006). Convention on the Rights of Persons with Disabilities. Treaty Series, 2515, 3.

Ustawa z 20 lipca 2018 r. – Prawo o szkolnictwie wyższym i nauce (Dz. U. z 2020 r. poz. 85 z późn. zm.). [Act of July 20, 2018 - Law on Higher Education and Science (Journal of Laws of 2020, item 85, as amended).].

Ustawa z dnia 18 marca 2011 r. o zmianie ustawy – Prawo o szkolnictwie wyższym, ustawy o stopniach naukowych i tytule naukowym oraz o stopniach i tytule w zakresie sztuki oraz o zmianie niektórych innych ustaw (Dz.U. 2011, nr 84, poz. 455). [Act of 18 March 2011 amending the Act - Law on Higher Education, the Act on Academic Degrees and Academic Title and Degrees and Title in Art and amending some other acts (Journal of Laws 2011, No. 84, item 455)].

Wytyczne bezpiecznego funkcjonowania uczelni i innych podmiotów systemu szkolnictwa wyższego i nauki w okresie epidemii (2021), Ministerstwo Edukacji i Nauki, Warszawa. [Guidelines for the safe functioning of universities and other entities of the higher education and science system during the epidemic (2021), Ministry of Education and Science, Warsaw.

Chapter 11

DISABILITY AND THE DIVERSITY FRAMEWORK IN THE POST-PANDEMIC WORKPLACE

Courtney Mullin, Robert Gould, Sarah Parker Harris and Robin Jones

ABSTRACT

Purpose: *In this chapter, we explore the role of disability-based employee resource groups (ERG) in implementing large organizations' disability inclusion strategies and how pandemic responses shaped the workplace treatment and inclusion of disabled employees.*

Methods/Approach: *We conducted semi-structured interviews with disability-based ERG members and diversity, equity, and inclusion (DEI) professionals in large corporate settings. Then, we analyzed how pandemic-induced changes in the workplace impacted disability inclusion efforts and experiences of disabled employees.*

Findings: *Results from our study revealed that workplace disability inclusion responsibilities shifted to disability-based ERGs during the onset of the pandemic. Participants detailed how organizational disability inclusion practices and policies expanded through increased awareness among some employee bases and were de-prioritized to the point of erasure in other situations. Within the context of the pandemic, members of disability-based ERGs played an integral part in both enhancing visibility of disability and responding to instances of ableism in their respective organizations.*

Implication/Value: *Findings provide context as to how shifting organizational contexts, such as pandemic related workplace policies, becomes disabling, and in turn illustrate the fluid nature of disability. By framing disability as an evolving (fluid) identity category and prioritizing the awareness of disabled*

Disability in the Time of Pandemic
Research in Social Science and Disability, Volume 13, 211–230

Published under exclusive licence by Emerald Publishing Limited
ISSN: 1479-3547/doi:10.1108/S1479-354720230000013012

perspectives, organizations can better support disabled employees in their future, overarching DEI strategies and approaches to workplace inclusion post-pandemic.

Keywords: Disability inclusion; pandemic; employee resource groups; diversity; equity; and inclusion

INTRODUCTION

The Office of Disability Employment Policy (ODEP), the United States federal agency responsible for promoting workplace success of people with disabilities, described the current pandemic as a cause of "unprecedented changes" to workforce participation and inclusion of disabled people (ODEP, 2020, p. 1). While the COVID-19 pandemic created universal uncertainty regarding the labor market and working conditions, from an employment perspective, people are not experiencing the pandemic in a universal way (McKinsey & Company, 2020). People from marginalized communities including women, people of color, and people with disabilities were more likely to experience unemployment, declined mental health, and other negative consequences compared to other groups (McKinsey & Company, 2020; ODEP, 2020). As the pandemic interrupted many of our regular ways of working, major global institutions such as the International Labour Organization (ILO) have highlighted the need to, "seize the opportunity for a more inclusive and better normal" (ILO, 2020, p. 6).

The systemic upheaval of workplace systems and traction from social movements have brought conversations of diversity, equity, and inclusion (DEI) to the forefront of social inquiry related to work. Exploring the implementation of workplace inclusivity initiatives is timely and relevant as organizations are increasingly being held accountable for their role in addressing the marginalization of various community groups. Improved understanding about disability inclusion is a key aspect of DEI efforts given the aging labor force, increasing disability related corporate social responsibility initiatives, and the elevated social awareness of DEI in corporate marketing and public relation endeavors (Moore et al., 2017).

This chapter draws from a multiyear research project that involved interviews with DEI professionals and disabled workers in the US to better understand how organizations include employees when disability is considered a diversity category in corporate workplaces. We considered the ramifications of changes to disability inclusion practices in the context of COVID-19 by synthesizing interviewee experiences with disability-based employee resource groups (ERGs), which were commonly described as a primary resource used by organizations to foster a sense of inclusion. Through an analysis of participant experiences, we observed how workplace practices related to disability inclusion are rapidly transforming in a variety of ways. Interviewees discussed how workplace disability initiatives both expanded and devolved because of changes to workplace culture, programs, and policies during the current pandemic. After presenting the project findings, we will describe how ongoing changes to the workplace may impact the treatment and participation of disabled people working in large organizations. First, we will consider the literature that informed our analytical approach, which includes diversity management theories and the framing of disability as a fluid and constantly evolving dynamic phenomenon (Barnartt, 2010).

Disability and Diversity Management Theory

Organizations have increasingly emphasized their support for employees who have "diverse" backgrounds, or differences in experiences, thoughts, and identities (Shore et al., 2011). Systemic and institutionalized discrimination has resulted in the overrepresentation of certain groups, namely able-bodied men and white people, in corporate settings, especially in leadership positions (Cook & Glass, 2014). The disproportionate representation has rendered almost all other groups and identities as "diverse." The enhanced focus on diversity in the workplace is a result of a multitude of changing social environments, such as globalization and pressure to address systemic inequalities (Roberson, 2019). A common organization strategy to facilitate recruitment and retention of employees with marginalized identities is the creation of DEI initiatives. DEI initiatives are described as ways for organizations to promote differences in employees while ensuring fairness in treatment across these differences (Meena & Vanka, 2017).

DEI practices have both shaped and reflected aspects of diversity management theory, referring to the body of research on how organizations increase representation, recognition, and feelings of inclusion and belonging among individuals from historically underrepresented groups (Yadav & Lenka, 2020). Much of diversity management research has focused on gender and race with limited exploration into other identity dimensions (Yadav & Lenka, 2020). While traditionally excluded from diversity management theory and practice, recent years have seen an influx of scholarly attention to disability as a diversity category (Yadav & Lenka, 2020) and the application of these theories to organizational practices, such as DEI planning (Fisher & Connelly, 2020; Gould et al., 2020). Though researchers have identified a growing number of organizations developing plans to support disabled employees (Gould et al., 2021), disability continues to be under-researched and under-synthesized in diversity management literature (Yadav & Lenka, 2020).

The increasing recognition of disability as part of diversity management may be viewed as a response to a variety of factors, such as access to an untapped labor source (Lengnick-Hall et al., 2008), the economic benefits of disability inclusion (Kalargyrou, 2014), the efforts of disability inclusion "champions" (Gould et al., 2021), and a multitude of others. However, disability holds a unique position in the overarching conceptualization of workplace diversity. For example, the heterogeneity across the disability community in terms of range of impairments, stakeholder groups, and its cross-cutting statuses makes disability distinct from other diversity dimensions (Chan et al., 2010). Furthermore, disability is described as a social category that people may "move in and out of" on a regular basis, which also differentiates disability when compared to other, more static categorizations (Kruse & Hale, 2003, p. 9).

Within diversity frameworks utilized by organizations, there tends to be little acknowledgment of the fluidity that exists along the spectrum of disability, nor how contexts and environments influence and are influenced by disability (Barnartt, 2010). As conceptions of disability shift over time and space, and experiences of disability are largely affected by surrounding environments, it is vital to explore the categorization within the milieu of a fluid identity (Altman, 2014). The complexity of disability's categorization in relation to work and intersectionality further positions disability as a unique facet of diversity, meriting critical exploration in organizational settings.

Employee Resource Groups

One common diversity management strategy is the formulation and engagement of employee resource groups (ERGs). ERGs offer important insights into the evolution and framing of disability as a diversity category as ERGs offer a potential "bridge" between individual and cultural identities and a person's position within an organization (McPhee et al., 2017, p. 1113). By engaging with ERGs, we can uncover how disability is included and considered within workplace settings.

Though ERGs may be known by several names, such as affinity groups, employee networks, and others, these groups tend to have similar goals. ERGs promote career development for employees with "diverse" backgrounds through social support, information sharing, and leadership development (Friedman & Craig, 2004; O'Neil et al., 2011). ERGs also offer opportunities for employees to connect with others who have similar experiences and create opportunities for mentoring and community building (Dennissen et al., 2018). Additionally, ERGs may act as learning communities and raise awareness to organizational leadership to better meet the needs of underrepresented employee bases (Green, 2018). While ERGs are common in practice, there is limited research regarding ERGs, especially those designated for employees with disabilities (Welbourne et al., 2017).

Investigation into disability-based ERGs is needed to contribute to evidence-based practices that encourage workplace acceptance for disabled employees. ERGs have been shown to facilitate an increased sense of inclusion and belonging for people from marginalized communities (Dennissen et al., 2018), but there is limited information on how this may be similar or different for disability. Other evidence suggests that disability-based ERGs may foster workplace disability inclusion by engaging in recruitment efforts and providing support for the business case for disability (Gould et al., 2021). However, many of these strategies are continuing to develop, and there is limited understanding of how ERGs may influence and sustain awareness of disability and workplace disability inclusion.

The Pandemic and the Workplace

As ERGs play a role in shaping workplace culture, especially for people with marginalized identities, members of these groups may offer insight into how organizations considered disability as they responded to, and employees experienced, the impact of the pandemic. Many employers transitioned to remote work, and there were significant impacts on both the physical environment and relationships between managers and employees (Schur et al., 2020). Changes caused by the pandemic influenced nearly all business strategies, including diversity management and ERGs. To encourage greater inclusion, it is important to understand how disabled employees navigated and managed the changing physical, social, and material aspects of their workplace environments (Altman, 2014). As these contexts shifted and are continuing to shift, so are the experiences of disabled employees.

Employees with disabilities were uniquely impacted by the transition to virtual work settings and the pandemic (Tang, 2021). While some have suggested that teleworking may enhance accessibility and promote work opportunities for people with disabilities (Jesus et al., 2020), others have been more critical of these positive assumptions, citing inaccessible technology and limited engagement with both personal and professional networks for people with disabilities during the pandemic (Koon et al., 2022; Schur et al., 2020). Furthermore, certain aspects of teleworking may have unintentionally excluded people with disabilities as some organizations overlooked disability rights laws when implementing emergency responses (Reid et al., 2020; Tang, 2021).

There is a small but growing body of research exploring how the pandemic has impacted the employment/unemployment rate of disabled workers (Schur et al., 2020). Toward the beginning of the pandemic and the implementation of public health restrictions, disabled people reported higher rates of reduced work hours, rates of unemployment, concerns about a lack of job security, and higher levels of financial stress compared to people without disabilities (Emerson et al., 2021; Houtenville et al., 2021; Maroto et al., 2021). Considering how disability inclusion practices and awareness of disability is evolving and the nuance of COVID-19 on employment disparities and outcomes, highlights the need to better understand how the pandemic is impacting the working lives of disabled people.

Next, we describe our study about workplace processes in the context of the pandemic. We then provide additional discussion about how the findings add to the understanding disability inclusion practices and awareness of disability, a fluid workplace category. The analysis emphasizes the importance of exploring disabled experiences during contextual changes, like that of the COVID-19 pandemic.

Study Overview

Given the challenges to integrating disability inclusion into DEI endeavors and the central role of employee groups in implementing such efforts, the research team explored the question: "What do the actions of disability-based ERGs reveal about disability inclusion practices in large corporate settings during the pandemic?" To gain insights into disability inclusion within this context, we conducted semi-structured interviews with members of disability-based employee resource groups and diversity, equity, and inclusion professionals who have experience in disability inclusion at their organizations. Disability-based ERG members and DEI professionals were sought out because of their personal and professional insights into disability inclusion in their workplace (Beatty et al., 2019). Ethical approval for this study was granted by the University of Illinois at Chicago Internal Review Board, protocol number 2018-0829.

METHODS

Sample/Recruitment

The research team used a purposive sampling strategy to recruit participants in collaboration with technical assistance (TA) specialists from the Americans with Disabilities Act (ADA) National Network (ADANN). The ADANN is comprised of 10 federally funded regional centers across the United States that provide training, information, and guidance to help implement the ADA in support of its mission to assure equality of opportunity, full participation, independent living, and economic self-sufficiency for individuals with disabilities (ADANN, 2021). The ADANN is not a regulatory body, which gives them unique insight in organizational practices and connections to key stakeholders who may otherwise be unknown to the research team (Fujiura et al., 2015). The sampling strategy was critical for this study to reach organizational "champions" who advocate for increased recognition and inclusion of particular groups (Colgan, 2011). The recruitment plan also may have resulted in an over-representation of participants who have more access to disability inclusion resources. Connecting with such champions was necessary to answer the primary research question "What do the actions of disability-based ERGs reveal about disability inclusion practices in large corporate settings during the pandemic?" as champions are uniquely positioned to share information about internal employer practices (Gould et al., 2020).

Inclusion criteria for this study is as follows: (1) 18 years or older, (2) worked at the organization for more than six months, (3) the organization employed more than 500 people, and (4) they were active members in a disability-based ERGs and/or a DEI professional with intimate knowledge disability inclusion within their organization. Other data collected about participants included: state where their office was located, disability status, caregiver/family member status, age range, gender, pronouns, race/ethnicity, and access needs for participation in the interview.

"DEI professional" for this project referred to a variety of positions with functional responsibilities promoting disability inclusion, such as: accommodations specialists, ADA coordinators, and DEI specialists. Many of these positions spanned multiple functions and departments to support disability as part of overarching DEI strategies and compliance with disability rights laws. Other participants who were not DEI professionals but were members of disability-based ERGs, also held a variety of positions, which represents the widespread impact and reach of ERGs and disability identities.

Recruitment began in June 2020 via emails sent by ADANN technical assistants (TAs) to relevant listservs. Potential interviewees were asked to contact the research team if interested in participating and a member of the research team replied with an information sheet and a link to an online survey to determine eligibility. A total of 38 people reached out to the research team with interest in participating. Of these, 21 final interviews were included in analysis based on participant eligibility. Most participants (13/21; 62%) identified as having or sometimes having a disability. Individuals' descriptions of their impairments varied, including chronic illness (e.g., diabetes), sensory disabilities (e.g., blindness and d/Deafness), and mental health conditions. In addition to the 62% of participants who described various states of identifying as a person with a disability in the survey, a small number of participants additionally disclosed having impairments, which might be considered a disability, during the interview process. This revelation in and of itself highlights the stigma of claiming a disability identity within the workplace, even when discussing organizational supports for disability inclusion. The sample overall was somewhat limited in terms of racial and ethnic diversity as a majority of those who disclosed a race or ethnicity, 79% (15/19; 2 did not disclose) identified as white (or variation e.g., Caucasian) alone. Participants worked at a mixture of large nonprofit, public, and private organizations representing multiple industries and functions. Examples include, hospital systems, public institutions, professional services firms, among others. The organizations were recommended by ADANN TA providers who identified these organizations as having progressive disability inclusion and DEI initiatives. This sample presented a broad range of rich perspectives and experiences from which to draw. Recruitment and data collection ended in August 2020 when the research team agreed that they had reached saturation during the initial analysis (Saunders et al., 2018). In this study, saturation was determined when researchers were able to independently identify the same concepts and discreet data points repeated across various organizations and contexts in relation to the research questions (Guest et al., 2006). More information about the sample is included in Table 1.

Data Collection

Data were collected through in-depth, semi-structured interviews focused on how the current pandemic influenced organizational disability inclusion practices. The research team developed an interview guide based on themes identified in previous project activities, information from key contacts, and existing literature (Kallio et al., 2016). Semi-structured guides helped provide connection across interviews while maintaining flexibility (Saunders et al., 2018). Questions in the guide facilitated conversation about workplace experiences since the onset of the COVID-19 pandemic and how this shift impacted diversity and disability inclusion strategies. Examples of questions included in the guide are: "What strategies did your organization use to encourage disability inclusion before the COVID-19 pandemic?"; "How have disability inclusion strategies influenced your/employee engagement with the organization?"; and "How has your workplace changed since the onset of the COVID-19 pandemic? What has this shift been like?"

Table 1. Participant Sample.

Organization Industry:	State Where Office is Located:	Do You Identify as a Person With a Disability?	Do You Identify as a Caregiver or Family Member of a Person With a Disability?	Age Range:	Self-Described Gender:	Self-Described Race/ Ethnicity:
Professional services	Virginia	Yes	No	61+	Female	White
Professional services	Pennsylvania	Sometimes	No	18–30	Female	White
Professional services	Illinois	Sometimes	No	51–60	Male	White
Professional services	New York	Yes	Did not disclose	41–50	Female	Did not disclose
Professional services	Illinois	Yes	No	41–50	Female	Black
Professional services	Pennsylvania	No	No	18–30	Female	White
Hospital system	Illinois	Yes	Yes	41–50	Male	White
Insurance	Illinois	No	Yes	31–40	Male	White
Hospital system	Illinois	Yes	No	18–30	Female	White
Hospital system	Minnesota	No	No	51–60	Female	White
Government agency	New York	Yes	No	51–60	Male	Canadian American
Government agency	Washington, D.C.	Yes	No	41–50	Male	Asian Pacific Islander
Hospital system	Illinois	No	No	18–30	Female	White, Puerto Rican
Agribusiness	Minnesota	Yes	No	18–30	Female	Irish, European
University	Michigan	Yes	Yes	51–60	Female	White
Government agency	Minnesota	Yes	No	31–40	Female	Caucasian
University	California	Yes	No	51–60	Female	Caucasian
University	Ohio	No	No	61+	Male	White
Government agency	Minnesota	Yes	Yes	61+	Female	White
Government agency	Michigan	No	No	31–40	Female	Black
Government agency	Iowa	No	Yes	41–50	Female	Did not disclose

Interviews were conducted by a member of the research team via the online video platform Zoom, lasted for approximately 60–75 minutes, and were video-recorded and auto-transcribed. Hosting interviews online was relevant for the context of the interviews as well as necessary during the time of the current pandemic (Roberts et al., 2021). Interviews began with a description of the research, statement of confidentiality, and confirmation of participant consent. All interviews had both a notetaker and interviewer who independently recorded observations using a field note guide. A field note guide was developed collaboratively by the research team to record observations, contextualize interviews, and capture interviewee responses (Phillippi & Lauderdale, 2018). Transcripts were edited and de-identified by the interviewer and notetaker as an initial stage of analysis. Neither names of participants nor names of organizations are included in this chapter. Additional documentation was also captured to support analysis, such as public facing diversity statements, descriptions of disability-based ERGs, and other supporting documents identified during the interview process, like ERG strategic plans.

Data Analysis

The research team utilized framework analysis to identify themes across the interviews. Framework analysis was selected as it is useful for analyzing data in organizational and policy contexts and is centered on personal observation and accounts of participants (Srivastava & Thomson, 2009). The analytical process included: data familiarization, data coding, developing and applying the analytical framework, charting data and summarizing themes, and interpreting results (Goldsmith, 2021). For this study, familiarization involved reading and editing transcripts and reviewing field note guides and supplemental documents. The field note guides included brief organization and interviewee descriptions, observations about the interview, and an area to identify potential themes.

Using data derived from field notes and supplemental documentation, two members of the research team engaged in an iterative process to develop a codebook for the data coding stage of analysis. Codes were organized into three main themes which served as the analytical framework: COVID-19 specific information, personal connections to disabling experiences, and DEI practices and strategies. The research team piloted the codebook in which two reviewers coded three transcripts independently using Atlas.ti version 8. There was a series of four codebook drafts, where codes were continually refined and the codebook was finalized when the research team was satisfied with the high level of intercoder agreement (Campbell et al., 2013).

As part of the charting and summarizing stage, the remaining transcripts were independently coded using the finalized codebook. Relevant quotes were copied into Microsoft Excel to be compared across interviews and memos were written as an application of the analytical framework (Goldsmith, 2021). Finally, results were interpreted through a collaborative writing process where findings were situated within existing literature and summative insights were derived, as discussed in the following section.

RESULTS

As people adapted to new ways of working due to the pandemic, structured groups like disability-based ERGs were a central force for driving workplace disability inclusion. Through interviews with disability-based ERG members and DEI professionals, we found that the pandemic and changed working environment also shifted how disability-based ERGs operated within large corporate settings. Interviewees described evolving organizational policies and practices related to disability inclusion during the pandemic in two key areas: (1) increased visibility of disability as access issues became more universal to employees with and without disabilities and (2) the de-prioritization of disability inclusion initiatives where the specific concerns of employees with disabilities were overlooked or ignored.

ERGs and Increased Disability Visibility

The changed work environment required people to navigate their jobs, interactions with coworkers, and multiple other aspects that comprise "the workplace" in a different way. Interviewees provided stories of their experiences around disability-based ERGs that showcased the heightened visibility of disability in relation to the following key subthemes: enhanced relevance of disability-based ERGs and increased connection to disability identities.

Enhanced Access and Relevance of Disability-Based ERGs

Many disability-based ERGs reacted to pandemic-induced shifts by increasing awareness of their role as a resource within their respective organizations. Prior to the pandemic, many of the ERGs facilitated learning opportunities related to disabled experiences. However, the contextual change of the pandemic also shifted what information employees most needed, and ERGs responded by changing how and what type of information they shared.

One interviewee, a Black woman who identified as a person with a disability and worked at a professional services firm, described how participation in disability-based ERG events grew during the pandemic,

> [ERG events have] become virtual... the audiences are bigger ... We're not having the distractions of being in the office. And so people are able to get work done or do things that maybe they would not have had time for before. ... So they're much more well attended than...when we were in person.

The transition to teleworking necessitated that disability-based ERGs host events in virtual settings. While using technology for ERG activities was novel for many interviewees, this mode of connection appeared to solve some of the ERGs' previous limitations, such as inaccessible spaces and geographical separation of ERG members. Many of the participants described an increase in engagement in ERG initiatives from across their organization because people could, as stated by one participant, "check in from anywhere." Without some of the confines of physical locations, as well as the increased availability of employees, disability-based ERGs were able to raise awareness and recognition of both their group and of disability overall.

Additionally, disability inclusion practices shared by ERGs appeared to be more relevant to a wider array of people due to the universalizing experience of the pandemic. The unique knowledge held by disabled employees was increasingly pertinent to others who may not have connected with disability-based ERGs previously, as one participant described "...we all need [these resources]." By driving this connection point, that disability resources and information shared by disability-based groups were relevant to employees broadly, more people considered disability within their organizations. Many participants detailed how disability-based ERG members offered unique insights that were especially useful as employees from across organizations navigated the changing work landscape. An example comes from a white woman who did not identify as having a disability and worked at a healthcare organization, who shared how awareness of the ERG positioned members as internal resources for accommodations processes:

> I think we tend to be kind of consultants at this time... I've had a couple of managers call and say... "This is happening with an employee that's deployed to home. This is their disability. Do you have any recommendations? Can you point me to the resources?" So, we're getting connected that way just because people...are aware of the ERG and that there are people that may have some information if you don't know the answers.

In the above example, members of the disability-based ERG fulfilled an important role as internal experts for individuals seeking to address access needs. With the changes in the workplace, like moving to remote environments, the needs of employees also changed. Employees, with varying disability identities, who previously may not have required accommodations were now needing to address workplace access in a new way.

Participants revealed that disability-based ERGs were positioned to support critical aspects of disability inclusion strategies and considerations. These expert insights into disability inclusion were important to ensure successful workplace transitions as part of organizations' crisis responses. Other examples of how disability-based ERGs became more relevant within organizations include: providing connection to outside resources, sharing information about COVID-19 as related to people with disabilities, and creating guidelines about accessible and inclusive remote work considerations. For example, a white man who identified as a caregiver or family member of a person with a disability who worked at an insurance company described how the ERG provided connections to outside resources to support disability inclusion during the pandemic,

> [Members of the ERG] wanted to say...how does this [the pandemic] impact someone's ability or a caregiver...We were able to share ... the COVID disability resources that [a Center for Independent Living] has on their page...[an] amazing list of all these different resources and connection points...

These efforts highlight the enhanced awareness of disability as there was a conscious effort in considering disability in the new work environment, driven by actions of disability-based ERGs and disability inclusion champions.

Increased Recognition of Connection to Disability

The enhanced visibility of disability through ERG efforts changed how some interviewees understood their own personal experiences with that of the larger collective of disability-based ERG members. A professional services firm employee (who identified as a person with a disability and did not disclose either their race or their gender) shared how they became involved with the disability-based ERG because of an informational session about mental health,

> ...[T]he Disability Resource Group was sponsoring [a seminar about mental health and working from home] ... And after I learned about them I've realized, hey, that could be a really great thing for me... I have my own personal disabilities...and I thought that might be a good way to connect.

The above quote highlighted not only how the changing environment connected more people to disability-based ERGs, but also how individual recognition of disability expanded during the pandemic. The fluid nature of disability was reified within the context of the pandemic as more people understood their own experiences through a disability lens. Individuals became more aware of how their personal experiences and impairments connected to a disability identity.

This was further exemplified by the way in which disability-based ERGs acted as a point of connection for members of these groups. ERGs appeared to be a support system for disabled employees who were navigating the changed work landscape. For example, a white man who identified as a person with a disability and worked at a health services organization explained how members of ERG's relied on connections through the group to harness collective knowledge about addressing work related issues,

> ... [P]eople were really missing the group and people really count on it ... some issues have come up in terms of meeting accommodations, since the pandemic hit ... some people are concerned about their health and working ... and so we decided to go ahead with the [ERG] meeting ... and it was something worth doing.

The example showcases how ERGs may act as a community of practice, where members are able to learn information from each other. Participants described disability-based ERGs as a place to "share common experiences" and "a safe space for folks to raise issues." This type of support may be broader than simply the logistics or technical aspects of navigating inaccessible environments, such as accommodation processes, and included insights about the emotional labor attached to these actions. Several of the interviewees discussed how ERG members felt less isolated during the pandemic because they were able to come together to discuss experiences and potential solutions to problems with peers. The changing environment of work necessitated a heightened role of disability-based ERGs within some organizations, and the above quotes and descriptions of how ERGs offered opportunities for connections highlight how these groups fit into overarching DEI strategies that foster feelings of inclusion for disabled employees.

This placed a spotlight on awareness of disability as employees needed support to address novel experiences resulting from the pandemic. This elevated position of disability-based ERGs represents the increased visibility of disability overall and reinforces the understanding of disabling experiences as ones that may shift over time and space.

De-Prioritization of Disability Awareness and Inclusion

While disability awareness efforts expanded within some organizations, interviewees also described the de-prioritization of disability recognition efforts in others. Corporate leaders in some organizations responded to the pandemic in ways that did not reflect nor include disabled perspectives. Interviewees discussed the de-prioritization of disability-centric policy across two key subthemes: devolving disability inclusion efforts and the obligation to respond to intensified ableist structures.

Devolving of Disability Awareness Initiatives

Interviewees provided descriptions of how disability inclusion efforts were minimized as policies intended to facilitate compliance with disability rights laws were negated, and there was waning support for disability inclusion endeavors. For example, due to the economic strains of the pandemic, many organizations were described as limiting spending to only "essential functions." Though workplace accommodations are protected civil rights within the US, interviewees shared how accommodation procedures, often a cornerstone of disability inclusion initiatives, became debated within their organizations. One participant, a white woman who identified as a person with a disability and worked at a university, gave a presentation about disability inclusion to her organization. She stated her surprise that,

> We kept getting the same question over and over ... "Are these accommodations, activities, considered essential?" Because the university actually cut out all non-essential spending... I'm like, yeah, it's essential.

The above quote exemplifies the simultaneous expansion of disability by hosting this type of event and raising awareness as well as a clear de-prioritization of disability inclusion. Some participants who relied on workplace accommodations expressed concern that their access needs were suddenly questioned as an unnecessary cost. One participant described this as a "sucker-punch," knowing that their civil rights might not be considered "essential" to some organizational leaders. Though disability was a celebrated aspect of many of DEI strategies, there was still a need to prove that disability inclusion and creating accessible workplaces was worthwhile considering the pandemic.

Responses to Intensified Ableist Structures
In addition to needing to prove the value of disabled perspectives during the pandemic, many participants described how ERG members felt obligated to identify and address workplace barriers. Interviewees reported feeling added responsibility for rectifying instances of exclusion as ableist structures became more prevalent due to the de-prioritization of disability inclusion within organizational crisis responses. In some organizations disability inclusion activities devolved to a point that disability policy was seemingly invisible, except through the efforts of individual champions and disability-based ERGs.

One participant shared that organization leaders are, "not going see the problems even exist without … advocacy." Because decision makers were not always aware of disabled perspectives, members of the disability-based ERGs felt responsibility to bring these needs to the forefront. The lived experiences of ableism provided a foundation to recognize inaccessibility, and therefore members of disability-based ERGs were called upon to identify ableist structures. The de-prioritization of disability awareness on an organizational level resulted in the amplified need for disability inclusion.

Within some of these organizations, ERGs became a place for mobilizing and collectively advocating for changes as a response to the de-prioritization of disability inclusion and pandemic-related barriers within various workplaces. One participant, a white man who identified as a person with a disability and worked at a public social services agency, shared that during the pandemic, his organization transitioned to new computer system that did not have captioning capabilities even for those who required captioning to do their work. As a response to this clear access concern, the disability-based ERG responded with,

> … a position paper … saying all of these things have happened during this pandemic … are not appropriate, not ethical and we sent that to upper management. I think we got some traction … I think people heard us. I don't know if that's going to make any difference unfortunately…

Even though there were doubts of the outcome of these advocacy actions, the above quote highlights how ERGs provided an opportunity for employees to feel like they can affect organizational change. ERGs connected employees to leadership in ways that may not otherwise exist for individuals. However, this linkage was described by one participant as a "tightrope." The precarity of balancing advocacy and not being overly adversarial with leadership was felt deeply during the pandemic, as new work environments necessitated new ways of working. Due to the de-prioritization of disability inclusion, disabled employees and disability-based ERGs were moved to advocate and address the enhanced ableism present in their workplaces.

DISCUSSION

Findings provide useful answers to our research question "What do the actions of disability-based ERGs reveal about disability inclusion practices in large corporate settings during the pandemic?" Employee accounts of experiences with disability-based ERGs and descriptions of employer responses to disability inclusion revealed how organizations simultaneously shifted to advance the recognition of disabled employees while also, at times, failing to deliver needed support for access and inclusion during the pandemic. Disability-based ERGs offer a useful vantage point from which to observe and explore these shifts and how the pandemic impacted disability inclusion in the workplace. The unique role of ERGs as shared and collective spaces to spearhead advocacy has been largely unexplored in relation to disabled employees. Findings contribute to the growing body of literature detailing how disability is incorporated into overarching DEI efforts and disability inclusion at work (Fisher & Connelly, 2020; Gould et al., 2021).

The simultaneous expansion and de-prioritization of disability inclusion highlights how shifting environments became disabling, further exemplifying the fluid nature of disability experiences (Barnartt, 2010). This study offers insight into the connections among impairment, environment, and functionality which reifies the dynamic understanding of disability and conceptualizes this identity as being neither "fixed nor given" (Barnartt, 2010, p. 2). Framing disability as a fluid category, especially in work settings, is an important consideration for future disability inclusion policies and practices to be reflective of transformative experiences and will continue to be important as companies more forward with fostering workplace inclusion post-pandemic.

ERGs and Disability Visibility

Our analysis demonstrates how ERGs play a vital role in make disability more included or visible within organizations. These findings align disability-based ERGs with that of the intended outcomes of overarching DEI strategies, as ones that enhance representation and feelings of inclusion for employees from marginalized backgrounds (Yadav & Lenka, 2020). By creating opportunities to promote representation and awareness of disability-based ERGs, the results offer additional evidence in support of engaging disability within organizational DEI strategies as a vehicle to enhance disability inclusion at work (Gould et al., 2021). Though seeking out disability inclusive practices shows a recognition of disability, this does call into question the potential overreliance on ERGs, and specifically individual champions within ERGs, to facilitate DEI initiatives (Katz & Miller, 2020). Engaging champions as the primary driving force behind raising awareness of disability may limit the effectiveness of long-term organizational change. There are still many unknowns regarding the lasting impacts of DEI initiatives on workplace culture, especially regarding sustained outcomes of disability inclusion efforts in the context of the pandemic.

Key findings in this study also highlight how the conceptualization of disability was further expanded as people became more aware of their individual connections to disability identities. As ERG efforts enhanced the visibility of disability, some participants described how they understood their own personal experiences within that of the larger collective of disability-based ERG members. ERGs played an increasingly important role in creating a "safe space" for disabled employees to connect and share their experiences. While this is somewhat surprising given the literature and understanding of disability as a heterogenous category (Chan et al., 2010), it is also in alignment with other findings on ERGs as ways to decrease social isolation (Dennissen et al., 2018), which was particularly important in the time of the current pandemic as isolation was required to adhere to public health concerns and disabled people had decreased access to social and professional networks (Koon et al., 2022). The increased recognition of disability highlights how shifting environments and subsequent changes in individual functions or workplace roles is connected to the fluid nature of disability (Barnartt, 2010). Broadening how disability is understood in this way also further reinforces disability as a dynamic experience, as people who had previously not ascribed to a disability identity, sought out disability-based ERGs as their environments changed due to the pandemic.

De-Prioritization of Disability Inclusion and Awareness Initiatives

While the expansion of disability played a central role in some participant experiences, other perspectives further illuminated how disability inclusion initiatives devolved during the pandemic and the increased responsibility felt by members of disability-based ERGs to address inaccessibility. Participants described how disability-based ERGs were tasked with proving the value of and advocating for disability inclusion in the workplace, which was exacerbated during the pandemic. These experiences of exclusion reinforce other, emerging literature regarding disability inclusion at work, where workplace changes resulting from the pandemic were not fully accessible (Ocean, 2021). In the present study, some participants expressed shock that regular workplace accommodations, often fundamental to fostering disability inclusive workplaces, were not always considered "essential." This aligns with other critiques that have highlighted how emergencies like the current pandemic can potentially render disability laws and inclusion practices as "optional and aspirational" (Reid et al., 2020, p. 2). As a result, disabled employees and members of disability-based ERGs described how they were obligated to address inaccessibility in their workplaces. The increased awareness and forced response to disabling workplace conditions in the context of the pandemic created the need for dialogue to address access in key areas that impact disabled people's labor such as telework, flexible scheduling, and employee wellbeing initiatives.

Disability-based ERGs held a prominent role in addressing inequality and inaccessibility faced by disabled employees as a reaction to the de-prioritization of disability inclusion. Though the outcomes of these efforts were largely unknown, this mindset that disability-based ERGs offer a collective voice to influence leadership decisions, coincides with previous literature regarding ERGs as informing perspectives of organization leaders (Green, 2018). Participants further complicate this role of ERGs as they described the precarious position that disability-based ERGs are in when attempting to address issues regarding disability inclusion. The "tightrope" of advocating for change without antagonizing leadership, may potentially detract from efforts to include disabled employees.

LIMITATIONS

While this study contributes significantly to the understanding of workplace disability inclusion during the pandemic, it is not without limitations. One limitation of this study is the lack of representation among the sampled participants. The overrepresentation of white participants compared to other identities is a persistent concern in literature regarding disability and disability inclusion policies overall (Wiener, 2021). Furthermore, most of the participants identified as women, which is reflective of other literature that notes the overrepresentation of female participants in qualitative research on management and organizational practices (Ashmos Plowman & Smith, 2011). The overrepresentation could also reflect the fact that women are more likely to participate in organizational DEI efforts compared to men (McKinsey & Company, 2020). Similar to other qualitative studies with relatively limited sample sizes, there are concerns about applying findings more broadly (Boddy, 2016). However, the sample of this study aligns with original study purpose, and results may act as an initial foundation for future engagement.

CONCLUSION

Overall, this study demonstrates important insights into the conceptualization of disability as part of organizational DEI strategies, the role of disability-based ERGs, and experiences of disabled employees within the context of the pandemic. The shifted environment caused by the pandemic altered workplaces, ways of working, and organizational resources. These transitions resulted in an enhanced awareness and increased visibility of disability as well as a de-prioritization of disability inclusion. Our findings support the understanding of disability as not a static, binary experience or identity but is instead fluid and consistently evolving (Barnartt, 2010). More time is needed to assess the long-term impact of the pandemic and changes in the workplace and the influence these factors have on disabled experiences. However, we are at a critical juncture as organizations continue to reconfigure their workplaces. Organizational leaders must consider leveraging the shifting environment to further enhance and promote a sustained commitment to include disabled employees both now and in the future.

ACKNOWLEDGMENTS

This research was conducted under a grant from the National Institute on Disability, Independent Living, and Rehabilitation Research (NIDILRR grant number 90DP0091). NIDILRR is a Center within the US Administration for Community Living (ACL), Department of Health and Human Services (HHS). The contents of this manuscript do not necessarily represent the policy of NIDILRR, ACL, HHS, and you should not assume endorsement by the Federal Government.

REFERENCES

ADA National Network (ADANN). (2021). Learn about the national network. https://adata.org/national-network

Altman, B. M. (2014). Introduction: Environmental contexts and disability. In B. M. Altman & S. N. Barnartt (Eds.), *Environmental contexts and disability* (pp. xiii–xxii). Emerald Publishing Limited.

Ashmos Plowman, D., & Smith, A. D. (2011). The gendering of organizational research methods: Evidence of gender patterns in qualitative research. *Qualitative Research in Organizations and Management: An International Journal*, *6*(1), 64–82. https://doi.org/10.1108/17465641111129399

Barnartt, S. N. (2010). Disability as a fluid state: Introduction. In S. N. Barnartt (Ed.), *Disability as a fluid state* (pp. 1–22). Emerald Publishing Limited.

Beatty, J. E., Baldridge, D. C., Boehm, S. A., Kulkarni, M., & Colella, A. J. (2019). On the treatment of persons with disabilities in organizations: A review and research agenda. *Human Resource Management*, *58*(2), 119–137. https://doi.org/10.1002/hrm.21940

Boddy, C. R. (2016). Sample size for qualitative research. *Qualitative Market Research: An International Journal*, *19*(4), 426–432. https://doi.org/10.1108/QMR-06-2016-0053

Campbell, J. L., Quincy, C., Osserman, J., & Pedersen, O. K. (2013). Coding In-depth Semistructured Interviews: Problems of unitization and intercoder reliability and agreement. *Sociological Methods & Research*, *42*(3), 294–320. https://doi.org/10.1177/0049124113500475

Chan, F., Strauser, D., Gervey, R., & Lee, E.-J. (2010). Introduction to demand-side factors related to employment of people with disabilities. *Journal of Occupational Rehabilitation*, *20*(4), 407–411. https://doi.org/10.1007/s10926-010-9243-7

Colgan, F. (2011). Equality, diversity and corporate responsibility: Sexual orientation and diversity management in the UK private sector. *Equality, Diversity and Inclusion: An International Journal*, *30*(8), 719–734. https://doi.org/10.1108/02610151111183225

Cook, A., & Glass, C. (2014). Women and top leadership positions: Towards an institutional analysis. *Gender, Work and Organization*, *21*(1), 91–103. https://doi.org/10.1111/gwao.12018

Dennissen, M., Benschop, Y., & van den Brink, M. (2018). Diversity networks: Networking for equality? *British Journal of Management*, *30*(4), 966–980. https://doi.org/10.1111/1467-8551.12321

Emerson, E., Stancliffe, R., Hatton, C., Llewellyn, G., King, T., Totsika, V., Aitken, Z., & Kavanagh, A. (2021). The impact of disability on employment and financial security following the outbreak of the 2020 COVID-19 pandemic in the UK. *Journal of Public Health*, *43*(3), 472–478. https://doi.org/10.1093/pubmed/fdaa270

Fisher, S. L., & Connelly, C. E. (2020). Building the "business case" for hiring people with disabilities: A financial cost-benefit analysis methodology and example. *Canadian Journal of Disability Studies*, *9*(4), 71–88. https://doi.org/10.15353/cjds.v9i4.669

Friedman, R. A., & Craig, K. M. (2004). Predicting joining and participating in minority employee network groups. *Industrial Relations: A Journal of Economy and Society*, *43*(4), 793–816. https://doi.org/10.1111/j.0019-8676.2004.00362.x

Fujiura, G., Groll, J., & Jones, R. (2015). Knowledge utilization and ADA technical assistance information. *Journal of Rehabilitation*, *81*(2), 19–25. https://www.nationalrehab.org/journal-of-rehabilitation

Goldsmith, L. (2021). Using framework analysis in applied qualitative research. *Qualitative Report*, *26*(6), 2061–2076. https://doi.org/0.46743/2160-3715/2021.5011

Gould, R., Mullin, C., Parker Harris, S., & Jones, R. (2021). Building, sustaining and growing: Disability inclusion in business. *Equality, Diversity and Inclusion: An International Journal*. Advance online publication. https://doi.org/10.1108/EDI-06-2020-0156

Gould, R., Parker Harris, S., Mullin, C., & Jones, R. (2020). Disability, diversity, and corporate social responsibility: Learning from recognized leaders in inclusion. *Journal of Vocational Rehabilitation*, *52*(1), 29–42. https://doi.org/10.3233/JVR-191058

Green, W. M. (2018). Employee resource groups as learning communities. *Equality, Diversity and Inclusion: An International Journal*, *37*(7), 634–648. https://doi.org/10.1108/EDI-11-2016-0085

Guest, G., Bunce, A., & Johnson, L. (2006). How many interviews are enough?: An experiment with data saturation and variability. *Field Methods*, *18*(1), 59–82. https://doi.org/10.1177/1525822X05279903

Houtenville, A. J., Paul, S., & Brucker, D. L. (2021). Changes in the employment status of people with and without disabilities in the United States during the COVID-19 pandemic. *Archives of Physical Medicine and Rehabilitation*, *102*(7), 1420–1423. https://doi.org/10.1016/j.apmr.2021.03.019

International Labour Organization. (2020). COVID-19 and the world of work: Ensuring the inclusion of persons with disabilities at all stages of the response. https://www.ilo.org/wcmsp5/groups/public/—ed_emp/—ifp_skills/documents/publication/wcms_746909.pdf

Jesus, T. S., Landry, M. D., & Jacobs, K. (2020). A 'new normal' following COVID-19 and the economic crisis: Using systems thinking to identify challenges and opportunities in disability, telework, and rehabilitation. *Work*, *67*(1), 37–46. https://doi.org/10.3233/WOR-203250

Kalargyrou, V. (2014). Gaining a competitive advantage with disability inclusion initiatives. *Journal of Human Resources in Hospitality & Tourism*, *13*(2), 120–145. https://doi.org/10.1080/15332845.2014.847300

Kallio, H., Pietilä, A.-M., Johnson, M., & Kangasniemi, M. (2016). Systematic methodological review: Developing a framework for a qualitative semi-structured interview guide. *Journal of Advanced Nursing*, *72*(12), 2954–2965. https://doi.org/10.1111/jan.13031

Katz, J. H., & Miller, F. A. (2020). ERG's can't do it alone: Traps to successful organization change efforts. *Organization Development Review*, *52*(2), 18–22. https://www.odnetwork.org/page/odreview

Koon, L. M., Greiman, L., Schulz, J. A., Goddard, K. S., Nzuki, I. M., & Hall, J. P. (2022). Examining the effects of the COVID-19 pandemic on community engagement for people with mobility disabilities. *Disability and Health Journal*, *15*(1, Suppl.), 101212. https://doi.org/10.1016/j.dhjo.2021.101212

Kruse, D., & Hale, T. (2003). Disability and employment: Symposium introduction. *Industrial Relations*, *42*(1), 1–10. https://doi.org/10.1111/1468-232X.00273

Lengnick-Hall, M. L., Gaunt, P. M., & Kulkarni, M. (2008). Overlooked and underutilized: People with disabilities are an untapped human resource. *Human Resource Management*, *47*(2), 255–273. https://doi.org/10.1002/hrm.20211

Maroto, M. L., Pettinicchio, D., & Lukk, M. (2021). Working differently or not at all: COVID-19's effects on employment among people with disabilities and chronic health conditions. *Sociological Perspectives*, *64*(5), 876–897. https://doi.org/10.1177/07311214211012018

McKinsey & Company. (2020). Diverse employees are struggling the most during COVID-19—Here's how companies can respond. https://www.mckinsey.com/featured-insights/diversity-and-inclusion/diverse-employees-are-struggling-the-most-during-covid-19-heres-how-companies-can-respond

McPhee, D., Julien, M., Miller, D., & Wright, B. (2017). Smudging, connecting, and dual identities: Case study of an aboriginal ERG. *Personnel Review*, *46*(6), 1104–1119. https://doi.org/10.1108/PR-10-2015-0270

Meena, K., & Vanka, S. (2017). Developing an empirical typology of diversity-oriented human resource management practices. *The Journal of Management Development*, *36*(7), 915–929. https://doi.org/10.1108/JMD-02-2016-0031

Moore, K., McDonald, P., & Bartlett, J. (2017). The social legitimacy of disability inclusive human resource practices: The case of a large retail organisation. *Human Resource Management Journal*, *27*(4), 514–529. https://doi.org/10.1111/1748-8583.12129

Ocean, M. (2021). Telework during COVID-19: Exposing ableism in U.S. higher education. *Disability & Society*, *36*(9), 153–1548. https://doi.org/10.1080/09687599.2021.1919505

Office of Disability Employment Policy. (2020). Employment for persons with a disability: Analysis of trends during the COVID-19 pandemic. https://www.dol.gov/sites/dolgov/files/OASP/evaluation/pdf/ODEP_Employment-for-PWD-AnalysisofTrendsDuringCOVID_Feb-Sept.pdf

O'Neil, D. A., Hopkins, M. M., & Sullivan, S. E. (2011). Do women's networks help advance women's careers? *Career Development International*, *16*(7), 733–754. https://doi.org/10.1108/13620431111187317

Phillippi, J., & Lauderdale, J. (2018). A guide to field notes for qualitative research: Context and conversation. *Qualitative Health Research*, *28*(3), 381–388. https://doi.org/10.1177/1049732317697102

Reid, B. E., Vogler, C., & Alkebsi, Z. (2020). Telehealth and telework accessibility in a pandemic-induced virtual world. *University of Colorado Law Review Forum*. https://papers.ssrn.com/abstract=3651535

Roberson, Q. M. (2019). Diversity in the workplace: A review, synthesis, and future research agenda. *Annual Review of Organizational Psychology and Organizational Behavior*, *6*(1), 69–88. https://doi.org/10.1146/annurev-orgpsych-012218-015243

Roberts, J. K., Pavlakis, A. E., & Richards, M. P. (2021). It's more complicated than it seems: Virtual qualitative research in the COVID-19 era. *International Journal of Qualitative Methods*, *20*. https://doi.org/10.1177/16094069211002959

Saunders, B., Sim, J., Kingstone, T., Baker, S., Waterfield, J., Bartlam, B., Burroughs, H., & Jinks, C. (2018). Saturation in qualitative research: Exploring its conceptualization and operationalization. *Quality and Quantity*, *52*(4), 1893–1907. https://doi.org/10.1007/s11135-017-0574-8

Schur, L., Ameri, M., & Kruse, D. (2020). Telework after COVID: A "silver lining" for workers with disabilities? *Journal of Occupational Rehabilitation*, *30*(4), 521–536. https://doi.org/10.1007/s10926-020-09936-5

Shore, L. M., Randel, A. E., Chung, B. G., Dean, M. A., Holcombe Ehrhart, K., & Singh, G. (2011). Inclusion and diversity in work groups: A review and model for future research. *Journal of Management*, *37*(4), 1262–1289. https://doi.org/10.1177/0149206310385943

Srivastava, A., & Thomson, S. B. (2009). Framework analysis: A qualitative methodology for applied policy research. *Journal of Administration and Governance*, *4*(2). https://ssrn.com/abstract=2760705

Tang, J. (2021). Understanding the telework experience of people with disabilities. *Proceedings of the ACM on Human-Computer Interaction*, *5*(CSCW1), 30:1–30:27. https://doi.org/10.1145/3449104

Welbourne, T. M., Rolf, S., & Schlachter, S. (2017). The case for employee resource groups. *Personnel Review*, *46*(8), 1816–1834. https://doi.org/10.1108/PR-01-2016-0004

Wiener, D. R. (2021). Dis/ability and critical cultural studies. In *Oxford research encyclopedia of communication*. Oxford University Press. https://doi.org/10.1093/acrefore/9780190228613.013.1006

Yadav, S., & Lenka, U. (2020). Diversity management: A systematic review. *Equality, Diversity and Inclusion: An International Journal*, *39*(8), 901–929. https://doi.org/10.1108/EDI-07-2019-0197

Printed and bound by CPI Group (UK) Ltd, Croydon, CR0 4YY

13/09/2026

14961061-0002